Evolution of Radiation Oncology at Massachusetts General Hospital

Herman D. Suit · Jay S. Loeffler

Evolution of Radiation Oncology at Massachusetts General Hospital

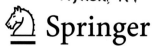 Springer

Herman D. Suit
Department of Radiation Oncology
Massachusetts General Hospital
Boston, MA, USA
hsuit@partners.org

Jay S. Loeffler
Department of Radiation Oncology
Massachusetts General Hospital
Boston, MA, USA
jloeffler@partners.org

ISBN 978-1-4419-6743-5   e-ISBN 978-1-4419-6744-2
DOI 10.1007/978-1-4419-6744-2
Springer New York Dordrecht Heidelberg London

Printed on acid-free paper

Springer is part of Springer Science+Business Media (www.springer.com)

Preface

The undisguised goal of the Massachusetts General Hospital [MGH] Department of Radiation Oncology is to work intensively to progressively and substantially increase the proportion of patients who are free of tumor and of treatment-related morbidity. There is acute awareness of the high incidence of cancer and the fact that we do not achieve our goal in a non-trivial proportion of patients. We are definitely sensitive to the fact that there are many questions to be posed and that the answering of those questions requires imaginative and thoughtful laboratory and clinical research. Importantly, there is no ambiguity that time is moving forward without the slightest delay for any person on this planet. This means posing critical questions and moving energetically to the generation of answers. The clear importance of questions and the relentless progress of time are illustrated by the image of the question mark and hour glass in Fig. 1.

A history of radiation oncology at the Massachusetts General Hospital (MGH) is a history of one component of the hospital and it will be considered in the context of the history of the hospital. This extends from 1811 to the present. Similarly, the hospital evolved out of the long history of medicine and science. Selected developments/events during that pre-MGH era will be discussed briefly.

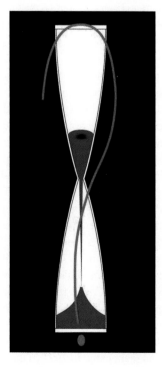

Fig. 1 Questions abound and are to be answered and time does not wait

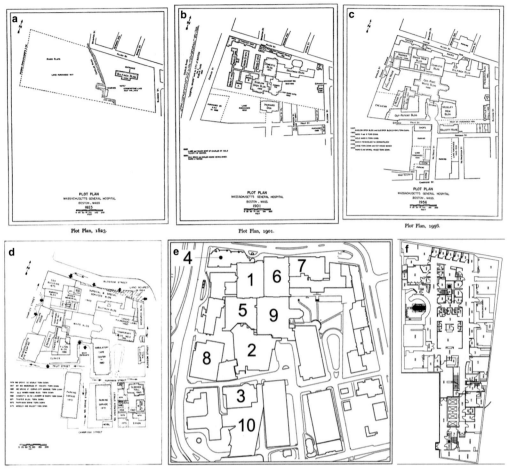

Fig. 2 (**a–d**) Footprints of the MGH in 1823, 1901, 1956, and 1980. (**e**) Footprint of the MGH as of 2011. Notice buildings 2, 3, 4, and 10 are the Third Century, the Francis Burr Proton Therapy center, the Cox, and the Yawkey, buildings, respectively. Buildings numbered 1, 6, 7, 5, 9, and 8 are Blake, Grey, Jackson, Ellison, White, and MEEI, respectively. (**f**) Floor plan of Cox Ground clinical radiation area

We describe the creation of the MGH in 1811 and its subsequent growth and its contributions to advancing medicine, its staff and physical size. For the latter, look at the increasing MGH footprint vs time, 1823, 1901, 1956, 1980, and 2011; the floor plan of the Cox Ground floor is included, Fig. 2a–f. The present complex is illustrated by the aerial view, a view from across the Charles River, the new Yawkey, and the Third Century Building nearing completion are shown in Fig. 3a–d. In 2004 the Yawkey building was opened and added 440,000 ft^2 for hospital programs and an additional 530,000 ft^2 is to be available in 2011 in the Third Century Building. These do not show the Schimches building just across Blossom St. and the extensive complex in Charlestown. The present array is indeed substantial. Further, the sites of our radiation oncology programs at the Boston University Medical Center, Emerson Hospital, Newton Wellesley Hospital, and North Shore Center are not shown.

The Cox building, Fig. 4a, was opened in 1975 as the MGH Cancer Center, housing the radiation oncology program, viz., the clinical radiation equipment and treatment areas (ground floor), staff offices, and administration on Cox 3; physics, Cox 3; machine shop and engineers work space, Cox 4; and biology research laboratories and mouse colony, Cox 7 and half of Cox 6. In addition there were several multidisciplinary oncology clinics, office spaces for medical and surgical oncology staff. A significant expansion in our radiation biological research program occurred after R. Jain and team came in 1991 to the Steele Laboratories in Cox 7 and

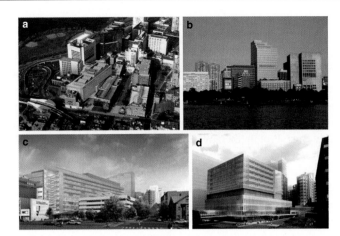

Fig. 3 (**a**) An aerial view of the MGH complex; (**b**) A view from across the Charles River; (**c**) The Yawkey building from Cambridge St (2004); and (**d**) The Third Century Building, to open 2011. This is on the site of the old Clinic Building and the Vincent Burnham Building

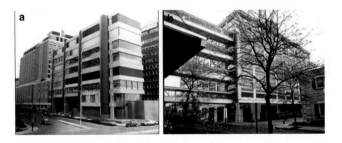

Fig. 4 (**a**) The Cox Building (1975). (**b**) Building 149, one of the Charlestown complex of MGH buildings

to substantial laboratory space in Building 149 in Charlestown, Fig. 4b. The MGH now has several large buildings in the Charlestown complex.

We operated the proton therapy program for 28 years at the Harvard cyclotron. In 2001 that program was transferred to the Francis H. Burr Proton Therapy Center, shown in Chapter 6. The Yawkey building was constructed around and above the MGH proton center. The plan is that the Third Century Building will house all of the photon and electron therapy units and related clinical functions. In addition, consideration is given to including an additional proton facility. Thus, all of the clinical activities of radiation oncology will be convenient for patients and staff to the array of oncology clinics and conferences in the Yawkey. The only remaining radiation oncology function in Cox is to be the Steele Laboratory. The labs in Charlestown are to continue.

The physical scale of the MGH is impressive. Specifically, the gross total floor space is 7,335,654 ft^2, the equivalent of ∼168 acres. These figures include all spaces, e.g., clinical, research, general operations, parking. Of this, 4,729,053 ft^2 are on the main MGH Campus.[1] Our Charlestown complex represents 1,680,000 ft^2. There are several properties at other sites.

---

[1]The area of the Clinics, Vincent and Tilton buildings were not included as they have been demolished in preparation for the construction of the Third Millennium Building for 2011.

Of the total, 6,166,212 ft^2 are owned and 1,169,442 ft^2 are leased by the MGH. These figures include all spaces, e.g., clinical, research, general operations, parking.

These figures do not include the building for the third century, scheduled to be completed in 2011. The gain in ft^2 will be 530,000 ft^2. This would raise the total to 7,865,000 ft^2 or a total of ~180 acres. In addition, MGH rents 348,000 ft^2 in the Simches building that is in the space toward the shopping mall, just beyond the Holiday Inn. This brings the total to ~8,200,000 ft^2.

The areas for radiation oncology in ft^2 are 24,414, 25,265, 3884, and 2062 for the Cox building, the Burr Proton therapy Center, Emerson building, and Harvard Gardens, respectively.[2]

The MGH is an exceptionally well-regarded institution internationally as providing the finest quality of medical care, advancing medicine by clinical and laboratory research and education of persons entering healthcare professions. The present size and scope of the hospital merit brief comment at this point. The number of beds started at 73 and is to be 1057 in 2011. The MGH now has 18,283 employees (2008), including 1625 M.D.s and 527 Ph.D.s. Importantly, the research budget for the hospital is $528 M. For some years, the research budget has been in the 22–26% of the hospital total budget. Of this total, 80% is for on-site programs. For research training and for clinical trials, the distribution has been 8 and 7%, respectively. Financially, the MGH is in good condition, at this point in time: the FY2007 income is budgeted at $2300 M and expenses of $2200 M, i.e., a surplus of $100 M. This reflects wise and prudent fiscal management combined with an undisguised commitment to providing continuously improving quality of medical care.

Over this 28-year period the department has enjoyed sustained medical, scientific, and educational success and is judged to be one of the very top radiation oncology programs on the global scene. These successes have been accompanied by continued growth in patient numbers and physical equipment and size. For example, the number of medical (M.D.) and science (Ph.D.) staff is now 46, with 19 physicians and 27 scientists. Of the Ph.D. full-time science staff 13 are in physics, 3 in biomathematics, and 11 in biology. This compares with four full-time clinicians and no Ph.D. scientists in 1970.

The total number of FTE employees is 258 and fortunately we are operating in the black. The number of patients treated per day has increased from ~90 in 1970 to ~270 by x-ray, electron, and proton beams. This includes ~11 pediatric patients treated per day.

In 1994, the MGH joined with the Brigham and Women's Hospital to create Partner's Health Care System. This organization has grown quite rapidly in the intervening 16 years to include a broad complex of eastern Massachusetts hospitals. Those owned by Partners Systems and are MGH related include Newton Wellesley, Spaulding, North Shore, and McLean Hospitals. Our department has responsibility for the clinical staffing and operation of radiation oncology programs at Boston University Medical Center and the Emerson Hospital. Further, the MGH has a very close affiliation with the Massachusetts Eye and Ear Infirmary. Despite ongoing speculation of a merger of the MEEI and MGH during the 40-year period of 1970–2010, the department continues to maintain extremely close collaborative working relations but remains generally independent. The MEEI cancer patients are seen collaboratively by MGH radiation and medical oncology staff and receive radiation treatment at MGH.

Similarly, the Brigham Women's Hospital (BWH) operates a clinical therapy unit in the Dana Farber Cancer Institute (DFCI). The Brigham works very closely with Boston Children's Hospital. It has working arrangements with several community hospitals also. Further, there is a complex interaction between the MGH, BWH, the Dana Farber Cancer Institute (DFCI), and the Beth Israel Deaconess Hospital (BID) to form the Harvard Cancer program. One benefit is

---

[2] This information was generously provided by David Ryan and David Hanitchak (Planning and Construction, real Estate and Facilities, MGH), personal communication, 2008.

a mechanism for planning and conducting Harvard-wide clinical investigations, clinical trials, and laboratory research. In addition, there is a Harvard-wide residency program.

At this time, the MGH is the largest component of the quite impressive and expanding Partner's Health Care System.

Recent and Present Leaders of Radiation Oncology at the MGH

Milford Schulz was the first MGH radiologist to practice almost full-time radiation therapy. He was on the staff from 1942 to 1976. Herman Suit was Chief of the Department of Radiation Oncology from June 1970 to October 2000. Jay Loeffler was then appointed as the new chief and is continuing effectively in that role. Figure 5a is a photograph of these three in the Fogg Museum of Fine Art of Harvard University at the evening function of a Science Festivity Day of the department. We work collaboratively with Jay Harris and his team at BWH and Mary Ann Stevenson and her team at the BID; see Fig. 5b.

MGH residents and fellows who have become chairs of academic departments of radiation oncology

Resident/fellow	Chief of radiation oncology	Resident/fellow	Chief of radiation oncology
Michael Baumann	University of Dresden, Germany	Thomas DeLaney	Boston University
Wilfred Budach	Düsseldorf, Germany	Sten Graffman	University of Lund, Sweden
Krzysztof Bujko	Marie Curie Cancer Center, Warsaw, Poland	Edward Halperin	Duke University University of Louisville as Dean
Arnab Chakravarti	Ohio State University	Eugen Hug	Dartmouth University, NH and at present Paul Scherrer Institute, Switzerland
Jurgen Debus	University of Heidelberg	Lisa Kachnic	Boston University
		Simon Powell	Washington University and at present Memorial Sloan Kettering Cancer
Larry Marks	University of North Carolina	Tyvin Rich	University of Virginia
Raymond Miralbell	University of Geneva, Switzerland	Joel Tepper	University of North Carolina
Rene Mirimanoff	University of Lausanne	Chris Willet	Duke University
Paul O'Kunieff	National Cancer Institute, Radiation Branch University of Rochester University of Florida	Takashima Yamashita	National Cancer Center, Tokyo, Japan
Marie Overgaard	University of Arhus		

Resident who became director of Cancer Research Center
Jens Overgaard   University of Arhus, Denmark

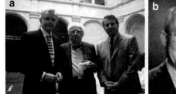

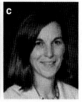

Fig. 5 (**a**) Milford Schulz with Jay Loeffler (*right*) and Herman Suit (*left*) in the Harvard Fogg Museum of Fine Art. (**b**) Jay Harris, chief at the Brigham, and (**c**) Mary Ann Stevenson, chief at the Beth Israel-Deaconess system

Physicists who have become chiefs of medical physics

Physicist	Head of medical physics	Physicist	Head of medical physics
Art Boyer	Stanford, CA	Clift Ling	George Washington, UC San Francisco, Memorial Sloan Kettering, NY
Ken Gall	Southwestern University, Dallas, TX	Marcia Urie	U Mass Worchester
Dale Kubo	UC Davis, CA	Lynn Verhey	UC San Francisco

One of the characteristics of the MGH program is the international character of its staff as is clearly illustrated in Fig. 6. The dots indicate the geographic origin of our faculty (blue) and residents, fellows, and students (red). This reflects our definite policy of seeking talent from the entirety of this planet. Our attitude has been "we have no interest in where you came from but only where you are going." This has definitely been a positive factor in the productivity of all sections of the department.

Of the full-time faculty at MGH as of this writing, the fraction who came from abroad are medical, 7 of 19; physics 11 of 16; laboratory research 7 of 11; or a total of 25 of 46.

Ed Halperin was chief at Duke and then associate dean. He was next appointed to be dean of the Medical School at Louisville, KY. Nancy Tarbell has been appointed as dean for Academic Affairs at Harvard Medical School.

Jens Overgaard is director of the Cancer Research program at Arhus.

Daniel Dosoretz is the most successful entrepreneur in American radiation oncology. He started with one center in Florida and now has more than 100 centers in the USA. He is credited with a model QA system yielding a quality operation.

Three of our former residents are now Editors in Chief of the three major journals in radiation oncology. These are Joel Tepper for Seminars in Radiation Oncology, Jens Overgaard for Radiotherapy and Oncology and Anthony Zietman for International Journal of Radiation Oncology, Biology and Physics. The impact factors are 4.1, 4.0 and 4.8. This is a unique achievement for residents from any single program.

Major books include (Underlined names are present or former MGH staff): George Holmes and Milford Schulz *Therapeutic Radiology*; CC Wang (Editor) and author, *Clinical Radiation Oncology: Indications, Techniques, and Results;* CC Wang, *Radiation Therapy for Head and Neck Neoplasms*; E. Halperin and co-editors L. Constine, Nancy Tarbell, and L. Kuhn (co-editors), *Pediatric Radiation Oncology* (in 5th edition); E. Halperin and co-editors C. Perez and L. Brady, *Principles and Practice of Radiation Oncology*; Peter Black and Jay Loeffler, *Cancer of the Nervous System*; Peter Mauch and Jay Loeffler, *Radiation*

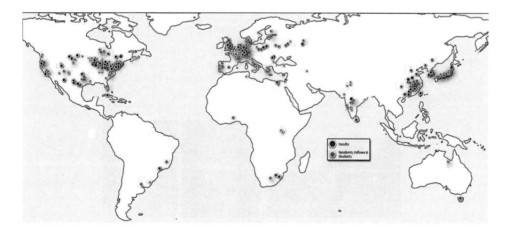

Fig. 6 Geographic distribution of the origin of our faculty (*blue*) and residents, fellows, and graduate students (*red*)

Oncology Technology and Biology; Dennis Shrieve and Jay Loeffler *Human Radiation Injury;* L. Gunderson and J. Tepper *Clinical Radiation Oncology*; Gunderson l, Willett C, Harrison L, Calvo P. *Intraoperative Irradiation.*

From the MGH, there have been five presidents of ASTRO: M. Schulz, H. Suit, J. Tepper, A. Zietman, and L. Gunderson. In addition, J. Overgaard and M. Baumann (former resident and fellow) have become presidents of ESTRO. T. Yamashita (former fellow) has severed as president of JASTRO.

Among ASTRO gold medalist are C.C. Wang, W. Shipley, C. Ling, J. Tepper, and H. Suit.

Presidents of MGH 1970–Present

During the history of the start of the planning for department and its operation to the present the MGH has had seven general directors/presidents. These are Dean Clark (1941–1962), John Knowles (1962–1972), Charles Saunders (1972–1981), J. Robert Buchanan (1982–1994), Sam Their (1994–1996), James Mongan (1996–2002), and Peter Slavin (2002–Present). The general directors/presidents with whom this department has interacted are shown in Fig. 7a–f. We have worked effectively and productively with each.

For the MGH radiation oncology department, virtually all of our staff, residents, and fellows, past and present, accept as a given that MGH stands for Man's Greatest Hospital. This decidedly immodest assessment is widely viewed among our group as being manifestly true and that perception is clearly reflected in a marvelous esprit de corp. Such an exceptionally

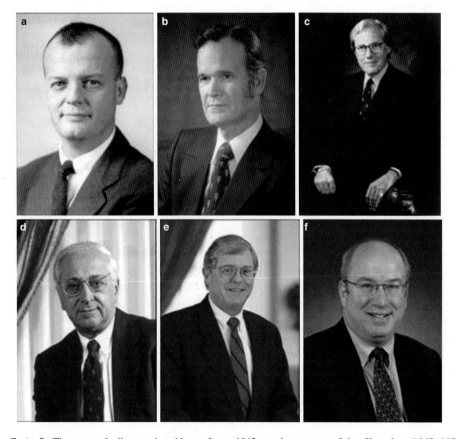

Fig. 7 (**a–f**) The general directors/presidents from 1962 to the present: John Knowles (1962–1972), Charles Saunders (1972–1981), J. Robert Buchanan (1982–1994), Samuel Their (1994–96), James Mongan (1996–2002), and Peter Slavin (2002–present)

positive attitude is solidly based on the judgment that the best possible care is provided for each MGH patient, i.e., the patient is, in fact, number one. Quite importantly, such an attitude is widespread throughout the hospital. Further, there is a deep pride in the contributions to the scientific advancement of oncology by this department.

Autobiographical Sketches of the Two Chiefs of the MGH Department of Radiation Oncology

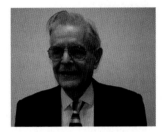

Fig. 8 Herman Suit

February 1929. I lucked into life in Houston, TX, by way of a C section by Dr. Herman Johnson, required because of a placenta previa. This was a very uncommon surgical procedure in Houston at that time. My parents were so relieved at the success that they named their new son Herman. My medical experience was just beginning as at 4 weeks I was operated by Dr. Judson Taylor for pyloric stenosis. After the procedure, my mother was told that there was no need to bandage the surgical scar as I could not survive. She insisted that I would survive and they had to provide care to that effect. Johnson and Taylor later became the first chairs of OB-Gyn and of Surgery, respectively, at Baylor College of Medicine after its move to Houston. My luck continued in that Herman Johnson took a long-term interest in me. This medical history and the interest by Johnson were important factors in my decision to want a career in science and medicine. My mother's wish was for me to become a concert pianist or orchestral conductor. My maternal grandmother articulated very serious disappointment in my not wishing to be a preacher (such was not even on my screen but certainly never mentioned to her).

I had a very good time as a student and greatly enjoyed the years in the public schools and was a regular user of the school libraries and the Houston public library. Libraries became a significant interest/hobby for my adult life. A most special time for a boy in Texas were my three summers (ages 11, 12, and 13) and one fall school term on my grandparents farm/ranch in New Mexico. This provided riding, shooting, and the life of a young cowboy. At 13, I had a New Mexico driver's license. This carried zero weight with my father when I returned to Houston and had to wait to age 16 before getting the keys to the family car. I had the most wonderful parents. They were extremely supportive and caring and there was a deep and mutual love.

WWII was a very big concern to all and I assumed that I would be drafted. My determination was to be an officer and not a "troop." Hence I went to summer school and took extra courses during the regular terms in order to be a university junior by age 18 and hence eligible for officer's training school. Fortunately, the war was over in 1945. I graduated in January 1946 and then had my B.Sc. at 19 from the University of Houston. The finest teacher in my life was Eby Nell McElrath from whom I took organic and then biochemistry. This enhanced my determination to be in a scientific field of medicine. My family had very modest finances and I worked as a sales person at a lady's shoe store, Saturdays all day and Thursday evenings. The earnings combined with living at home provided for all of my college tuition, books, etc.

This work stopped upon entering medical school. My contacts with Herman Johnson continued quite warmly. He invited me to meet the Dean of Baylor. Johnson told him that he really should admit Suit into the incoming class in 1948. If not, there would be an awkward situation as he, as chair of the Advanced Admission Committee, would admit me as a junior. Clearly, I had no worry re-admission. My class had 89 students. A definite positive was the school policy that there be at least four women per year.

My plan was to obtain an M.Sc. in biochemistry while at Baylor. The goal was to become an endocrinologist as I judged it the most scientific specialty in medicine. Early as a freshman, I met Prof. Joe Gast, chair of biochemistry. Although I had had 1 year of college physics and of math, he required that I take physics and math at University of Houston in the summer between years 1 and 2 and more math at night during the fall term of my second year. Then, I had to take courses in nuclear and atomic physics at University of Texas at Austin in the summer between years 2 and 3. This was an extremely exciting experience, viz., learning about the atom and nucleus, viz., some real science. As a medical student taking such courses was definitely uncommon, the professor suggested that I read two books dealing with radiation biology and take an exam for credit. The result was a very large surprise, i.e., learning that radiation was being used to cure patients of their tumor with preservation of anatomy and function. I changed my career plans to radiation oncology.

As a boy of ~11, I developed the opinion that Oxford University had the highest concentration of intellectual power on this planet and I wanted to go there. That was not a prospect. I was enormously thrilled when considering a center to go for research and clinical education in radiation oncology to learn that Oxford was indeed an absolutely top-rated center. I applied and was accepted to my huge surprise. I did not appreciate that there were practically no applicants to radiation oncology and that they were keen to get a young doctor, even an ex-colonial with research interest. That there had been no competition for the position was of no concern to me as I was actually at Oxford. The chief was Frank Ellis, a super role model as he was interested almost entirely in data and little interest in opinions. Further, there was an outstanding researcher L. Lajtha. He became my thesis advisor, really brilliant and a true scholar. I was most pleased to be surrounded by extremely impressive talent in many areas of human interest and activity. I was admitted as a D.Phil. student (Oxford and Cambridge do not use the designation Ph.D.) and a scholarship. The 3.4 years in Oxford were the most intellectually stimulating time of my life. There was constant questioning, offering of contrary opinions, disputations and all with real respect and courtesy. I did learn much in radiation oncology, lab research, and most certainly respect of data as the critical factor in assessing an interpretation of any phenomenon. One close colleague and long-term warm friend is Eric Hall.

This was followed by two excellent years at the radiation branch of the NCI with approximate half time in the lab and half in the clinic. As a young American physician with English boards and an Oxford D.Phil. even with only quite modest clinical experience, I was given responsibility for the radiation treatment of all patients at the NCI except for electron irradiation by a giant Van de Graaff unit. I declined the latter, as the machine was unreliable, having produced one fatal and one quite serious injury due to malfunction not long before I arrived at the NCI.

I was then recruited to MD Anderson by Warren Sinclair, head of physics, during the 1958 meeting of the International Society of Radiation Research at Burlington Vermont. He asked me to go for a swim out into Lake Champlain. There he discussed the MD Anderson and the opportunity to work in the clinic:lab on a 50:50 time basis and be the head of the to be formed section on experimental radiation therapy. I accepted and we swam back to shore. Several months later G. Fletcher was in Washington and confirmed the invitation.

I moved there in July 1957 and was assigned to work with Paul Chau in Gyn. Also close clinical colleagues were L. DelClos, E. Montague, R. Martin, W.O. Russell, and others. After about 2 years, I proposed studying the role of radiation for mesenchymal tumors based on the work of T. Puck, viz., showing that a wide spectrum of human tumor cell lines in vitro had similar radiation sensitivities. Thus, sarcomas might not have a different inherent sensitivity.

As a starter, the patients were those with extremity lesions and were treated under conditions of tourniquet hypoxia, to minimize the role of hypoxic cells. Due to the impressive success rate, this approach was extended to proximal extremity and torso sarcomas under conditions of normal blood flow. As a function of volume, TCPs of non-superficial sarcomas and epithelial tumors are now known to be similar. The time in the laboratory was extremely pleasant both in terms of the problems investigated and the people with whom I interacted, viz., R. Sedlacek, R. Withers, L. Milas, W. Dewey, Ian Tannock, A. Howes, and many others. Of special pleasure were the two Ph.D. students: Larry Thompson and Helen Stone. Fletcher was a highly effective leader and I really enjoyed working with him. See Chapter 4 re lab research while at MDACC.

After 11 years at MDACC, I had the excellent luck to be recruited to MGH and commenced work in 1970. To state that I have enormously enjoyed my years in medicine and at such incredibly fine institutions would be a serious understatement.

My wisest decision was to propose marriage to Joan and to have had the marvelous good fortune of her acceptance. We have had an extremely happy time together and are planning to celebrate our 50th anniversary this coming November (2010).

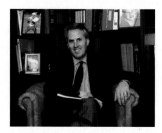

Fig. 9 Jay S Loeffler

I was born on December 27, 1955, in Carlisle – a lovely college town in south central Pennsylvania. My father was the first pediatrician in this region of the state and my mother was an English teacher in the public school system. I was the "baby" of the family with an older brother (John) and sister (Jan). While sports were my first love in life, I cannot remember a time when I was not interested in following my father's path into medicine. Even at a very young age, I would accompany dad to his office and observe him seeing patients and reviewing x-rays. On weekends, I would often round with him seeing neonates and children on the floor of our local hospital. At the age of 16, I was offered a job in the hospital laboratory drawing blood from patients and performing blood chemistries and hematology tests. When I would return from work in the evening, dad would explain how these tests were used in the management of patients. These lectures soon transformed into discussions of human physiology, endocrinology, pathology, pharmacology, biochemistry. This very early introduction into the field of medicine has had a profound effect on my career as a physician.

In ninth grade, I went off to boarding school following my brother's footsteps. I attended The Hill School in Pottstown, Pennsylvania, from 1970 until graduation in 1974. My main interests were in mathematics and biology and sports. I received 10 varsity letters during my time at The Hill and was the captain of the soccer and baseball team and received the coach's cup in both sports. I received two prizes at graduation for excellence in advanced placement biology and chemistry. I was accepted to Williams College early decision – again following my brother's path. At Williams, I immediately declared my major to be biology and began my pre-medical studies. I graduated with honors from Williams and was elected to the Purple Key Society – Williams' honors "club." Between my junior and senior year at Brown University School of Medicine, I was accepted to a summer fellowship program at the National Cancer Institute and was assigned to the Radiation Oncology Branch (ROB) under the leadership of Dr. Eli Glatstein. Other members of the ROB were Joel Tepper, Tim Kinsella, Allen Lichter,

Jim Schwade, Liz Travis, Jim Mitchell, and Dick Fraass. I was immediately impressed with the clinical and research talents I encountered and I decided to concentrate my efforts on seeking a career in radiation oncology. When I returned to Brown, I worked for Dr. Arvin Glicksman on several clinical projects as well as a lab project with Dr. John Leith. By the time I applied to residency programs, I had three peer-reviewed publications resulting from the work I had done at NCI and Brown. I applied to four residency programs – University of Pennsylvania, Yale, Joint Center for Radiation Therapy (JCRT), and the MGH. This was the time before the match and admissions were rolling in nature. By August of my senior year, I was accepted by Penn, Yale, and JCRT. I had only 2 weeks to make up my mind and I chose the JCRT based on my very favorable impression of Dr. Sam Hellman. Ironically, I never heard a word from the MGH until late October when Dr. Munzenrider invited me for an interview. I informed him that I had already accepted a position 2 months earlier at the JCRT.

Three months before I was to matriculate at the JCRT, Jay Harris sent me a letter announcing that Sam was leaving to become the physician-in-chief at Memorial Sloan-Kettering Cancer Center. Dr. Bob Goodman called me from the University of Pennsylvania later that week and offered me a "transfer" position explaining that it may take years for Harvard to replace Sam and my residency could be quite "disruptive." During my first 2 years at the JCRT, Jim Belli, Bob Cassady, Joel Greenberger, Les Botnick, Chris Rose, Bill Bloomer, Arnold Malcolm, Ralph Weichelbaum, and Itzak Goldberg all left to accept leadership positions at other institutions. This left only two senior attending physicians, Jay Harris and Peter Mauch, and a first year attending – Nancy Tarbell. During my residency, I spent a year in the laboratory of radiobiology at the Harvard School of Public Health under the leadership of Dr. Jack Little. I concentrated my efforts on mutagenesis research on TK6 lymphocytes after exposure to commonly used chemotherapeutic agents and radiations. I was involved in another project evaluating the intrinsic radiosensitivity of human fibroblasts derived from patients who demonstrated extreme acute reactions to modest doses of radiation – and showed a correlation. I also attended a molecular biology and genetics course at Harvard Medical School. Jack was a great mentor for me personally and professionally and remains a dear friend. I was awarded a Farley Prize from Children's Hospital that provided funds for me to travel to UCSF and spend time in neuro-oncology with the late Glen Sheline and Steve Leibel as well as neurosurgeons Phil Gutin, Mark Rosenbaum, and Charles Wilson. This was the period of my life when I clearly decided to enter the field of radiation neuro-oncology. I began my faculty time at the Brigham and Women's Hospital with the charge of building a neuro-oncology program. I was named the director of the Brain Tumor Center of Children's Hospital, Brigham and Women's Hospital, and the Dana-Farber Cancer Institute and Peter Black and I had the fortunate experience of recruiting Howard Fine from medical oncology, Patrick Wen from neurology, Eben Alexander and Phil Stieg from neurosurgery, and Malcolm Rodgers from psychiatry to build one of the largest and most respected brain tumor centers in the USA. At the same time, I was involved with the early development of stereotactic radiosurgery and stereotactic radiotherapy which shortly would change the practice of radiation neuro-oncology worldwide. As the principal clinical radiation oncologist involved in the development of stereotactic radiation, we analyzed the results of radiosurgery in the treatment of a wide variety of vascular, benign, and malignant brain lesions as well as an extensive analysis of factors (both clinical and physical) associated with acute and late effects. After the completion of these studies, it was clear to me that fractionated stereotactic delivery would be preferable for the treatment of larger and critically located lesions. The development of immobilization and delivery systems for stereotactic radiotherapy (SRT) was an enormous task. The result, however, was a significant reduction in toxicity. A great example was hearing preservation following the treatment of >2 cm acoustic neuromas – a feat not achievable with radiosurgery.

In 1996, after many attempts, Herman Suit successfully recruited me to the MGH to serve as the medical director of the Northeast Proton Therapy Center. I began my time at the MGH on 12/1/96. My best friend, greatest supporter, closest colleague, mentor, wife, mother of my two children joined us from Children's Hospital in the spring of 1997 to direct both the pediatric proton project and the first Director of Office of Women's Careers at MGH. In August 2000, I was chosen by the search committee chaired by Kurt Isselbacher to replace Dr. Herman Suit as chair of the department and the Andreas Soriano Professor of Radiation Oncology at Harvard Medical School. In retrospect, my decision to come to the MGH was second only to marrying Nancy as the wisest move of my life.

Boston, MA   Herman D. Suit
                                                                                   Jay S. Loeffler

Acknowledgments

The authors are extremely grateful to a very large number of talented and thoughtful members of the MGH, Harvard University, MIT, and other institutions. First credit is happily given to the many faculty and staff that cooperated in providing information for the preparation of the material in the many chapters. This includes the medical and science staff in the clinical, physics, and biology sections in addition to the radiation therapists, nurses, and social workers. Of real importance has been the support by administration. Importantly, we have had valuable assistance from the Photography Department, Treadwell Library, Archives, Architectural and Engineering Department. Important support has been given by the Countway Medical Library, Harvard Medical Rare Books Library, Widener Library, Harvard Physics Library, among others. The critical support was effectively provided by the Information Technology Unit. Special mention is made of large contributions from George Chen, Lance Munn, Tim Lehane, Saveli Goldberg, Khai Le, and David Ryan. We are very appreciative of the essential secretarial work on this book by Julie M. Finn, Dominique Jeudy, Tina Power, and Judith Wilson.

Contents

Chapter 1

Early Culture and Medicine to 1895 and the Creation of the MGH

1.1 Early Cultural, Medical, and Scientific/Technical Developments[1]

There is no certainty as to the origins of medicine. Well before recorded history, there was surely a wide spectrum of shamans with their sacred herbs and diverse procedures to relieve symptoms and make the "patients" more comfortable with their situation.

Beyond medicine, there were developing interests in activities that we associate with culture, viz., music as evidenced by musical instruments, and art as demonstrated by the impressive paintings in caves and rock walls. Several flutes that date from 35,000 BCE are in archeological collections and museums. Examples from southern Germany, near Ulm, area is a flute and a carved sculpture in ivory of "Venus" from ~34,000 BCE [7, 8] are shown in Fig. 1.1a, b. With little doubt, after language the most important development for modern culture was that of writing. This has made the transmission of knowledge to each succeeding generation vastly more efficient and comprehensive as it would be based on the extant knowledge at each generation. Without writing, the knowledge available to the young would be merely that transmitted orally by parents and tribe members. Writing developed in ~3200 BCE in Sumer or the Indus valley. This advanced quickly and was at a very useful level by 2900 BCE in Sumer (southern Iraq of today), as illustrated by the Philadelphia Tablet (Museum of U of Pennsylvania), Fig. 1.1c [29]. Thus, writing developed ~29,000 years later than these works of music and art.

1.2 Early Medicine

The oldest existing medical text is from Sumer at ~2100 BCE, Fig. 1.2a [37]. There is substantial written evidence

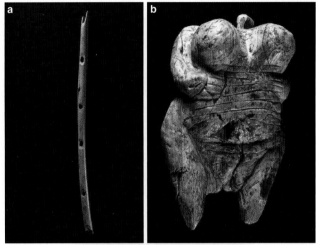

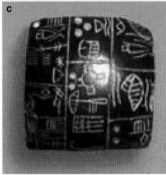

Fig. 1.1 (**a, b**) A flute made from the bone of a swan and a carved sculpture of "Venus" from ~34,000 BCE [7, 8]. (**c**) The Philadelphia Tablet with Sumerian script from ~2900 BCE [29]

of very active medical practice in ancient Egypt [13, 23, 33]. Imhotep is frequently cited as the first doctor and credited as the architect of the first pyramid, i.e., that at Saqqara. A doctor in Ancient Egypt was named *Sinw*. The prefix Met is added to form the noun, thus Metceni, from which the word medicine was derived. A female doctor was named *Sinw.t* (*t* is the feminine sign), i.e., there were female physicians in ancient Egypt. Perhaps the most important sources of information of the very early history of Egyptian medicine are the Ebers and the Edwin Smith Papyri of ~1600 BCE.

[1] General references on medical history for this chapter include references [1, 3, 6, 16, 17, 39].

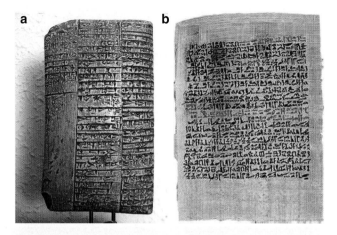

Fig. 1.2 (**a**) This is the oldest known medical text. This is from Sumer at ~2100 BCE [37]. (**b**) A segment of the Ebers papyrus, a medical text from ~1600 BCE [12]

The Smith papyrus is considered to represent a copy of documents of ~2700 BCE. The Smith papyrus was principally a general surgical text and included detailed accounts of the problems and management of 48 patients, Fig. 1.2b. The problems were traumatic, except for a few patients with infections and one apparent neoplasm. Emphasis is placed on a detailed history and physical examination with comments as to management. Case 45 appears to be that of a breast tumor. There are descriptions of approximation of edges of wounds by adhesive plaster and by sutures. Sutures were found closing the wound made by the embalmer in a mummy of 1100 BCE [23]. One common minor surgical procedure was circumcision. This was illustrated in a bas-relief of a youth and the surgeon ~2250 BCE in the tomb of Ankhmahor [23]. Presumably, wound infections were uncommon or not serious or this would not have been a standard practice in many cultures throughout that region.

Another medical text but of impressive length and of nearly the same vintage is the Ebers papyrus. This was primarily a medical text. It is very long, viz., 20.2 m and 30 cm high. There is discussion of a wide array of medicines, viz., herbals, minerals, animal parts, and a description of the circulatory system, and that the heart functions as a centre of the blood supply. These papyri were not textbooks for students, as they were extraordinarily expensive. Further, the required copying by hand meant not rare transcriptional errors.

The Hammurabi Code. The Hammurabi Code of 18th century BCE Babylon is the oldest known written code of laws [23]. The code was inscribed in stone. Several of its provisions stipulated fees for surgeons and the penalties for treatment-induced injury. These laws formalized the practice that the cost of medical care was dependent on ability to pay.

The Word Cancer. Hippocrates (460–370 BCE) is credited by some as originating the word cancer based on his observation of prominent swollen blood vessels surrounding the

tumor which were thought similar to the claws of crabs. He is also credited as the first to distinguish between benign and malignant tumors. Further, many rate him as the "Father of Medicine." The "writings" of Hippocrates and other Greek thinkers of 4th and 5th BCE held a central position in western thinking until the Enlightment.

First Hospital. The high likelihood is that some of the temples and religious sites of primitive societies provided accommodation for selected categories of supplicants. As such, certain of those facilities might be loosely classed as primitive or proto hospitals. The Greeks had established Asklepieia at Epidauros and other sites in the 5th century BCE. These provided sleeping quarters for those who came to have their dreams interpreted [17, 39]. Perhaps the oldest "record" of a special facility or hospital for medical treatment of the sick was in Sri Lanka. According to a 6th century history of Sri Lanka, the Mahavansa, and King Pandukabhaya built a series of hospitals (Sivikasotthi-Sala) in different regions of his country in about 300 BCE [36].

1.3 Early Hospitals that Later Developed Academic Radiation Oncology Programs

1.3.1 Santa Maria Della Scala in Siena

The origin of hospitals as specially constructed facilities for the care of the sick of Europe is not well defined. The oldest continuously functioning European hospital is perhaps the Santa Maria Della Scala in Siena, viz., 1091–1996. This hospital was immediately opposite to the site of a church that is now the famous cathedral of Siena. Siena was a popular resting and recovery point on the path of pilgrims from France and northern Europe to Rome. The hospital directed special attention to the care of orphans and had a reputation for highly competent patient care. Due to gifts and bequests from grateful persons it became very wealthy and progressively modernized. In 1930, the *Istituto di Radiologia e Terapia Fisica* of the hospital was inaugurated as the department of radiology of the U of Siena. The radiation therapy section included a ward for in-patients. Radiation therapy became an independent department in 1990 and in 1995 was moved to the new hospital on the outskirts of Siena. That new department is equipped with two linear accelerators (one with stereotactic accessories, including a dynamic MMLC), a simulator, and treatment planning systems connected online with a multi-slice CT unit, a 1.5 T MR unit, and a HDR brachytherapy unit.

The information on this most venerable hospital was kindly provided by Prof. Luigi Pirtoli of Siena and Prof. Santoni, a former clinical proton Fellow at MGH, now at Rome and the guide book of the Santa Maria de la Scala.

1.3.2 St. Bartholomew Hospital in London

Rahere, an Augustine monk and favorite of Henry I, made a pilgrimage to Rome in ~1120.[2] He contracted malaria and vowed to build a hospital for the poor were he to return to London. He was further motivated by a vision in which St. Bartholomew ordered him to build the hospital and a priory and the two to be named in his honor. This, Rahere did with enthusiasm and style. St. Bartholomew's Hospital was opened in London in 1123. St. Bartholomew's Hospital is the oldest continuously operating hospital in Britain. Physicians who have practiced there included William Harvey, Percival Potts, and James Paget.

The first radiation treatment at St. Bartholomew was in 1900 and the first supervoltage (1 MeV or greater) X-ray machine in Britain was at St. Barts 1939. Ernest Rutherford and Ms Sassoon officiated at the opening ceremony of the new unit in December 1936. The total cost, including the building was £12,823. The first patient treatment on the new machine was in April 1937. For 2 years the unit was operated at 700 kVp and in 1939 regular operation at 1 MeV was instituted. There were several episodes of drama during WWII. Despite the hospital receiving a direct hit by a bomb one night that inflicted major damage to the therapy suite, physicist George Innis and radiation oncologist R. Phillips worked throughout the night and managed to have the unit functioning by the time of the first patient appointment the following morning. Sources of these historical notes include Klaus Trott (personal communication, 2007) and the Web page of the hospital museum [35].

Dr. Trott has served as a Visiting Professor in our department on several occasions. This dept has a close connection to St. Barts in that Dr. Rita Linggood was recruited from St. Barts to our staff in 1976. She moved to Fall River and the Joint Center for Radiotherapy in 1993.

1.4 Status of Health Care at the Start of 19th Century

The extremely limited means for diagnosis and treatment of patients with virtually any disease in 1800 is difficult for a physician in 2009 to comprehend. The doctor in 1800 had only the history and physical examination. The latter was confined to the physician's sense of sight, touch, sound, smell and taste; examination of urine, sputum, and feces; and use of thermometry, pulse, respiration rate, and knowledge of anatomy, and blood circulation. The stethoscope was not invented until 1816. There were extremely few but some effective medicines, e.g., quinine for malaria, limes to treat and prevent scurvy. Autopsy studies had demonstrated the specific diseased organ as the cause of the patient's symptoms and dismissed the famous humors as causative factors. Not insignificant was the introduction of effective vaccination against the scourge of smallpox. There were no imaging techniques, histopathological diagnoses, and amputation was the major surgical procedure.

The lack of effective medicines is made strikingly clear even though an overstatement by O.W. Holmes. In 1860, he commented *Excluding opium 'which the Creator himself seems to prescribe', wine which is a food, and the vapors which produce the miracle of anesthesia and I firmly believe that if the whole material medica, as now used, could be sunk to the bottom of the sea, it would be all the better for mankind—and all the worse for the fishes* [27]. This was the opinion of a nationally prominent writer, a former staff physician at the MGH, a Dean of the Harvard Medical School from 1847 to 1853, a professor at the school, and the author of a paper in 1843 on the transmission of puerperal fever by physicians.

1.5 Life Expectancy vs. Time

Understanding of disease and availability of effective medicine developed quite slowly. This is strikingly evident by the relative constancy of life expectancy from ~30,000 BCE to ~1850. That is, life expectancy varied between ~20 and ~40 years during that period for which there are life expectancy data [38]. This short human life span over this long period reflected the high fatality rate from infectious diseases, very poor public sanitation, poor and highly variable food supply, trauma, etc., combined with minimally effective medicine. As cancer is a disease predominantly of older people, it was not a major problem.

From 1850 to 1890 and to 1900 life expectancies for US white males at birth were 38.3, 42.5, and 48.2 years. Almost at the turn of the century, the increase became rapid, viz., at 1950 and 2004, life expectancies were 66.3 and 75.7 years, respectively. These increases were largely due to lessening of fatal infectious diseases. In contrast, there has been only a small increase in life expectancy of 80-year-old men between 1850 and 2004, viz., 5.9 to 8.1 years. That is, the gain during those 154 years for the 80-year-old men was only 2.2 years as compared to 37.4 years for the newborn males [40].

At approximately 1850, general health commenced to improve at an impressive rate. This was principally the consequence of gains in public sanitation, availability of clean water, adequate nutrition for larger proportions of the people,

---

[2] The dates of this pilgrimage are only approximate.

Fig. 1.3 (**a**) The Broad Street water pump on Broad St., London [5]. (**b**) US death rate from tuberculosis and pneumonia and cancer, 1900–2001 [28]

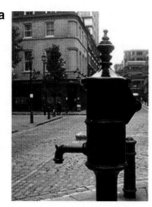

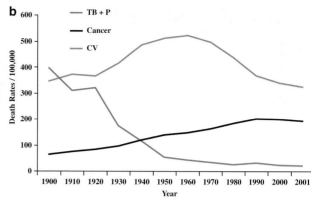

etc. A central event was the determination by Dr. J. Snow that the spread of cholera in the serious epidemic of 1854 in London was via contaminated water [5]. He had the Broad Street water pump closed after determining that it was in a very heavily involved section of London. There was a dramatic decline in incidence of cholera. His work is accepted by many as the foundation of epidemiology. A recent photograph of the famous pump is shown in Fig. 1.3a. Today this is a tourist attraction in London.

An important factor in the gain in life expectancy was the precipitous drop in death due to TB, pneumonia, and influenza, generally attributed to the public sanitation measures and more recently to drugs and antibiotics. By 2005, the mortality due to TB and pneumonia had decreased ∼ by 99.9 and ∼90% from the levels in 1900, respectively, as demonstrated in Fig. 1.3b. As would be readily predicted, cancer mortality began to increase with aging of the population. Over that period death due to cancer increased from 64 to 189 per 100,000 populations [28].

1.6 Creation of the Massachusetts General Hospital 1800–1821[3]

1.6.1 Boston and Its Medical Community at ∼1800

Dr. Samuel Fuller was a passenger on the Mayflower that landed at Plymouth in December 1620. He served as physician and pastor or deacon until his death in 1633 from smallpox [42]. The colony expanded with arrival of

additional ships loaded with pilgrims. They established several new towns, among which was Boston in 1630, i.e., not quite 400 years ago.

Several medical facilities for the public had been in operation in Boston well prior to the birth of the MGH. Among the first was an Almshouse erected in 1662, at the corner of Park and Beacon Street. Reflecting its significance to the lives of many, Beacon Street was frequently called *The Way to the Almshouse*. In 1717, a smallpox hospital commenced operation on Spectacle Island in Boston harbor. A dispensary was founded in 1796, which provided outdoor medical relief for the very poor. In addition there was a US Marine hospital in Charlestown, which opened in 1804 to provide medical care for seamen [11, 42].

After functioning for more than 100 years, the Almshouse was replaced by a new Almshouse on Leverett St., Fig. 1.4a. Charles Bulfinch was the architect of the Almshouse, one of his early major commissions. This handsome building opened in 1800. Although of substantial size, medical function was quite modest, a capacity for only eight patients[4] and a minimal dispensary. The number of applicants greatly exceeded capacity.

At the start of the 19th century, the culture and high ambitions of New England were derived principally from its highly successful maritime fleets and the associated worldwide trading activities, especially with China. Boston was quite prosperous and thought rather well of itself. By the conclusion of the War of 1812, the position as Number 1 in US commerce began to decline relative to New York, Baltimore, and Philadelphia.

The physicians of the Boston region were quite aware of their relatively disadvantaged situation, i.e., no general hospital. There were two major hospitals in the country. Benjamin Franklin had been active in founding the Pennsylvania Hospital in Philadelphia, which had opened in

---

[3] References [4, 16, 18, 24–26, 42, 45] were used for Sections 1.6–1.10. Importantly, Jeff Mifflin, Director of the MGH Archives, has been extremely helpful and provided substantial information and photographs [24].

[4] The most common diagnosis was "insanity."

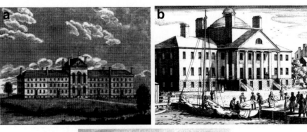

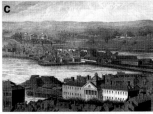

Fig. 1.4 (**a**) The Boston Almshouse, 1800. (**b**) The Bulfinch building as it appeared in 1821. (**c**) The Bulfinch after the symmetrical lengthening of each wing in 1837 [24]

1756. Thirty five years later, 1791, the Bellevue Hospital of New York City commenced operations. The Boston physicians were concerned that the quality of their medical care was less than optimal as they did not have the option of longer patient observation and the utilization of the standards of practice they had learned during their tenure in European medical schools and hospitals. Paris and Vienna were the most frequent centers for study by our physicians at that time. French culture and science were quite highly regarded and additionally there was a great affection for France, in part due to its decisive support during our war for independence. An additional point was the huge impact that a general hospital would have on the quality of the education of young doctors. Only some of the privileged few could manage the needed time for completion of their education in the highly regarded European medical centers. Not of little significance was the necessity of a hospital and an asylum for Boston to continue its status as a national leader.

Support for a hospital also came from the founding of the Harvard Medical School in 1782. The ceremony was presided over by John Warren, Professor of Anatomy. He was the father of John C. Warren, one of the principals in the creation of the MGH and its first four decades of operation.

An additional impetus for a hospital was the growing concern regarding the incidence of epidemics in Boston and neighboring coastal towns. These were commonly assumed to be secondary to the wide prevalence of poverty and the large numbers of persons passing through as an inevitable component of the maritime business.

In 1800, the social unit was primarily the family, rather than the individual. The family accepted responsibility for the care of all members, viz., the young, old, infirm, unmarried or widowed women, as well as the sick and disabled. In addition, families were expected to aid and care for servants.

This was obviously not a uniformly successful arrangement and many difficulties were clearly evident. By 1810 the concept of responsibility had begun to transcend the family and be accepted in part as a community responsibility. The need most clearly recognized was that for an asylum for the insane. There was no acceptable place even for the members of affluent families needing such care.

In 1784, a petition to the Overseers of the Poor of Boston Almshouse to permit faculty and students of the Medical Department of Harvard College to attend the sick and poor in the Almshouse was denied. The application was resubmitted in 1810. This time approval was granted, provided no expense would be charged to the town. The Professors of Harvard College in October 1810 voted that the patients of the Almshouse were to be classed as surgical or medical and placed under the charge of Drs. John Warren and James Jackson, respectively. This arrangement was continued at the MGH at its opening in 1821, where they became the Chiefs of Surgery and Medicine, respectively, and each served in that capacity for several decades with much distinction.

Drs. Warren and Jackson were graduates of Harvard Medical School and had spent considerable time studying in Europe. They were principals in the founding of the *New England Journal of Medicine* in 1812. They each served 1 year as Dean of the Harvard Medical School. Dr. Warren was the surgeon in the first publicized use of ether as anesthesia in 1846. Pertinent to this book, he wrote the first American treatise on tumors [44].

1.6.2 The Initiation of the Process by the Reverend John Bartlett to Create an Asylum and a Hospital

Reverend John Bartlett was Chaplain at the Almshouse from 1807 to 1811. He became very distressed at the conditions in which patients were held at the Almshouse, especially those classed as insane. This motivated him into a well-designed strategy to effect a correction. To assess the situation, he personally examined the hospitals in Philadelphia and New York City and read of the operation of hospitals in the cities of Europe. He then devised his plan to obtain a hospital for Boston. His initial effort was to invite Drs. Warren and Jackson, the two most highly regarded physicians in Boston, Dr. John Gorham, Peter Brooks (the most wealthy man of Boston), and John Phillips (later mayor of Boston) to a meeting at Conant Hall on March 8, 1810, for a discussion of the need for and means to realize an asylum. See Appendix Item 1 for a letter by Rev Bartlett to his son recalling this meeting [30]. The letter sent by Bartlett to several friends to consider his plan for a hospital is included in the Appendix as item 2.

At the meeting, Bartlett described as entirely unsatisfactory the conditions for patients at the Almshouse in comparison with the treatment of such patients in European countries, especially France. There was evidently no disagreement as to his description of conditions. Drs. Warren and Jackson proposed expanding the plan to include a general hospital in addition to an asylum. This was well received after initial concern that they risked getting neither by requesting "too much." They concluded the meeting by planning to circulate a letter to a substantial number of wealthy citizens and inviting them to become supporters of their scheme. When this had been achieved, they would then submit a petition to the legislature for a Charter for a general hospital and an asylum for the insane. Drs. Warren and Jackson were to lead this project.

Warren and Jackson circulated their letter on August 20, 1810, to many of the wealthy men of Boston and neighboring towns. The first few sentences are reproduced here:

> Sir- It has appeared very desirable to a number of respectable gentlemen, that a hospital for the reception of lunatics and other sick persons should be established in this town. By the appointment of a number of these gentlemen, we are directed to adopt such methods as shall appear best calculated to promote such an establishment. We therefore beg leave to submit for your consideration proposals for the institution of a hospital, and to state to you some of the reasons in favor of such an establishment.
>
> It is unnecessary to urge the propriety and even obligation of succoring the poor in sickness. The wealthy inhabitants of the town of Boston have always evinced that they consider themselves as treasurers of God's bounty; " and "in countries where Christianity is practiced, it must always be considered the first of duties to visit and to heal the sick. When in distress, every man becomes our neighbor, not only if he be of the household of faith, but even though his misfortunes have been induced by transgressing the rules both of reason and religion. For the entire letter, see Item 2 of the Appendix.

Their letter had appeal to the wealthy strata of society as the asylum would be a convenient place for members of their own class who became insane and for general medical care for their wards of various categories. In other words these new institutions could be viewed, as special purpose extensions of their homes. Warren and Jackson did emphasize that since this was an institution that would provide care for far more than the residents of Boston, this should not be an initiative by only Boston but by the entire Commonwealth. They had effectively argued that efforts to transform the Almshouse would be insufficient but that two new hospitals were necessary.

There was precedent in the history of the commonwealth for corporations charted by the state to achieve public purposes without requiring the establishment of tax supported public institutions. Instead, public incorporation of volunteer associations would be invested with semi-governmental power and accordingly required to follow approved rules and regulations. Further, there was a mechanism for formal monitoring by the state. This was to an important extent modeled on practices in England. Establishment of such corporations constituted an attractive means by which communities could achieve goals judged to be of benefit to many citizens.

1.6.3 The Legislature Grants the Charter for the MGH

Warren and Jackson's letter was highly successful and they obtained the written support of a total of 56 "worthy gentlemen" for the petition. Among these were John Adams, John Quincy Adams, Generals W. Heath, and H. Dearborn as well as representatives of important families, viz., Cabot, Coolidge, Gray, Green, Lowell, and Thorndike. The petition was prepared and submitted to the Legislature. Amazingly, the Legislature promptly granted a Charter to Mr. James Bowdoin and 55 gentlemen on February 25, 1811. See Appendix Item 3, for our charter. These men were designated the Incorporators. They were predominantly merchants and lawyers with a few physicians and clergymen.

The process thus moved with extraordinary rapidity, i.e., the initial meeting was called by Rev Bartlett on March 8, 1810; the letter of Warren and Jackson circulated on August 20, 1810, and the Charter granted on February 25, 1811, viz., less than 12 months. The Charter provided for the appointment of a Board of Visitors to be composed of the Governor, Lt Governor, President of the Senate, Speaker of the House, and Chaplains of both houses. Direct management of the institution was to be by a Board of 12 Trustees with 4 appointed by Board of Visitors. The Board of Visitors was charged to inspect the hospital at regular intervals and to examine and disallow or annul any of its bylaws, rules, and regulations. As enthusiasm for the project developed there was easing of these strictures. By 1818 the charter had been modified such that the Board of Visitors' powers to alter or annul the corporation's bylaws or repeal the corporate charter were withdrawn.

John Adams served as moderator of the first meeting of Corporation on April 23, 1811. For financial support, the state gave the hospitals: (1) the Province House property. This was built in 1679 on a 0.5-acre plot fronting on Washington Street. It was quite close to the Old South Meeting House and served as the residence for the provincial governor up to the revolution and then as a Government House until it was transferred to the MGH. This was valued at $40,000; (2) for construction of the hospital, the stone and the labor for cutting the blocks of granite into correct sizes. This represented a value of ~$35,000; and (3) hospital officers were exempted from military duty.

One severe requirement was that the Incorporators must raise $100,000 within 5 years, a not inconsiderable sum in that era. Due to the problems consequent on the War of 1812, progress on the two hospitals was delayed. There was an extension of time for raising the $100,000 by an additional 5 years. A gift by Mr. Phillips was made on condition that the Hospital be sited within the limits of Boston. The MGH is in Boston and the Asylum was constructed in Somerville.

The Incorporators found initially that there was less keenness to contribute to the hospital than the asylum, since the hospital would clearly be more expensive. An additional consideration was the common perception that there was a less severe need for a hospital. A major fund raising appeal was initiated in 1814 which achieved a modest success. There were 1047 subscribers, residing in Boston, Salem, Plymouth, Charlestown, Hingham, and Chelsea (including a few residents elsewhere). Of this number, 245 became members of the Corporation, by a gift of at least $100. Despite this level of success, the incorporators were short of funds and they petitioned the legislature for a license to sell spirited liquors. This was denied.

They were, however, provided a richer and more appropriate source of income. An Act of February 24, 1814, authorized the MGH to sell insurance. The Massachusetts Hospital Life Insurance Company was chartered in December 1818. There was a close connection between this insurance company and its "parent" institution, i.e., the MGH and the men working with it. For a while William Philips served simultaneously as the president of both the MGH and the insurance company. Messrs. Quincy, Francis, and Lowell became vice presidents and directors of the insurance company. The hospital subscribed to 10% or $50,000 of the first stock issued in 1823. The purchase of this stock was financed through a mortgage on the Province House estate. As an aside, Drs Warren and Jackson were among the initial stockholders. This insurance business did provide a valuable source of revenue for the hospital for a sustained time period in the form of interest, stock dividends, and 1/3 share of profits. Later the business was expanded to include trust accounts, which proved to be highly profitable.

1.6.4 Acquisition of Sites for the Asylum and the MGH

For the site for the Asylum, the Joseph Barrel estate of 18 acres on a hill near Lechmere Point in Somerville was purchased in December 1816. This was directly across the Charles River from future site of the MGH. Charles Bulfinch was the architect for the building program there. The Asylum admitted its first patient on October 6, 1818. As a result of gifts of $120,000, in total, by the Boston merchant John McLean, the Asylum became The McLean Hospital in 1825.

Mr. Warren Phillips increased his father's legacy of $5 K–$20 K. This large donation had a powerful stimulatory effect on other patrons and accelerated fund raising. By January 5, the amount received had reached $93,969. Purchases of small plots of land at the potential site of the hospital commenced.

On October 6, 1817, the corporation acquired Prince's pasture, a 4-acre field on the bank of the Charles River for $20,000. This was called the North Allen Street property. That site on the Charles River provided the major advantage of making the hospital readily accessible to the patients from coastal New England who would come by boat. To facilitate the arrival of these patients, a pier was added to the hospital. Although this location was convenient for the wealthy living on Beacon Hill's south side, some viewed it negatively due to the proximity to the "drunkards, harlots and spendthrifts and outcasts of the country" on the north side, adjacent to the site of the planned hospital.

The design of the MGH seal was accepted on November 30, 1817. This featured an Indian with a bow in one hand and an arrow in the other. On the right side is a star encircled by the inscription, Massachusetts General Hospital, 1811.

Charles Bulfinch was commissioned to serve as the architect of the new hospital. In preparation for his work on the hospital, he visited hospitals in New York and Philadelphia. In March 1817, Bullfinch submitted his plan. He was then commissioned to arrange the construction of the MGH. On December 7, 1817, a decision was made that the building would be "of stone and of that kind called granite." The new Board formally adopted the plan by Bulfinch on February 1. A relatively uncommon design feature was the provision of the building with central heating and plumbing.

Reflecting the high importance of the Bulfinch building to the history of our hospital, several comments on the architect may be of interest [22]. Charles Bulfinch (1763–1844) was connected with medicine, viz., his father was a prominent Boston physician. Charles was a graduate of Boston Latin School and Harvard College with B.A. and M.A. degrees. This was followed by 2 years in Europe and for part of the time; he had the great good fortune to have Thomas Jefferson as a mentor. Among his buildings were the first theater in New England; the Massachusetts state capital; 1795–1797; the Almshouse, 1801; Faneuil Hall, Boston, 1805; Harvard University Hall, 1813–1814; and the Asylum, 1818. Then came the MGH in 1821. He exercised an important additional role in the city, as evident by his long service as a member of the Board of Selectman, starting in 1797. Later important works included the rotunda of the national capital during his tenure as Commissioner of US Public Buildings, 1818–1830. Also, he was the architect for the state capitals in Connecticut and Maine. Thus, our first building was designed by America's foremost architect.

1.7 The Massachusetts General Hospital 1821–1895

1.7.1 The MGH Opens

The name of our hospital, the Massachusetts General Hospital, implies that it is owned and operated by the state of Massachusetts. This name is based on the state charter permitting its establishment. The MGH has not been operated by the state either initially or at any point in its history. The hospital was created on February 25, 1811, by a Charter granted by the Massachusetts Legislature or General Court. The MGH has been operated as a private philanthropic institution for just short of 200 years by the generous and intelligent effort of many public spirited citizens.

On July 4, 1818, the ceremony for laying the cornerstone of the MGH featured an address by Josiah Quincy with the Governor in attendance. Three years later, August 21, 1821, letters were sent to John Warren and James Jackson stating that the hospital would quite soon be ready to accept patients.

The appearance of the original MGH Bulfinch Building is illustrated in Fig. 1.4b. The hospital site on the Charles River with a wharf provided ready access to patients from along the river and the coast. An important point is that there were provisions for the treatment of outpatients from the opening of the hospital. The first patient was admitted on September 3, 1821, a 30-year-old sailor. Neither his diagnosis nor the outcome of this admission is mentioned in the accounts of the early history reviewed. Not until September 20 was the next application made for admission. Six free beds were established; three each for medicine and surgery. By October, there had been 7 female and 12 male patients in hospital. There were some of the usual behavioral problems, e.g., in 1824 a patient was dismissed "for having introduced liquor privately." The bed capacity in 1823 was 73 beds [4]. There was satisfaction and pride in Boston in that the care provided at the MGH was assessed by the staff as comparable to that at the Pennsylvania and Bellevue hospitals. The demand for hospital service exceeded capacity and in 1837 both wings of the Bulfinch building were expanded to their present dimensions, Fig. 1.4c.

A mummy from Thebes was received as a gift in 1822. The hospital leased this mummy for exhibition in other cities for a period of 1 year. In September of that year, profits from exhibits of the mummy were reported as $1500. This mummy is presently on exhibit in the Ether Dome.

The Harvard Medical School moved to a new building on North Grove St., adjacent to the MGH 1846–1875. One gain for the school was an increment in space by a factor of 2. This provided for large lecture halls, a chemical laboratory, rooms for surgical and pathological demonstration, and the school library. Importantly, the building was heated and well ventilated [20].

During the period 1849–1895, there were at least 10 buildings added to the MGH complex. To appreciate the scale of this expansion, review the changing MGH footprint as illustrated in the Introduction, Figs. 1–5. Among the new buildings was the Thayer building in 1883 on the site that would be used in 1975 for the Cox building, the first MGH cancer center.

1.7.2 Early Medical Advances at MGH

1832 Henry Bowditch introduced the method of thoracentesis.
1835 Bigelow's Essay on Self-limited Diseases essentially eliminated the common but futile bleeding, purging, etc., categories of "therapies."
1843 O. Holmes proposed that puerperal fever was contagious, *vide infra*
1846 Anesthesia first used. *Vide infra.*
1886 Pathologist R. Fitz proposed the pathogenesis of appendicitis and the cure by surgery.
1891 The Dalton Scholarship program was created. This served as the birth of basic science at MGH.

1.8 Major 19th Century Medical Advances that Impacted Oncology

1.8.1 Anesthesia. October 16, 1846

Humphry Davy proposed in 1800 that nitrous oxide "appears capable of destroying physical pain, it may probably be used with advantage during surgical operations." Several dentists employed nitrous oxide with mixed success to reduce or eliminate the pain of dental procedures. Eighteen years after the suggestions of Davy, Michael Faraday suggested the potential control of pain by breathing the vapors of sulfuric ether. The first use of ether for anesthesia for a surgical procedure was in March 1842 by Crawford Long, practicing in a small community in Georgia, for excision of a neck tumor. William Morton began using sulfuric ether, mixed with oil of orange to reduce unpleasantness of dental procedures. Henry Bigelow, a young member of Warren's team, observed several dental procedures on patients under ether anesthesia by Morton. He arranged for Morton and Warren to meet. They met and discussed the potential of anesthesia for larger surgical procedures. Morton was invited by letter to come to the MGH and demonstrate the efficacy of his agent. On October 16, 1846, William Morton administered ether anesthesia to patient Mr. Gilbert Abbott for John C. Warren to remove a tumor of the neck. Mr. Abbott experienced no pain. The famous comment to the crowd in the amphitheater of Warren after the procedure was "Gentlemen, this is no Humbug."

That this procedure was performed by the most famous surgeon of the country and at the Massachusetts General Hospital had an immediate and dramatic impact. Anesthesia became available for surgery worldwide in a remarkably short time. This made for major expansions of surgery. Prior to October 1846, the number of surgical procedures per week at the MGH was 1–3, only one lightly used operating room. Anesthesia constitutes one of the greatest advances in all of medicine [1, 6, 14]. A large and quite impressive painting of this historic event hangs in the Ether Dome. The artist is Warren Prospero.

1.8.2 Puerperal Fever

That puerperal fever was a contagious disease was clearly stated by A. Gordon of Aberdeen in 1795. This concept was accepted with quite remarkable reluctance by the medical community until late in the 19th century. In 1843, O. W. Holmes published evidence that child bed fever was a contagious disease and often the result of physicians coming from examining patients or attending an autopsy of patients with puerperal fever [21]. The evidence he provided had slight effect. I. Semelweiss demonstrated in 1848 at the First Obstetrics Clinic of the University of Vienna that the washing of hands with chlorinated lime before entering the obstetrics wards reduced childbirth mortality from 18% in April 1847 to 2.4% for June and 1.2% for July. This rate was comparable to that in the Second Obstetrics Clinic managed by mid-wives who did not participate in postmortem examinations. Despite this clear success, his findings were rejected at his institution, despite acceptance by a few colleagues. Further, his appointment was not renewed and he returned to Hungary in 1850. There he continued to achieve the very low mortality rate while death of women at Vienna continued at the earlier high rate [3]. Change in clinical practice was slow until almost the time of Pasteur and Lister. Today, the risk of death due to infections at delivery is $\sim 10^{-4}$.

1.8.3 Antiseptic Surgery

Joseph Lister was the Professor of Surgery at Glasgow. Knowing that Pasteur had shown that heat sterilized objects, Lister decided to test chemicals in preparation of the surgical field. He used carbolic acid which had been shown effective in disinfection of sewage in Carlisle, England. On August 12, 1865 he treated the room and operative site for a compound tibial fracture with carbolic acid. The almost invariable infection did not develop. In March 1867, he published his experience with disinfectant agents and the clear success. His work was widely acclaimed and initiated intensive study of methods of disinfection. Lister fully extended credit to Semelweiss and Pasteur. Achievement of sepsis free

surgery on anesthetized patients was a medical advance of the highest importance [43]. However, surgical gloves did not become widely used until late in the 1880s. The surgical mask came on the scene in 1898, due to largely to the work of Mikulicz-Radecki in Wroclow, Poland.

1.8.4 Endocrine and Chemotherapy

Hormone therapy for breast carcinoma commenced in 1895 by Beatson of Edinburgh who performed the first oophorectomy as treatment [2]. There is a report that castration was used in 1898 for prostate cancer patients by Dr. J.W. White in Philadelphia [10]. Chemotherapy for cancer patients started in the 1940s with the use of nitrogen mustard and related agents that had produced severe bone marrow toxicity during WWII [19]. The discovery of X-rays by Röentgen brought into the medicine radiological imaging and treatment methods.

1.9 Wilhelm Konrad Röentgen and the Discovery of X-Rays

The announcement of the discovery of X-rays by Röentgen of Würzburg on December 28, 1895, introduced an entirely new modality into oncology [9, 15, 32]. The start of the year 1896 brought an intense interest for technological and clinical advancement of diagnostic and therapeutic radiology. Amazingly, within 5 years, discoveries of the electron, alpha, beta rays, and the gamma rays were announced [31]. Then in 1919 and 1932 the proton and neutron were discovered, respectively. These constitute the technical basis for our discipline.

Röentgen was born in 1845 in Lennep, Germany, not far from Düsseldorf [9]. At 3 years of age, Röentgen and his family moved to Apeldoorn, the Netherlands where he lived until age 17. At that time he entered Utrecht Technical School. He was an excellent scholar and wrote a section in one of his professor's chemistry textbooks and did work as an instructor in chemistry. Despite these successes, when Wilhelm refused to give the name of a fellow student who wrote a negative caricature of one of the professors on a blackboard he was expelled. Because of this incident, which many would not characterize as a negative personal characteristic, he was denied admission to Utrecht University. This is the basis for his going to Zurich Polytechnikum. There he studied Mechanical Engineering and at age 24 was awarded the Ph.D. degree. Röentgen was promptly offered a position in physics in Zurich by Professor Kundt. Within a year (1870), Kundt went to Würzburg as chair of physics and then 2 years later to the Kaiser Wilhelm's University of Strasburg. Röentgen moved with him. An offer to Röentgen in 1879 of

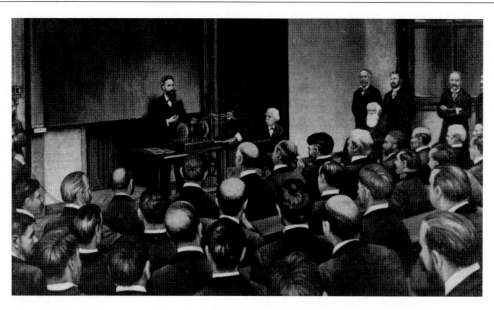

Fig. 1.5 Wilhelm Konrad Röentgen [9]

the professorship of physics at the University of Hessian was accepted. After 10 years of productive research, he accepted the invitation to be the Chair of Physics and directorship of the Physics Institute of the University of Würzburg, Fig. 1.5.

In the spring of 1894 Wilhelm Röentgen commenced his own series of experiments seeking to understand the cathode rays using Hittorf-Crookes tubes. During an experiment on Friday, November 8 1895, using a Crookes[5] tube that featured a high vacuum, he covered the tube with cardboard and tinfoil. While passing a high tension discharge through the tube, he happened to notice a reflection from a mirror. This was quite unexpected and he determined that the light had originated from a barium platinocyanide coated piece of paper at a distance of approximately 1 m from his Hittorf-Crookes tube. By observing the light and repeatedly discharging the tube, the source of the agent activating the barium platinocyanide was readily proven to be the tube. He appreciated that this could not be due to cathode rays as their range in air was far too short. He observed that magnets that easily deflected cathode rays did not affect the propagation of these rays and that they moved in straight lines. Further, there was no detectable refraction by lenses. The intensity of the rays decreased with the square of the distance. As his experimentation continued, he learned that metal was not transparent to the rays while they readily penetrated rubber and wood. At one point while the tube was active, he noticed a shadow of one of his fingers on the paper while he

placed objects in front of the paper. This was the first radiographic image of human anatomy. Next he recorded images of diverse objects on photographic film. On December 22, he took the first radiograph of a human anatomic part, his wife's hand. His manuscript was given to the Würzburg Physical and Medical Society on December 28, 1895. See Appendix Item 4. The title of his paper was *Ueber eine neue Art von strahlen* or a new kind of rays. He requested that the rays be called X-rays as their physical nature was still little studied. He later resisted their being called Röentgen rays. A translation of his paper is reproduced in the Appendix as Item 5. He sent a letter to several physicists to inform them of his experimental findings. This received wide newspaper coverage almost immediately. He made a presentation to the Kaiser on January 14. His first public lecture was January 23, 1896. To the consternation of several physicists who had been working with the same or similar tubes, there was the realization that they had missed a most important phenomenon. These included Lenard, Hertz, Crookes.

The radiograph of his wife's hand clearly demonstrated the details of her ring, bony details, and outline of the soft tissues. The implications for high accuracy of diagnosis of the site of bone fracture and foreign objects were not subtle.

This report had a huge, immediate, and growing impact on medicine, physics, and the general public. Röentgen's investigation of this problem is a model of care in planning, thoroughness of experimental procedure, speed in completion of a definitive investigation and understanding of a newly recognized phenomenon of nature, and submission of a report of his findings for publication in a mere 7 weeks. The stimulus for intensive investigation by scientists, engineers, and physicians of these newly observed radiations and their medical applications was powerful.

---

[5] There is variability of the details of the actual experiment. Roentgen requested that all of his experiment records be burned after his death. Apparently for this series of experiments, he used a Crooke's tube although earlier he had used Hittorf and Lenard tubes extensively.

Fig. 1.6 (**a**) A Sunday Afternoon on the Island of La Grande Jatte by G. Seurat, 1885 [34]. (**b**) The Abstract Plant Composition of 1892 by H. Van de Velde [41]

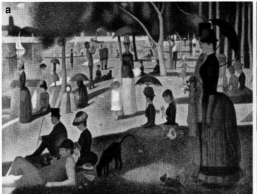
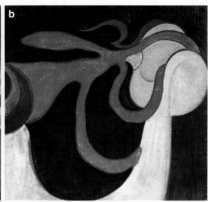

1.10 The World that Received the News of Röentgen's New Rays

These medical and scientific advances were concurrent with the industrial revolution that was rapidly effecting dramatic changes in the lives of persons in all continents. These induced a spirit of optimism and a sense that the future would bring to humanity a continuing series of real gains. This spirit perhaps contributed to the extreme alacrity with which Röentgen's announcement of his new Rays was accepted. That is, the traditional attitude had been that which was "good enough for our fathers is good enough for us" was increasingly replaced by the attitude that we can and should improve on the standards of our fathers. We have noted the failure of physicians in the USA and in Europe to act on the findings of Holmes and of Semelweiss re the infectious nature of puerperal fever. Society had moved into a much more positive response pattern regarding new concepts and technologies.

This more ready acceptance of the new and different is reflected by the radically new art that began to be produced at the end of the 19th century. Two examples are included here. The *A Sunday Afternoon on the Island of Le Grand Jatte* by G. Seurat in 1885 illustrating a happy afternoon by the greatly expanded middle class, Fig. 1.6a [34]. As an example of the interest in the radically new is one of the very earliest of the abstract art, viz., the 1892 painting by H. van de Velde, titled Abstract Plant Composition, Fig. 1.6b [41].

References

1. Adler R. Medical firsts: from Hippocrates to the human genome. Hoboken, NJ: Wiley; 2004.
2. Beatson GT. On treatment of inoperable cases of carcinoma of the mamma: suggestions for a new method of treatment with illustrative cases. Lancet. 1896;2:104–7.
3. Bender G. Great moments in medicine. Detroit, MI: Parke Davis; 1961.
4. Bowditch N. A history of the Massachusetts General Hospital. Boston, MA: John Wilson & Son; 1851.
5. Broad Street Pump. http://en.wikipedia.org/wiki/File:John_Snow_memorial_and_pub.jgp. Accessed on 2009.
6. Camac CN. Classics of medicine and surgery. New York, NY: Dover; 1959.
7. Conard NJ. Palaeolithic ivory sculptures from southwestern Germany and the origins of figurative art. Nature. 2003;426(6968):830–2.
8. Conard NJ. Tubingen University Museum. With permission.
9. Del Regato JA. Radiological physicists. New York, NY: American Institute of Physics; 1985. With permission.
10. Dodson JL. A century of oncology. Greenwich, CT: Greenwich Press; 1997.
11. Eaton LK. New England Hospitals. Ann Arbor, MI: University of Michigan Press; 1957.
12. Ebers Papyrus. http://en.wikipedia.org/wiki/Ebers_Papyrus. Accessed on 2009.
13. Estes JW. The medical skills of ancient Egypt. Canton, MA: Science History Publications; 1989.
14. Fenster JM. Ether day: the strange tale of America's greatest medical discovery and the haunted men who made it. New York, NY: Harper Collins; 2001.
15. Gagliardi R, Wilson JF. A history of radiological sciences: radiation oncology. Reston, VA: Radiology Centennial; 1996.
16. Garland J. Every man our neighbor: a brief history of the Massachusetts General Hospital. Boston, MA: Little, Brown & Co.; 1961.
17. Garrison F. An introduction to the history of medicine. Philadelphia, PA; WB Saunders; 1929.
18. Gerteis M. The Massachusetts General Hospital, 1810–1865: an essay on the political construction of social responsibility during New England's early industrialization. Boston, MA: Tufts University; 1986.
19. Goodman LS, Wintrobe MM, Dameshek W, Goodman MJ, Gilman A, McLennan MT. Landmark article Sept. 21, 1946: nitrogen mustard therapy. Use of methyl-bis(beta-chloroethyl)amine hydrochloride and tris(beta-chloroethyl)amine hydrochloride for Hodgkin's disease, lymphosarcoma, leukemia and certain allied and miscellaneous disorders. JAMA. 1984;251(17):2255–61.
20. Harvard Medical School Countway Library. Center for the History of Medicine. Harvard Medical School. Harvard Medical School Buildings and Grounds, Early Locations. Images, ca. 1824–1975: Finding Aid. October 2004. Available at http://oasis.lib.harvard.edu/oasis/deliver/~med00018. Accessed on 2009.
21. Holmes OW. The contagiousness of puerperal fever. N Engl Q J Med Surg. 1843;1:503–30.

22. Kirker H. The architecture of Charles Bulfinch. Cambridge, MA: Harvard University Press; 1969.
23. Manjo G. The healing hand. Cambridge, MA: Harvard University Press; 1975.
24. Massachusetts General Hospital Archives 2005–2008.
25. MGH. Massachusetts General Hospital Memorial and Historical Volume (together with proceedings of the centennial of the opening of the Hospital.) Boston, MA: Griffith-Stillings Press; 1921.
26. Myers GW. History of the Massachusetts General Hospital: June 1872–December 1900. Boston, MA: Griffith-Stillings Press; 1929.
27. Neuhauser D. Oliver Wendell Holmes MD 1809–94 and the logic of medicine. Qual Saf Health Care. 2006;15(4):302–4.
28. Pearson Education, Inc. Death rates by cause of death, 1900–2005. Information Please^R Database. 2007. http://www.infoplease.com/ipa/A0922292.html. Accessed on 2009.
29. Philadelphia Tablet. Cuneiform Writing at the Philadelphia Museum of Archeology and Anthropology. With permission 2010.
30. Reed W. A memoir of the Reverend John Bartlett. Boston, MA: The Merrymount Press; 1936.
31. Reichen C. A history of physics. New York, NY: Hawthorne Books; 1963.
32. Roentgen WC. On a new kind of rays: translation of a paper read before the Würzburg Physical and Medical Society. Nature. 1895;53:274–6.
33. Ruiz A. The spirit of ancient Egypt. New York, NY: Algora Publishing; 2001.
34. Seurat G. A Sunday afternoon on the Island of La Grande Jatte.1885. Chicago Institute of Art. With permission.
35. St. Bartholomew Hospital. http://www.hiddenlondon.com/stbartsmus.htm. Accessed on 2009.
36. Sri Lanka Hospitals. Wikipedia. http://en.wikipedia.org/wiki/Hospital. Accessed on 2009.
37. Sumerian Medical Text. Museum of the University of Pennsylvania. With permission 2010.
38. Time line for Humans. Life expectancy from pre-historic era to present. Wikipedia. Available at http://en.wikipedia.org/wiki/Life_expectancy#Life_expectancy_over_human_history. Accessed on 2009.
39. Thompson J, Goldin G. The hospital: a social and architectural history. New Haven, CT: Yale University Press; 1975.
40. U.S. Department of Commerce, Bureau of the Census, Historical Statistics of the United States. Life Expectancy by age, 1850–2004. Information Please® Database. 2007. Available at http://www.infoplease.com/ipa/A0005140.html. Accessed on 2009.
41. Van de Velde H. Abstract Plant Composition. Stichting Kröller-Müller Museum. Otterlo. NK. With permission 2010.
42. Viets HR. A brief history of medicine in Massachusetts. Boston, MA: Houghton Mifflin; 1930.
43. Wangensteen OH, Wangensteen SD. The rise of surgery. Minneapolis, MN: University of Minnesota Press; 1978.
44. Warren JM. Surgical observations on tumours, with cases and operations. Boston, MA: Crocker & Brewster; 1837.
45. Washburn F. The Massachusetts General Hospital: its development, 1900–1935. Cambridge, MA: Houghton Mifflin Riverside Press; 1939.

Chapter 2

Radiation Oncology and the MGH 1896–1945

2.1 The Almost Instantaneous Acceptance of X-Rays into Medicine

Radiology literally erupted onto the medical and scientific community following publication of the paper by Wilhelm Conrad Röentgen on December 28, 1895, describing the discovery of new rays. The immediacy of the impact on the world was strikingly evident by the speed with which physics laboratories, hospitals, and clinics began assembling equipment. Within a year there was a substantial and positive experience using radiographs for diagnosis and a beginning of testing of their very low kVp beams as treatment for superficial lesions. Reflecting the literally fantastic excitement in medicine and physics generated by Röentgen's paper were the >1000 scientific papers and ~50 books during 1896 on the new rays [6].

The first documented medical use of x-rays in the USA was that by Edwin Frost, an Assistant Professor of Physics at Dartmouth College on February 3, 1896, and reported in *Science* on February 14,1896 [10]. This article did not include a medical radiograph. The patient was provided by Frost's brother, a Professor of Medicine at the medical school. The patient, a young man, was proven by this x-ray to have a Colles' fracture of the left ulna as presented in Fig. 2.1 [19]. That February 14 issue of *Science* had several articles on these rays, including a 5-page article by W. Röentgen.

Francis Williams, a physician of Boston City Hospital, began to investigate the potential of the new x-ray images concurrently. For his initial studies, he took patients for imaging studies to the physics laboratory of R. Lawrence and C. Norton at MIT. A radiograph of the hand demonstrating "anomalies of the phalanges" was published on February 20, 1896, in the *Boston Medical and Surgical Journal*[1] [44]. MGH began use of x-rays in March 1896 along with large numbers of American and European hospitals [11].

That the new rays could injure normal tissues became quite clear within a month of the Röentgen discovery. Perhaps the earliest instance of radiation injury to human tissues was that of Emil Grubbe, an electrical engineer [7, 11]. He was examined at the Hahnemann Medical College of Chicago by three physicians for a "suppurating erythema" of the left hand on January 27, 1896, viz., 1 month after Röentgen's paper was published. He reportedly had tested his x-ray beam by examining the image of his hand multiple times per day. At that visit, the physicians suggested that the radiations might be effective therapeutically. One day later, Grubbe was referred a patient with post-surgical recurrent breast cancer whom he claimed to have treated. He was evidently among the first to employ radiation therapeutically for malignant disease. There has been no published description of the result. Grubbe sustained grievous radiation injuries, some requiring surgery. Elihu Thomson published in *Electrical Engineer*, New York on March 4, 1896 [38], a warning of the potential of injurious effects of these new rays and described protection by enclosing the machine head in a box with only a small aperture for the beam.

The number of severe skin reactions being reported was accepted as proof of a biological effect of these new rays and indicated a potential for these new rays in the treatment of one or more human diseases. Actually, the new rays

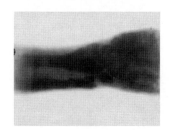

Fig. 2.1 Perhaps the first medical x-ray taken in the USA (February 3, 1896). This demonstrated a Colles' fracture [19]. With permission

---

[1] This article did not give the author but did state that the picture "is taken from a patient at Boston City Hospital, by the kind co-operation of the Department of Physics at the Massachusetts Institute of Technology with gentlemen connected with the hospital." Williams was a physician at Boston City Hospital, a graduate of MIT, had connections with the physicists, and almost immediately became a specialist in this emerging specialty.

H.D. Suit, J.S. Loeffler, *Evolution of Radiation Oncology at Massachusetts General Hospital*,
DOI 10.1007/978-1-4419-6744-2_2, © Springer Science+Business Media, LLC 2011

were rapidly being assessed for therapeutic efficacy against virtually the entire spectrum of diseases. Note that the basic nature of most diseases was unknown, the efficacy of available remedies low, and the biological action of the rays on tissues quite unstudied. Hence, a major medical "fishing expedition" ensued.

Although the name of the person(s) who first used radiation with therapeutic intent is not certain, there is clarity of the essentially immediate acceptance of a therapeutic potential of the new x-rays.

The leading academic radiologist in Boston in 1900 was Francis Williams [7], a graduate of MIT (chemistry) and then Harvard Medical School (HMS), in 1877. This was followed by 2 years in Vienna and Paris. Upon return, he practiced medicine at Boston City Hospital. In 1884, Williams was appointed to the faculty of HMS. Williams maintained his connections at MIT. As noted above he was among the first to employ x-rays for medical imaging. Williams was a friend of Elihu Thomson and was rare among radiologists at that time in his acceptance of Thomson's warning, viz., he enclosed his x-ray tubes in lead-lined boxes with only a small aperture. We have no information as to why this simple method was not implemented at MGH. Of interest is that Williams employed fluoroscopy extensively and lived to the age of 84 years. No injurious effect of his radiation exposure is mentioned in the accounts of Williams reviewed.

In 1901, Williams published a landmark book in radiology: *The Röentgen Rays in Medicine and Surgery* [45]. This most impressive book has 658 pages and 390 figures, principally of radiographic images. William's book has been reprinted in a special edition in 1988 by the Classics of Medicine Library and a photograph of the book is in Fig. 2.2.

The book opens with 58 pages on technical aspects of radiology. There are 63 pages on radiation therapy, with 22

patient photographs. Williams employed tin foil or white lead painted masks to achieve shaped treatment fields and thereby reduce dose to normal tissues.

The industry, organizational skills, and efficiency to collect and organize this vast quantity of material, write the text, *sans* computer, submit for publication, and have the book on sale within 6 years of the discovery of Röentgen must be rated as most exceptional. This book is recommended for those interested in the start of radiology by a fine clinician and serious scholar.

Photographs of complete response of a patient with a squamous cell carcinoma of the lip is presented in Fig. 2.3a, b. Quite unrelated to present-day medicine, patients were treated by radiation for lupus vulgaris (TB of the skin). Evidently, complete responses were not uncommon. Figure 2.3c, d illustrates such a patient, from William's book [45]. The response was almost certainly not the consequence of bactericidal action of the low dose of radiation. Similar results on lupus patients at many clinics served as a stimulus for radiation treatment of patients with pulmonary TB, but evidently not at Boston City Hospital. The treatment was not effective against the pulmonary disease.

As evidence of the tendency to try radiation as treatment for nearly all diseases, examine Fig. 2.4, a photograph of patients treated for epilepsy in 1904 at the Philadelphia Hospital [11] by irradiation of the head. The one clear effect was epilation.

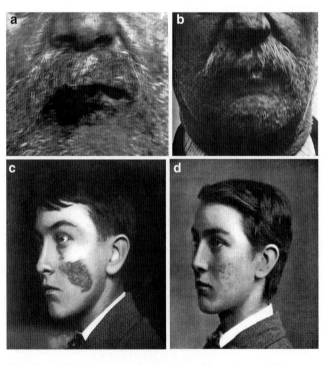

Fig. 2.3 (**a, b**) Squamous cell carcinoma of lip before and following x-ray therapy. (**c, d**) Lupus vulgaris of the cheek in a young man before and following x-ray treatment [45]. With permission

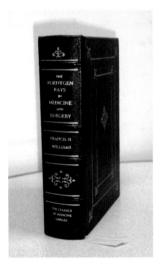

Fig. 2.2 *Röentgen Rays in Medicine and Surgery* by F. Williams published in 1901 [45]

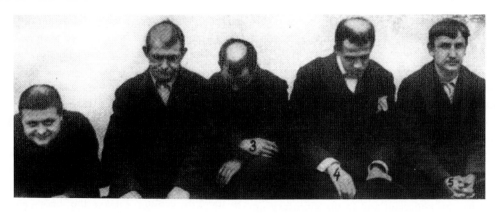

Fig. 2.4   Epilation after irradiation of the scalp for epilepsy at the Philadelphia Hospital, 1904 [11]. With permission

2.2 The First Experiment in Radiation Biology. *Lancet*. 22, 1896

Grover Lyon suggested that Röentgen rays might have therapeutic use against bacteria in a brief note in *Lancet* of February 1, 1896 [22]. In the February 22 issue of *Lancet* [23], he reported negative results for irradiation of an "impure culture of diphtheritic bacilli" in a test tube at 35° for 12 h. He observed that "considerable growth took place during these 12 hours." "A pure cultivation of tubercle bacilli exposed at the same time showed a vigorous power of growth afterwards." He concluded "experiments like these are not, of course final. Increased knowledge and improved apparatus may place the cure of disease by radiant energy within the possibility of the future." He was referring to bacterial infections. The x-rays were almost certainly of low energy and delivered at a low dose rate to bacteria in a test tube. Estimation of the dose delivered is not feasible due to absence of technical details of the radiation generator, the test tube wall thickness, target test tube distance, etc. Surely the doses were far less than that required to sterilize a test tube loaded with bacteria. At present, ionizing radiations are used extensively in industry to sterilize food and many items. In this department, all of the feed for our mouse colony comes as radiation sterilized by a single dose of 35,000 Gy.

Lyon was a Senior Assistant Physician at the Victoria Park Chest Hospital, London. The alacrity with which he acted after reading of a quite different radiation, planned and performed an experiment, analyzed results, wrote and submitted a paper, and had it published in *Lancet* in less than 8 weeks is clearly impressive.

2.3 Advances in Physics, 1895–1900

A fascinating aspect of the manifestly impressive record of multiple and significant advances in physics during the 19th century is the conclusion by a few very highly regarded physicists that there was little to no prospect for further advances. As an example of such a negative opinion for the future of physics, in 1900 Lord Kelvin, perhaps the most highly regarded physicist at the close of the 19th century, is quoted by multiple sources as stating to a meeting of the British Association for the Advancement of Science: "There is nothing new to be discovered in physics now. All that remains is more and more precise measurement"[2] [39]. This was not a unique view of the future of physics at that time, see the footnote.[3] Even at present, not dissimilar views are articulated by prominent science writers, e.g., Horgan in his book *The End of Science* of 1996. [16]

With significant discoveries popping up at an incredible frequency, pessimism of any physicist is not easily comprehended.

1895: Röentgen discovered x-rays.
1895: Perrin found that cathode rays are negative particles.
1896: Becquerel discovered natural radioactivity in uranium ore.
1897: J.J. Thomson discovered electrons, the first subatomic particle demonstrated.

---

[2] We found no published statement by Kelvin to this effect.

[3] Albert A. Michelson, in his speech at the dedication of Ryerson Physics Lab, U. of Chicago, 1894, is quoted as saying "The more important fundamental laws and facts of physical science have all been discovered, and these are now so firmly established that the possibility of their ever being supplanted in consequence of new discoveries is exceedingly remote.... Our future discoveries must be looked for in the sixth place of decimals" [27]. Max Planck commented in a 1924 speech: "When I began my physical studies [in Munich in 1874] and sought advice from my venerable teacher Philipp von Jolly... he portrayed to me physics as a highly developed, almost fully matured science ... Possibly in one or another nook there would perhaps be a dust particle or a small bubble to be examined and classified, but the system as a whole stood there fairly secured, and theoretical physics approached visibly that degree of perfection which, for example, geometry has had already for centuries" [30].

1898: Marconi achieved transmission of signals across the English Channel.

1898: The Curies discovered radium and polonium.

1898 Rutherford discovered α- and β-radiation.

1900: Planck formulated Planck's constant.

1900: Villard discovered γ-rays.

Thus, from December 1985 through 1900, x-rays, the electron, alpha, beta, and gamma rays were discovered [33]. This had to be, without equivocation, quite a remarkable 5 years for physics. The ease of separating these radiations by a magnetic field was an important tool in the discovery of these particles and is illustrated in Fig. 2.5 [12].

This fantastic pace of discoveries in physics continued without abatement. Below is a quite abbreviated listing of advances in physics, 1901–1920 [33].

1902: Rutherford and Soddy formulated a theory of transmutation by radiation and were the first to use the term "atomic energy."

1904: Nagaoka proposed the planetary model of the atom.

1905: Einstein announced his concept of special relativity plus his proposal of the equivalence of mass and energy.

1908: Geiger, Royds, and Rutherford identified α-particles as helium nuclei.

1912: Wegener proposed and presented substantial evidence for tectonic plates.

1913: Bohr utilized quantum theory to explain electron orbits in atoms.

1915: Einstein announced his theory of general relativity; he predicted the gravitational power of a star to bend light.

1919: Rutherford demonstrated the proton in the atomic nucleus.

1920: Rutherford proposed existence of the neutron and proposed its name.

The term photon was not proposed until 1926 in the article in *Nature* by G. Lewis [20]. The neutron was discovered in 1932 by J. Chadwick [4] while working in Rutherford's

laboratory.[4] Thus, the three prominent atomic constituents, electron, proton, and neutron, had been discovered by 1932. These are critical players in accelerating advance in nuclear physics. These shortly led to nuclear fission and then the atomic bomb. For medicine, an important result was the availability of a large and expanding number of radioactive isotopes (e.g., ^{60}Co, ^{137}Cs, ^{125}I, ^{131}I) for radiology, diagnostic and therapeutic.

Due to space constraints, the advances in biology chemistry and medicine are not considered here. Mention has to be made of two of the most significant developments in biology in the 19th century. First is the theory and extensive supporting data for evolution of life forms by Charles Darwin, 1859. Second is the work of G. Mendel who published in 1866 [8] results of cross-breeding of hybrids of peas and the basic laws of heredity. His important report was not appreciated until his work was "re-discovered" in 1900, after 34 years. He shortly became famous and is ranked as the Father of Genetics.

2.4 The Start-Up of Radiology and Radiation Therapy at the MGH: The Walter Dodd Era

2.4.1 Walter James Dodd, 1869–1916. The Developer of Radiology at MGH

This section is taken largely from Macy's *Biography of Dodd*, 1918 [24], and from [21, 25, 26, 43]. The initiator and developer of diagnostic radiology and of radiation oncology at the Massachusetts General Hospital was Walter J. Dodd (WJD). Despite being disadvantaged as a youth, he did achieve an impressive education, largely on his own. He was widely described as possessing exceptional personal charm, initiative, enthusiasm, and well-directed energy. That is a formidable combination and clearly served him well in his efforts to propel the MGH to a rapid entry into radiology at the start of 20th century medicine.

Walter Dodd (see Fig. 2.6a, b) was born in London in 1869. His father was a metal roofer and also quite active in the labor movement. However, he died when Walter was only 8 years old. Due to an insufficient family support system, the boy was sent to Boston to live with a married sister.

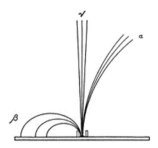

Fig. 2.5 The effect of a magnetic field on the path of α-, β-, and γ-rays

---

[4] For a thoroughly fascinating biography of Chadwick, read the book *The Neutron and the Bomb: A Biography of Sir James Chadwick* by Andrew Brown [2]. This book received a full page very positive review in *Nature*. Brown is a radiation oncologist. He had 2 years as a fellow in this department and is now working at the Kennedy School of Government and at a clinic in New Hampshire.

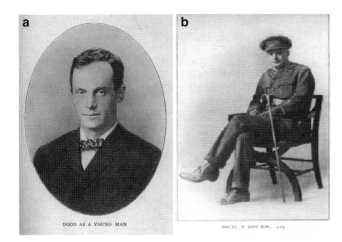

Fig. 2.6 (**a**) Walter J. Dodd as a young man. (**b**) Walter Dodd in his military uniform, 1915 [24]

She did manage for him to attend a public school to age 13, but then he had to "Drop Out." Dodd worked for almost 5 years at the Oriental Tea Co. as an office boy. He attended a Unitarian Sunday school at the Bulfinch Chapel. There he made a quite positive image for himself due in part to his success as an actor, especially as a comic in the Church theatrical program. His Sunday school teacher was a Ms. Bullard. At age 18, Walter professed interest in life as a seaman and world traveler. However, his sister was opposed to such a life for her brother. Ms. Bullard concurred and arranged for her cousin, Charles Eliot, the President of Harvard College, to meet Walter. Eliot rated the young man favorably and invited him to accept a job as an assistant janitor at a chemistry laboratory. Young Dodd judged this to be more attractive than the sea and accepted Eliot's offer. He worked there for 5 years, until 1892. WJD was intensely curious about the science discussed in the lectures and laboratory procedures. Reflecting his enthusiasm and obvious intelligence, he was granted permission to sit-in on lectures and to perform the experiments in the general chemistry course. Professor Hill of Harvard wrote of Dodd "While he was in our laboratory, Mr. Walter J. Dodd attended the lectures given in general chemistry and performed all of the experiments required of our students under the direction of one of our assistants. In the following year he was in my own course in Quantitative Analysis. His experimental work was unusually good and he also passed with credit the two written examinations of the course. I think that he profited more from the instruction in the two courses than most of our matriculated students."

In 1892, he was successful in applying for a position as Assistant Apothecary at the MGH. Almost immediately, Dodd took further chemical courses and became a registered pharmacist. The apothecary was responsible for the hospital's photography program that had been started by a gift of $100 in 1887 to provide pictorial records of patients

and their course in hospital. Dodd learned photography readily. These combined experiences were important to his MGH career as pharmacist, photographer, and then radiologist.

Dodd's work was progressing happily when the attention of much of the medical and scientific worlds became highly focused on the December 28, 1895, paper by Wilhelm Röentgen. Dodd was instantly excited by these incredible "pictures" of human bones in patients. He and his assistant, Mr. Joseph Godsoe, immediately commenced development of the technical devices for taking such pictures. Their enthusiasm was shared by many staff at the hospital. Due to his reputation as a photographer, Dodd was given responsibility for implementation of the new technology at the MGH, i.e., a quick shift from photographer to radiographer. Their first radiograph was made in approximately March 1896. This was, of course, simultaneously occurring at hospitals throughout the world. WJD took the first radiograph at MGH according to a later account by George Holmes and by J. Godsoe. However, H. Cushing did claim that he and Codman, very famous physicians at the MGH, made the first MGH radiograph.

From 1896 onwards, WJD and Godsoe made or assembled a series of x-ray generators from bits and pieces of equipment, secured from throughout the hospital. A photograph of an x-ray tube used by Dodd near the start of radiology at the MGH is shown in Fig. 2.7 [15].

In 1897 a Dr. Weld gave an x-ray apparatus to the hospital, a substantial assist in this new program. The röentgenology unit was moved through a series of locations, due to the steeply expanding range of activities. In reality, Dodd was functioning as a "radiologist" prior to becoming a physician. We have no record of WJD knowing of or attempting to interact with Williams at BU or the physicists at MIT or at Harvard.

There is little written record of this early period at MGH in contrast to the book by Williams at Boston City Hospital. Do note that Williams was an established physician from a medical family (his father was the first professor of ophthalmology) and he had the finest education available in this country plus post-graduate education in Europe. In contrast, Dodd was largely self-taught, not a member of an important family, and a recent graduate from pharmacy

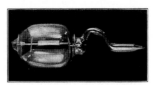

Fig. 2.7 One of the very early x-ray tubes employed by Dodd and Godsoe [15]

school. Perhaps, this partially explains the lack of knowledge by Dodd of Williams' work.

The MGH archives do not reveal records of the MGH early radiation treatments. Almost certainly, Dodd and colleagues were using the new rays against a variety of diseases, especially benign and malignant lesions of skin. Certainly, Dodd was highly active in the use of the new machines. By summer of 1898, he required skin grafting for radiation injury. In 1902, the department had three x-ray machines, viz., clearly a growing program. The work was intense, i.e., many patients but quite limited staff and space.

The following are from unpublished notes by Milford Schulz [36]: "the earliest hospital record of probable use of x-rays for therapy is a note in the Treasurers report of 1900 'expenditures of $125.24 for x-ray apparatus, $203.90 for x-ray tubes and $1062.54 for beer and ale.' In the records of surgical procedures done that year, there appears an item *repair of ulceration and X-ray burns.* 1901 surgical records include one case of x-ray burns. In 1902, two patients were treated for X-ray burns (one of the abdominal wall and one of the groin." In 1909 Dr. C.A. Porter published a paper "Surgical Treatment of X-ray Carcinoma" [31].

The MGH was very much alive and increasing its range of activities. This was reflected in statistics of growth in the number of patients and the population base. In 1900, the MGH had 260 beds and the medical program was almost exclusively for the care of the economically disadvantaged. These factors changed rapidly, viz., by 1935, there were 765 beds and medical care was provided to persons of all income levels.

Dodd was sensitive to the rate and scale of change in the practice and that he must increase his medical knowledge base to interact with physicians more effectively. In 1900, he entered HMS for 1 year, but then decided that he had to transfer to Vermont Medical School in order to concentrate on his studies, i.e., to be out of reach of the pressures of the work load at the hospital. On graduation in 1908, he was made röentgenologist (skiagrapher) at MGH. The Röentgenology Department was established, with WJD as Chief, a position he held until his death in 1916. Thus, he had no residency, as they did not exist. His appointment as Chief came almost as a graduation present. Dodd was given the academic rank of Instructor in Röentgenology in 1909, the first appointment in radiology at HMS. The clinical demand was rapidly expanding and there was a series of moves to progressively larger quarters. WJD was active in virtually all areas of radiology. WJD collaborated with the famous Walter B. Cannon in contrast examinations of the GI tract, using bismuth.

There was public appreciation of this new endeavor by physicians and physicists in radiology. Perhaps of interest is Fig. 2.8 [5], the self-portrait by G.A. Chicot in 1907. He was a French painter of substantial repute and a pioneer in

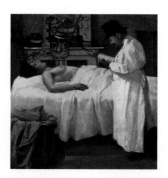

Fig. 2.8 G. Chicot's self-portrait of the artist treating the breast of a woman, 1907 [5]. With permission

radiology, i.e., a two-career man. In this painting, he portrays himself administering radiation to the breast of a female patient. This 1908 self-portrait is the only painting of a physician administering radiation to a cancer patient known by Dr. Luther Brady, an established art critic (Personal communication, 2007).

1911. WJD received a Dalton Scholarship to investigate radiological images of the GI tract.

1912. Dodd's stated in his annual report "There is great need for some simple but accurate standard of dosage in radiotherapeutic work – we believe that this can be accomplished by the new apparatus recently installed. The great importance of this can only be appreciated by those engaged in this work." Holmes, vide infra, was commended for his efforts to measure radiation dose. The Trustee's Report gave encouragement to increase the utilization of radiation postoperatively. Special emphasis was placed on breast cancer. The report also urged that more patients be treated by radiation. By 1912, the department had imaged and/or treated 6574 patients. Of special interest is that despite an extremely small staff, radiology service was available 24 h/day, 7 days per week. The first machine obtained specifically for radiation therapy was a 140 kVp unit.

Although the USA did not enter WWI until 1916, Walter Dodd volunteered in 1915 for service with the Harvard Medical Unit (in the British Expeditionary Force) in France. This reflected his character as a man who had to be involved as a participant, not as an observer. Another contributing factor could well have been his birth in England. He departed for France with recent and incompletely healed extensive surgery on an arm and chest wall. Figure 2.6b is of Dodd in uniform while on duty. He worked with a military unit from June to ~ October 1915.

Walter J. Dodd died on December 18, 1916, of metastatic cancer secondary to multiple radiation cancers. He had had his first in-hospital treatment in 1898, skin grafts for radiation dermatitis of the hands. This was followed by more than 50 surgical procedures with no major infections mentioned in the records (antibiotics were, of course, not available).

Dodd was an early martyr, but not the first in diagnostic and therapeutic radiology [3], but one very close to us. He was exceptionally respected and held in much affection in the hospital.

2.5   Advances in Radiation Therapy, 1917–1942, the George Homes Era

Dodd made a brilliant recruit to his staff in George Holmes from Tufts in 1910. Holmes was a graduate of Tufts medical school (1906) and had worked with F. Williams at Boston City Hospital, Fig. 2.9.

1914. The first radiation physics paper from the MGH was "Some Experiments in the Standardization of X-ray Dosage" by G.W. Holmes [13]. Although most of Holmes' work was in diagnosis, his interest in therapy was at a high level. His last paper was "Therapeutic Radiology" and that appeared in *Radiology* in 1946 [14]. The number of radiation treatments administered were 923 in 1914 and 1220 in 1915. Due to this expanding clinical load, there were yearly requests for new and better equipment and additional space.

1915. The First Resident in Radiology in the USA was in 1915 and at MGH. This is discussed in Chapter 10 on Education. From 1917 onwards, the MGH department was very active in the organization and teaching of radiology to medical students under G. Holmes. Although one could sub-specialize in diagnostic or therapeutic radiology and be credentialed by the American Board of Radiology as of 1939, the first to do so at the MGH was not until the late 1960s.

1916. Holmes emphasized the need for a lead-lined room and his desire to combine x-ray therapy with radium, which was not then available. Probably the first MGH paper on clinical outcome of radiation therapy was that by Malcolm Seymour in the *Boston Medical and Surgery Journal* "Treatment of Grave's Disease by the Röentgen

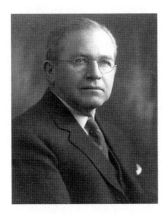

Fig. 2.9 Dr. George W. Holmes. MGH Chief of Radiology, 1917–1942 [21]

Ray" [37]. This was followed by a paper by Holmes and Merrill in 1919 on 262 patients treated for thyrotoxicosis using 140 kVp units.

1917. George W. Holmes was appointed as successor to Walter J. Dodd as röentgenologist [21]. He continued in that role until his retirement in 1942. Portable x-rays in the operating rooms were introduced that year. There was much interest in use of radiation post-operatively. The Phillips House (private patients) was opened and fitted with a diagnostic unit. A radiation therapy unit was not installed until 1924.

1919. Holmes organized special clinics for thyroid and skin diseases, antecedents of the Tumor Clinic.

1922. MGH was given $31,000 by Ms. W. Grove to provide for radium therapy. These funds were given to D. Barney, Chief of Urology and not Radiology, but were to be available to the MGH staff beyond Urology. In 1924 a Radium Committee was formed with the Chief of Röentgenology (George Holmes) as the Chair. The radium was stored in a lead safe in the radiology department. At the MGH, there were 40 mg in needles and a small amount in plaques. However, some 500 mg of radium was stored in solution at the Huntington Hospital. The emanation (radon) was available on 48 h notice from the "radon pump" under the control of the physicist, Duane [6]. This program continued until the closure of the Huntington in 1942, when the radium inventory came to the MGH with Milford Schultz. Duane was the first Professor of Biophysics at Harvard and in the USA [6]. At the MGH, surgeons had the responsibility for brachytherapy and intracavitary application while dermatologists used radium in surface applicators. Radiologists functioned merely as advisors until ~1950. Duane was among the first to measure ionization of air by x-rays and to develop instruments for dose measurements, a precursor of first international unit of radiation dose, the R (Röentgen), Fig. 2.10 [6].

1924. The first of several high-energy machines (220 kVp) based on the air cooled, hot cathode, and high vacuum Coolidge tube was obtained. Shielding was by a $\frac{1}{4}$ inch layer of lead. Treatments were given at 50 cm SSD. This was judged a marked improvement. Note that the dose at 10 cm depth was higher at 35%. These tubes were the sole basis for "deep therapy" at the MGH until 1940 when the new 1.2 Van de Graaff became operational. .

1925. The First Tumor Clinic in the USA. The special tumor clinics initiated by Holmes in the Radiology Department in 1919 developed into the Tumor Clinic in 1925. Many patients were referred directly to Holmes. He soon developed the practice of asking a surgeon or dermatologist with interest in the problem presented by the individual patient to come to the department and examine the patient with him. The start of the program was primarily a consultation service for skin disorders and thyroid diseases.

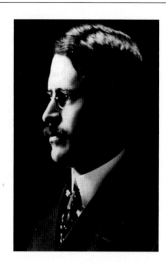

Fig. 2.10 William Duane, Professor of Biophysics, Harvard University [6]

This rapidly expanded to include cancer patients. As his clinics were working well, he concluded that there would be a gain for patients to be seen jointly by the radiologist and the appropriate surgeon or dermatologist.

Holmes and his partner in this development was surgeon Robert B. Greenough who had been an assistant to John C. Warren. He and Holmes were convinced of a clinical benefit by concentration of medical talent and facilities at one locus in the hospital. Holmes insisted and prevailed for the Tumor Clinic to be sited within the Radiology Department. Clinic hours were 9:00 to noon Monday through Saturday, with different patient categories seen on each of the 6 days. That is, the patient would experience *one* appointment in *one* setting. This was judged to be beneficial for patient care and resulted in the formation of the Tumor Clinic in April 1925, the first such clinic in the USA. There was the important gain of a central record for each patient. Referring or bringing patients to this clinic was entirely voluntary.

Specialties participating included internal medicine, pathology, GU, neurosurgery, and nose/throat surgery. From the various accounts, the clinic operation was pleasant and effective. A large fraction of the patients were from the House Service and the Out-Patient Department. At the opening of the White Building in 1939, the Tumor Clinic was transferred to space adjacent to the radiation therapy area.

1928. Holmes described the department in the summer issue of *Methods and Problems of Medical Education*, a publication of the Rockefeller Foundation. Parts of his report are reproduced here [21]:

> The department is on the ground floor of one of the older buildings of the hospital, occupying 7000 square feet of space. Located in a part of this space is a clinic for diagnosis and follow-up work in connection with the treatment of tumors. The protection of the operator is obtained by enclosing the tube, and

by the use of a small screen in front of the control board. No special operating booths are considered necessary. On the opposite side of the waiting room are examining booths for the observation of patients receiving treatment and for the follow-up of such cases as require it. Near these booths, separated by a corridor, are two rooms for preparation and application of radium, one of which is equipped for minor surgery.

About 20 percent of the patients who are seen come for treatment or observation. In the therapeutic division there are three machines capable of delivering a maximum current of 10 milliamperes at a voltage of 220 kVp. These much higher energy machines were based on inventions of the hot cathode and high vacuum tube by W D Coolidge. His machine achieved a major increment in operating voltage and the tubes had a long life and were relatively stable.

They also developed or obtained special apparatus for the measurements of Röentgen-ray and radium dosage. The measuring instruments employed are the ionization chamber of Duane, the electroscope developed by Dessauer-Bach, and the ionization chamber recommended by Weatherwax. There are also special standard milliampere and voltmeters which were used as controls.

During the year the entire department has been rewired and the current for energizing the x-ray machines had been changed from direct to alternating; this allowed us to do away with rotary converters. There was then a constant source of trouble and risk, and has given us a more stable power supply.

An important advance for all uses of x-rays and γ-rays was the adoption of the R or Röentgen as the internationally accepted unit of radiation dose by the International Congress of Radiology in 1928. The Röentgen, the R, was defined as "the quantity of X or gamma radiation such that the corpuscular emission per 0.001293 gram of air produces, in air, ions carrying 1 esu of quantity of electricity of either sign." The mass of 1 cm^3 of dry atmospheric air at 0°C and 760 mmHg pressure is 0.001293 g [12].

This was an era of quite dramatic discoveries in all of science and medicine. Among these in physics were the uncertainty principle (Werner Heisenberg), 1926; the cyclotron (E. Lawrence), 1929; the expanding universe (E. Hubble), 1929; the Van de Graaff accelerator (Van de Graaff), 1931; the neutron (Chadwick), 1932; fission of lithium by accelerated protons (Cockcroft and Walton), 1932; and an extensive array of other important discoveries. There were also many discoveries beyond radiation oncology, e.g., insulin (Banting and Best), 1922; penicillin (Fleming), 1929; and the first vaccines for tuberculosis and for yellow fever (1927 and 1932). The science of genetics became a very serious research area. The arts were advancing into quite new concepts and styles in painting, sculpture, and architecture. As one example of this remarkably free spirit, examine Fig. 2.11. This is a 1926 painting by Juan Miro, "Harlequin's Carnival." This is a dramatically new and different form of artistic expression. This is included as an example of the exploration and acceptance of new thinking.

Returning to the progress in radiation oncology at MGH by years:

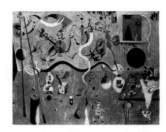

1929. Reports on the radiation treatment of patients with angina pectoris, carcinoma of the prostate, and carcinoma of the breast were published. That radiation would have been given to patients for angina pectoris certainly gets our attention and gives pause to consider the extent of counterproductive procedures in medicine in general. At HMS, radiology was transferred to the Department of Medicine from the Department of Surgery.

1930. At the Clinical Congress of the American College of Surgeons in Philadelphia, Dr. Greenough presented a paper describing the origin of the Tumor Clinic and how it had operated in the previous 5 years. The Baker Memorial Building was opened and the radiology section was equipped with a therapy unit.

1931. In a GEC report, the comment was made that cancer clinics similar in concept and function to the MGH Tumor Clinic have been established in many hospitals around the country.

The department staff consisted of three full-time radiologists (George Holmes, Aubrey Hampton, William C. Martin) and three part-time radiologists (Richard Dresser, John Meachen, and Robert Vance) and one consulting physicist, Howard Stearns.

1937. Gay ward was demolished to provide space for the new White building scheduled to open in 1939. Radiology was allotted a substantial new space for expansion of its programs. A new 1 MV or higher energy x-ray machine was planned to be installed in the new building.

In the late 1930s, Carl T. Compton, President of MIT, was enthusiastic to assess the clinical value of the uses of some of the radioactive isotopes in medicine, with special interest in isotopes of iodine. He arranged for discussions with Howard Means of the MGH Department of Medicine. The result was that the MGH was one of the first in the medical use of artificial radioisotopes. This close work between MGH clinicians and MIT scientists led to the establishment of Scientific Advisory Board in 1947, with Dr. Compton as the first chairman. Additionally, MIT Professor Francis O. Schmitt was appointed to the MGH Board of Trustees.

2.6   Robert J. Van de Graaff and His Accelerator

Van de Graaff (VdG) was born in 1901 in Tuscaloosa, AL [18, 34], from which he graduated with BS and MS degrees in mechanical engineering. After 1 year with the Alabama Power Company, he received a grant from the state that he combined with personal savings to study at the Sorbonne from 1924 to 1925. There he attended lectures and demonstrations by M. Curie and other notables in physics. While there he won a Rhodes Scholarship to Oxford University where he did well and was awarded the D.Phil. (the Oxford designation of the Ph.D.) in physics in 1928. During this period, he became familiar with the work of Rutherford and team at the Cavendish Laboratory, Cambridge University. His interest was greatly stimulated by their concepts of the potential of causing disintegration of atomic nuclei by the impact of energetic particles on atomic nuclei. Were there to be success, this would lead to increased understanding of atomic nuclei. This was a provocative concept and Van de Graaff commenced planning for a particle accelerator.

Young VdG was again fortunate in 1929 in winning a National Research Fellowship to join the Palmer Physics Laboratory at Princeton University and work in the laboratory of Karl Compton. He promptly commenced his project and within the year had assembled a special electrostatic accelerator; this Mark I device developed 80,000 V. This was a powerful encouragement for him and his supporters to initiate building a series of accelerators of increasing energy.

Compton was recruited to the Massachusetts Institute of Technology as President in 1930. The next year he brought Van de Graaff to MIT as a research associate. At the time of the inaugural meeting of the American Institute of Physics in November 1931, VdG exhibited his most recent model. That machine achieved energy levels above 1,000,000 V. This was a signal success for his career and for the smartly advancing field of nuclear physics. Figure 2.12 is a photograph of VdG with one of his early machine.

At MIT, Van de Graaff proceeded to construct an exceptionally powerful and quite large unit. This was built in an aircraft hangar. It featured two polished aluminum spheres, each 15 ft in diameter. These were mounted on insulating columns that were an impressive 6 ft in diameter and 25 ft in height. At its debut on November 28, 1933, the performance was a huge success and received national attention. Namely, the *New York Times* for November 29, 1933, report on the machine was titled "Man Hurls Bolt of 7,000,000 Volts" [41]. That Van de Graaff was thinking deeply

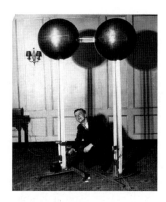

Fig. 2.12 Robert Van de Graaff, the inventor of the Van de Graaff accelerator [42]

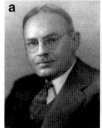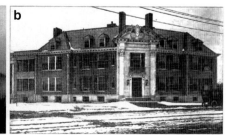

Fig. 2.13 (**a**) Richard Dresser was the Chief of Radiology (major interest in therapy) at the Huntington Memorial Hospital and part-time staff at the MGH [21]. (**b**) Huntington Memorial Hospital of the Harvard Cancer Commission [17]

regarding the potential of nuclear reactions and forces can be seen from the footnote.[5]

By the time of Robert Van de Graaff's death in January 1967 more than 500 Van de Graaff particle accelerators were in use in more than 30 countries. Of these, ~53 were used for radiation therapy.

2.7 The 1 MV Van de Graaff Accelerator at Huntington Hospital in 1937

A lecture on the clinical needs of improved radiation sources was given by G. Holmes at MIT in 1932. Van de Graaff and his assistant John Trump did not attend the lecture but learned that there would be serious clinical interest in their high-energy machines for treatment of cancer patients. Thus stimulated, they arranged to meet with George Holmes to discuss such an option. Holmes was interested in such a

machine for the MGH but had no space. He was anticipating adequate space in the new White Building in 1939.

Richard Dresser was a radiologist who had a major interest in radiation therapy (Fig. 2.13a). He had a part-time staff position at the MGH and his main appointment was at the Huntington Memorial Hospital. He learned of the meeting and the machines that had been built by Van de Graaff. He arranged to meet John Trump and discussed a generator of ≥400 KeV to be used in the Huntington Memorial Hospital. Trump replied "make it 1 MV and we might be interested" [35]. Dresser obtained a Hyams Trust grant of $25 K to build a 1 MV generator. Dresser and Trump began work in 1935 on a new class of clinical x-ray therapy machine at the Huntington Memorial Hospital, the cancer research hospital of the Harvard University. Trump and Van de Graaff described their design for the 1 MV machine in 1937 [40]. It had 25 beds, major laboratories, and was sited on the corner of Huntington Avenue and Shattuck Street[6] (Fig. 2.13b).

Patient treatments began in April 1937 [36]. The scale of this Van de Graaff machine is evident by its six charging belts of 1 m width that carried negative charges to the dome at 4000 ft/min or 45 mph. Surely, this was not a quiet machine. The machine was definitely impressive in size. There was ample space to walk inside and examine or repair as needed. The interior was air insulated and maintained at a constant temperature. The operation was based on clever manipulation of electric charge: charge is applied to the belts at the lower level and transported rapidly to the top of the

---

[5] VdG wrote this letter to Karl Compton on March 20, 1931, "homogeneous beams of protons at voltages that may be expected from the present work could be used for many simple experiments of fundamental nature. Among them would be the investigation of the effect of their impacts on uranium and thorium. These nuclei are already unstable, and it would be interesting to see if an impacting proton of great speed would precipitate immediate disintegration. On the other hand, it might be that the proton would be captured by the nucleus, thus opening up the possibility of creating new elements of atomic number greater than 92." "Near the other end of the series of atomic numbers is lithium. Now suppose that a proton is shot into the ^{7}Li nucleus, supplying the second component for the second alpha particle group. A consideration of Aston's curve and Einstein's law shows that a nuclear reaction might take place as follows: $VLi+ aH \sim 2\ 4He+ 16$ MV energy."

In his obituary of VdG, Peter Rose wrote, "This was one year before Cockcroft and Walton split the atom by bombarding ^{7}Li with protons and eight years before element 93 was artificially produced in an accelerator! He once told me that he wanted to include in his 1931 letter his belief that useful amounts of nuclear energy might be liberated by the disintegration of uranium or thorium, but he felt Compton would think this too bold!" [35]. See also the obituary by L. Huxley [18].

[6] The Huntington Hospital developed from the impact of the gift of $100,000 by a Ms. Croft that resulted in the establishment of the Harvard Cancer Commission. This was followed by an additional gift, viz., Ms. Collis Huntington gave $292,000. These were sufficient to commence the planning and construction of the small hospital for cancer research and patient care in 1912 by the commission. This hospital had the first 1 MV machine for clinical use [40]. Additionally, Duane was the world's first to devise the method for "pumping radon or as he called it emanation from a solution of radium salts" into glass capillary tubes which were then inserted into tumors. This pump was brought to the MGH by Schulz in 1942.

run. Negative charges from corona points are accelerated in the run-down to the target [12]. The dose rate was considerable for machines of that era, viz., of 40 R/min at 80 cm [36]. The first clinical treatment in April 1937 was a historic point in the development of radiation oncology, viz., the first clinical use of an x-ray beam of 1 MV. One of the first patients treated by the 1 MV beam at the Huntington in 1937 was a dentist with bladder cancer. According to Milford Schulz, the patient was alive and well 4 years later. This was the site of the first "supervoltage" clinical machine in the world, a 1 MV Van de Graaff.

In 1938, a 1 MV resonant transformer machine was installed at Memorial Hospital, New York. St. Bartholomew Hospital in London began treatment with an x-ray machine designed to operate at 1 MV but was operated at 0.7 MV from 1937 to 1939, then the unit was upgraded and commenced treatments at 1 MV.

2.8 The 1.2 MV Van de Graaff Machine at the MGH

The Hyams Trust supported development of a 1.2 MV Van de Graaff accelerator for MGH in the new space for radiology on the second floor of the White Building. Van de Graaff and Trump worked on this installation. This new machine was the first clinical unit to operate at more than 1 MV. Also of practical importance, it was vastly reduced in all dimensions relative to the Huntington unit and delivered 80 R per minute at 1 m. Installation was in 1940 with no full-time physicist on the MGH staff.

In that year, the department had the 1.2 MV Van de Graaff, four orthovoltage units (two in the White building, one each in the Baker and Founders buildings) and radium. Some 5000 treatments were administered in 1940. Dispersal of important equipment around the hospital appears to have been an inefficient operation and was prejudicial to sub-specialization.

We move to another big event in our history, viz., the appointment of Milford Schulz to the MGH staff in 1942 (Fig. 2.14). Milford started life in Sister Bay, WI, in 1909 and moved to Chicago for his medical education and residency in radiology at Northwestern. James T. Chase was the chief, a very highly regarded radiologist. Milford's interest in the most modern radiation therapy was evident in his move in 1939 to the Huntington Hospital to work with the 1 MV x-ray beam. At that time there were only three 1 MV machines: Boston, New York, and London.

The Huntington Hospital closed late in 1941 and virtually the entire research and clinical staff moved to the MGH at the beginning of 1942, at the time of US entry into WWII. These included Milford Schulz, Joseph Aub, Ira Nathanson, Rita Kelly, and Paul Zamecnik. Each was to be central player

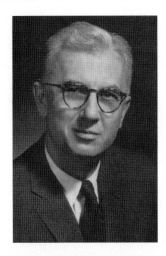

Fig. 2.14 Milford D. Schulz. Radiologist at MGH, 1942–1970. Radiation Oncologist, 1970–1976

in the development of oncology at MGH. Milford's arrival was indeed a fortunate event for the MGH, viz., obtaining one of the extremely few radiologists with substantial experience with 1 MV x-ray beams and whose principal medical interest was therapy. This obvious good luck was not fully appreciated as evidenced by a letter from A. Hampton, Chief of Radiology, to Faxon, the General Director of the MGH. Hampton made the appointment temporary, with the proviso that Milford might be dismissed at the end of the war with the return of staff from military duty. This was despite the near certainty that the patient load would continue to increase and that none of the returning staff were even remotely comparable to Milford in experience with high-energy x-ray therapy. The reality was that many of the returning radiologists moved to other hospitals. Milford was definitely needed and he remained.

Milford was one of the few to work at the hospital throughout WWII, as he did not pass the army physical examination. During WWII, most of the department staff had joined the military leaving the MGH quite depleted of radiologists. The military recruitment policy during WWII was that the most experienced physicians were recruited and the least experienced left to care for the civilians. As Robbins was the "boy" or the youngest among the staff, he was left at the MGH. At the end of the war in 1945, many of the returning staff retired or moved to other hospitals. Larry was rewarded for his good service under war time conditions by being made Chief of Radiology in February 1946.[7]

---

[7] The contributions to diagnostic radiology by Larry Robbins were very well regarded as evidenced by these honors: Gold Medals of ACR and RSNA; President of ABR; Chancellor of ACR; director and president of James Picker Foundation. Additionally, he wrote the eighth edition of *Röentgen Interpretation* in 1955. He retired in 1971 with the appointment of Juan Taveras as his successor.

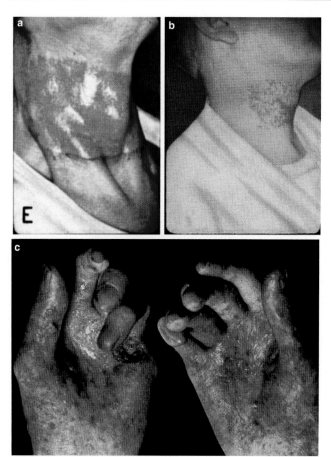

Fig. 2.15. (**a**) Acute and (**b**) late skin reaction after high-dose irradiation by orthovoltage x-ray beams. (**c**) The extremely severe late skin changes after low dose per fraction treatment of eczema that resulted in slight to no acute reaction [15]

The rationale for the enthusiasm for radiation beams of ≥ 1 MV photons was remarkably straightforward. There are four critical advantages for the 1 MeV relative to orthovoltage beams: (1) surface dose (skin dose) ~ 40 vs 100%; (2) marked increase in depth dose; (3) sharply decreased differential absorption of radiation between muscle, lung, and cortical bone; and (4) much reduced penumbra width.

The severe moist skin reaction that developed in virtually all patients treated to radical dose levels by orthovoltage machines is illustrated by Fig. 2.15a [15]. The patient was at ~ 2 weeks after treatment. These reactions required nontrivial nursing care and constituted a serious discomfort for the patient. The late reaction in a different patient treated by orthovoltage radiation is that of prominent telangectasia and contraction/fibrosis, Fig. 2.15b. For supervoltage x-irradiation, the acute skin reaction is usually that of a dry dermatitis and occasionally a patchy short-lived moist change followed by minimal to modest fibrosis. That severe late reactions can develop following minimal acute reactions is powerfully illustrated by Fig. 2.15c.

In other centers there had been use of γ-beams of ~ 1 MV from radium teletherapy units, "Radium Bombs." These had important disadvantages, viz., very low dose rate, short source surface distances, small field sizes, large source size, and wider penumbra than high-energy x-ray machines.

Milford could not limit his practice to radiation therapy as sub-specialization was not permitted. Although there was no designated radiation therapy section within the department, Schulz functioned as the de facto head of the therapy activities. G. Holmes, the Chief, was quite active in radiation therapy and supported Milford.

In 1944, there was a serious radiation accident. During work on the installation of the 1.2 MV Van de Graaff, several workers got into the path of the cathode beam. There were no fatalities but a few persons developed significant injuries. Use of the newly available antibiotics was credited for some of the success in caring for the injured.

The four war-time years provided few to no opportunities for innovation due to shortage of staff and essentially all manufactured goods. Despite these constraints, there were serious considerations for post-war improvements. One impressive result was the effort by Milford and Larry Robbins that led to the purchase, installation, and then the start of treatment in 1948 on a 2 MV Van de Graaff machine. Figure 2.16 is a photograph of such a machine. The MGH machine was in clinical service from 1948 to 1975. This was one of the first clinical units that operated at 2 MV. However, in that same year, a patient was treated at University of Illinois on the first clinical Betatron, a 22 MV machine.

The MGH 2 MV VdG was installed with no full-time physicist on the staff. There was an extraordinary problem in its installation. Lead was a protected item during the war and even by the time of the installation of this machine, lead was difficult to obtain and was pricey. The MGH arranged for a large quantity of lead from the storage unit at MIT to be used as shielding. From that newly acquired lead, 20 tons were stolen. After some protracted discussion, the lead was returned. In 1950 Holmes and Schulz published an

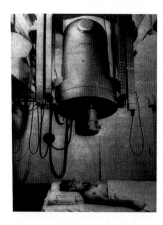

Fig. 2.16 A photograph of a 2 MV Van de Graaff [11]

extremely fine and lucid textbook on therapeutic radiology. They opened with 73 informative pages on physics and radiation biology. The Holmes and Schulz book had 347 pages with 111 figures. Their book was the first MGH book on radiation oncology and was one of three widely used radiation therapy textbooks in English of that era (1950). The other two were *The Treatment of Malignant Disease by Radium and X rays* in 1948 by R. Paterson of the Christie Hospital and Holt Radium Institute, Manchester, UK, and *Clinical Therapeutic Radiology*, edited by U. Portmann, of the Cleveland Clinic, in 1950 [29, 32].

Despite the large number of patients and minimal support staff, Milford made regular contributions to radiation oncology. Milford was a member of the group that revised the staging system for laryngeal carcinoma, authored papers on staging and end results for carcinoma of the thyroid, radiation in management of myasthenia gravis, spinal cord compression, advanced lung cancer, and radiation secondary sarcoma. He designed applicators for treatment of scleral lesions. Additionally, he commented on ethical issues in advertisements.

Milford was the only MGH radiologist working near full time in therapeutic radiology 1942–1953 when C.C. Wang joined him. Then some 15 years later, Melvin Tefft and George Zinninger also joined his team. The patient load progressively enlarged but no increase in space or equipment after 1956, when Milford oversaw the removal of the 1.2 MV Van de Graaff and installation of a 55 cm SAD ^{60}Co unit.

Milford Schulz enjoyed a very high reputation as a clinician and one very well informed in physics and technology. As evidence of his national status these distinctions and awards are noted:

Member of Board of Chancellors of the American College of Radiology

President. American Radium Society, 1958–1959

Gold Medalist and Janeway Lecturer of the American Radium Society, 1974

Founding Member of American Society of Therapeutic Radiology and Oncology

President of American Society of Therapeutic Radiology and Oncology (1971–1972)

President. New England Röentgen Ray Society, 1962–1963

President. American Cancer Society, Massachusetts Division

Member of the International Commission of Radiological Units for many years

Shortly after creation of the department, Milford was promoted to Professor of Radiation Oncology at HMS

Chair of the Group of 75 C45 (Radiology) Committee for Revision of the American Standard definition of electrical Terms – American Institute of Electrical Engineers

Milford's Janeway lecture "The Supervoltage Story" was a serious and scholarly account of the diverse actors and devices in the development of x-ray machines that produced beams of >1 MV [35]. The transition from 250 kVp to ≥ 1 MV is really a fascinating and central technical development in our specialty.

For the MGH program in radiation oncology, Milford was an energetic, articulate, and effective force in moving the hospital to recognize the necessity of a quite major upgrading of the space and facilities for the radiation therapy program. His memoranda to the administration on these needs for radiation oncology were not ambiguous in the least. See his letter to the MGH General Director of 1963 reproduced in Chapter 3. He had strong support from Benjamin Castleman (Chief of Pathology) and Howard Ulfelder (Chief of Gynecology). In the 1960s there was an increasing appreciation of the positions articulated by Milford that contributed to the decision to build a cancer center and establish a separate department of radiation therapy.

2.9 Nobel Prize to an MGH Staff

In 1944, Fritz Lipmann discovered co-enzyme A and its role in intermediary metabolism. For this he was awarded the 1953 Nobel Prize. This was shared with Hans Krebs of the UK.

In 2010, Jack Szostak received the Nobel Prize Physiology or Medicine for his role in the discovery of the mechanism by which telomeres and the enzyme telomerase protect chromosomes.

2.10 Establishment of the National Cancer Institute (NCI)

Laboratory and clinical research of our department has been generously funded by the NCI. This is also true for nearly all US cancer research centers. The NCI was the first of the institutes of the NIH. The accomplishments of the NCI in the US program in cancer research and education constitute a national record of achievements of which not only US citizens but all humans can be intensely proud.

Several steps in the US government involvement in health matters and the formation of the NCI are listed [46].

1836: The Library of the Office of the Surgeon General was established (the present National Library of Medicine).

1879: The National Board of Health was created by law, the first, national medical research effort of the US government.

Fig. 2.17 (a) Explosion of a test atomic bomb on July 16, 1945, near Alamogordo, NM [1]. (b) A spontaneous kiss in Times Square reflecting the intense excitement at the news of the end of WWII [9]

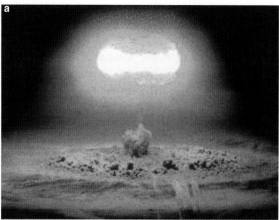
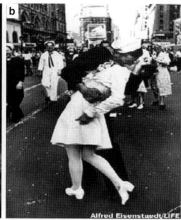

1912: The Public Health and Marine Hospital Service became the Public Health Service (PHS).

1930: The Ransdell Act redesignated the Hygienic Laboratory as the National Institute of Health, authorizing $750,000 for construction of two buildings for NIH, and creating a system of fellowships.

1937: The National Cancer Institute Act was signed on July 23.

1938: The National Advisory Cancer Council recommended approval of the first awards for fellowships in cancer research.

1938–1942: Ms. Luke Wilson made a series of 5 gifts of land to the NIH, for a total of 92 acres in Bethesda, MD. Her gifts constitute the nucleus of the NIH present site of 306 acres. NIH moved to Bethesda in July.

1946: The Research Grants Office was formed at NIH to operate a program of extramural research grants and fellowships.

Of special interest to us is the fact that the first application to the NCI was in 1937 from a Harvard scientist for "cancer research"; the amount requested was $4350 and was not funded. The first application funded was to Louis F. Fieser of Harvard on November 27, 1937, for $27,550. He had proposed to investigate the structure and carcinogenic activity of several chemicals. Grant number was 1C3 (Personal communication, Frank Mahoney, 2007).

2.11 The End of WWII

We come to the end of the 50-year period, 1895–1945. WWII ended almost immediately after the explosion of an atomic bomb on Hiroshima, August 6, 1945, and on Nagasaki, August 9, 1945. The destructive power of an atomic bomb is illustrated by the first test explosion that occurred on July 16, 1945, at 05:29 AM, in the Jornada del Muerto (Journey of Death) desert 210 miles south of Los Alamos,

near Alamogordo, NM, Fig. 2.17a [1]. There ensued a most powerful and broad interest in nuclear physics not only for military applications, but also for medicine and biological research.

The uninhibited joy that greeted the news of the end of World War II is powerfully illustrated by the Eisenstadt photograph of a sailor grabbing and kissing a nurse in New York, Fig. 2.17b. This was published on the cover of *Life* magazine issue of August 14, 1945 [9]. A statue of that impulsive kiss was erected in Times Square in August 1995, i.e., the 50th anniversary of the kiss and the end of the war.

References

1. Atom Bomb Test. July 16, 1945. Trinity Site. 1945. With permission of Oxford University Press.
2. Brown A. The neutron and the bomb: a biography of Sir James Chadwick. Oxford, England: Oxford University Press; 1997.
3. Brown P. American martyrs to science through Röentgen rays. Springfield, Ill: Charles C Thomas; 1936.
4. Chadwick J. Possible existence of a neutron. Nature. 1932;129:312.
5. Chicot G. Self portrait. 1907. Rijksmuseum. Stichting Kröller-Müller. With permission, 2010.
6. Del Regato JA. Radiological physicists. New York, NY: American Institute of Physics; 1985.
7. Del Regato JA. Radiological oncologist: unfolding of a medical specialty. Reston, VA: Radiology Centennial; 1993.
8. Druery CT, Bateson W. Experiments in plant hybridization. R Hort Soc. 1901;26:1–32.
9. Eisenstadt. The Kiss. Life Magazine. August 27, 1945. With permission, 2010
10. Frost EB. Experiments on the x-rays. Science. 1896;3(59):235–6.
11. Gagliardi R, Wilson J. A history of the radiological sciences. Reston, VA: Radiology Centennial; 1996.
12. Glasser O. Physical foundations of radiology. New York, NY: Hoeber; 1952.
13. Holmes G. Some experiments in standardization of dosage for Roentgen therapeutics. Am J Röentgenol. 1914;1:298–302.
14. Holmes G. Therapeutic radiology. Radiology. 1946;47(6):602–7.
15. Holmes G, Schulz M. Therapeutic radiology. Philadelphia, PA: Lea and Febiger; 1950. With permission from Wolters Kluwer, 2010.

16. Horgan J. The end of science. Reading, MA: Helix Books/Addison-Wesley; 1996.
17. Huntington Memorial Hospital, Boston, MA. Boston Med Surg J. 1912;166:888–9.
18. Huxley L. Dr. R.J. Van de Graaff. Nature. 1967;214(5084):217–8.
19. Klaas J. From Bavaria to Hanover: The early history of x-rays. Dartmouth Undergraduate J Sci Suppl. 2002;42–4.
20. Lewis G. The conversation of photons. Nature. 1926;118:874–5.
21. Linton O. Radiology at the Massachusetts general hospital. Boston, MA: General Hospital Corporation; 1996.
22. Lyon TG. Röentgen rays as a cure for disease. Lancet. 1896;74:326.
23. Lyon TG. Röentgen rays as a cure for disease. Lancet. 1896;147(3782):513–4.
24. Macy R. Walter Dodd: A biographical sketch. Boston, MA: Houghton Mifflin; 1918.
25. Massachusetts General Hospital Archives.
26. MGH. Massachusetts General Hospital Memorial and Historical Volume, together with the Proceedings of the Centennial of the Opening of the Hospital. Boston, MA: Griffith-Stillings Press; 1921.
27. Michelson A. Speech at the dedication of Ryerson Physics Lab, University of Chicago 1894. In: Beaty W, editors. Science hobbyist: the end of science. Available from http://amasci.com/weird/end.html. Accessed on 2009.
28. Miro J. Harlequin's carnival. 1925. Albright Knox Art Gallery, Buffalo, NY. With permission.
29. Paterson R. The treatment of malignant disease by radium and x-rays. London, England: Edward Arnold and Co.; 1948.
30. Planck M. Wikipedia http://en.wikipedia.org/wiki/Philipp_von_jolly warning to M Planck 2010. Accessed on 2009.
31. Porter CA. The surgical treatment of x-ray carcinoma and other severe x-ray lesions, based upon an analysis of forty-seven cases. J Med Res. 1909;21(3):357–414.
32. Portman U. Clinical therapeutic radiology. New York, NY: Thomas Nelson and Sons; 1950.
33. Reichen C. A history of physics. New York, NY: Hawthorne Books; 1963.
34. Rose R. In memoriam: Robert Jemison Van de Graaff. Nucl Instrum Methods. 1968;60:1–3.
35. Schulz M. The supervoltage story. Janeway Lecture, 1974. Am J Roentgenol Radium Ther Nucl Med. 1975;124(4):541–59.
36. Schulz M. Unpublished Notes. Boston, MA: MGH Archives.
37. Seymour M. Treatment of Grave's disease by the Röentgen rays. Boston Med Surg J. 1916;175:568–9.
38. Thompson E. Note in electrical engineer. 1896;89–90.
39. Thomson LWT (Lord Kelvin). Statement to physicists at British Association for the Advancement of Science. 1900. Available from http://www.pet.cam.ac.uk/student/kelvin/LordKelvin.html. Accessed on 2009.
40. Trump J, Van de Graaff RJ. Design of the million-volt x-ray generator for cancer treatment and research. J Appl Phys. 1937;8:602–6.
41. Van de Graaff RJ. Man Hurls Bolt of 7000000 Volts. New York Times. November 29, 1933.
42. Van de Graaff Image. MIT Archives. With permission.
43. Washburn FA. The Massachusetts General Hospital. Its Development, 1900–1935. Cambridge, MA: Houghton Mifflin Riverside Press; 1943.
44. Williams F. Rare anomalies of the phalanges shown by the Roentgen process. Boston Med Surg J. 1896;134:198–9.
45. Williams F. The Röentgen rays in medicine and surgery. London, England: Macmillan; 1901. With permission.
46. US Department of Health & Human Services. NIH Almanac-Historical Data. Chronology of Events Series. 2007. Available from: http://www.nih.gov/about/almanac/historical/chronology_of_events.htm. Accessed on 2010.

Chapter 3

The New Optimism After WWII and the Decision for a Cancer Center at MGH 1945–1970

3.1 The Optimism and Exuberant Confidence After the WWII

With the ending of World War II in 1945, Americans had a greatly enhanced sense of optimism that there would be a progressively improving world for themselves, their children, and all people. A central basis for that increased confidence was the reality that the USA was the world's "Superpower" in terms of its military, financial, diplomatic, industrial, scientific, and medical[1] status. Happily, this new position for our country was combined with the creation of the United Nations by a conference of 44 nations on July 26, 1945, in San Francisco. The permanent home of the United Nations headquarters was built on 17 acres on the river in New York City in 1950, Fig. 3.1 [23].

For the MGH and all of the Harvard community there can be pride in the role played by Harvard's Dumbarton Oaks, Washington, DC, in the establishment of the United Nations. The Dumbarton Oaks[2] Conference in September–October, 1944, defined the aims, structure, and functioning of the planned United Nations. This conference was a central event in the establishment of the United Nations. The United Nations was planned to serve as an effective organization for peaceful settlement of differences between nations and as a symbol for world peace.

The important concern for rights of each human being was articulated with great clarity in the United Nations Universal Declaration of Human Rights on December 10, 1948 [24]. Articles 1 and 2 are reproduced here:

Article 1. All human beings are born free and equal in dignity and rights. They are endowed with reason and conscience and should act towards one another in a spirit of brotherhood.

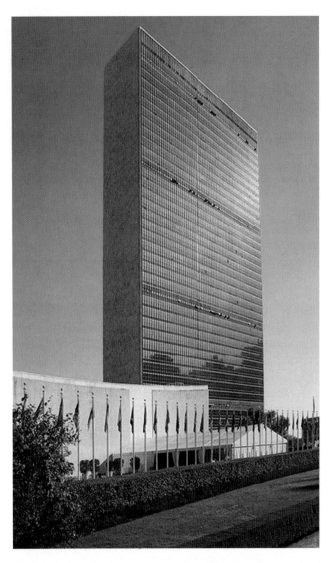

Fig. 3.1 The United Nations Building [23]. www.inetours.com/New_York/Pages/United_Nations.html Copyright Lee W. Nelson. With permission

---

[1] Radiation oncology was not in that rank and was definitely behind most of Europe at that point in time.

[2] Dumbarton Oaks is quite a beautiful place with extensive gardens and lawns and an excellent museum, especially for pre-Columbian Art. Absolutely this piece of Harvard is worth a visit. It is located in Foggy Bottom, viz., quite close to central Washington, DC.

H.D. Suit, J.S. Loeffler, *Evolution of Radiation Oncology at Massachusetts General Hospital*, DOI 10.1007/978-1-4419-6744-2_3, © Springer Science+Business Media, LLC 2011

Fig. 3.2 (a) Tensing Norgay at the peak of Mt. Everest as a guide to Edmund Hilary 1953 [12]. (b) The Guggenheim Museum [11]. (c) TWA terminal by the Finnish architect Eero Saarinen [22]

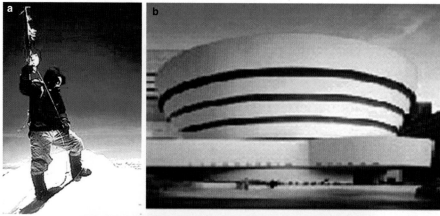

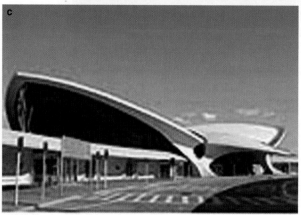

Article 2. Everyone is entitled to all the rights and freedoms set forth in this Declaration, without distinction of any kind, such as race, color, sex, language, religion, political or other opinion, national or social origin, property, birth or other status. Furthermore, no distinction shall be made on the basis of the political, jurisdictional or international status of the country or territory to which a person belongs, whether it be independent, trust, non-self-governing or under any other limitation of sovereignty.

In marked contrast to these noble aspirations, there was the strongly negative impact of the 41-year-long Cold War, viz., ~1948–1989. This had moments of extremely high tension, but fortunately remained a Cold War between the principal adversaries. Despite this exceptionally serious problem, there were numerous and quite important advances in medicine, science, and most areas of society. Among social actions by the USA, mention is made of only two: the Marshall Plan and Civil Rights legislation.

As relief from the intense political concerns, there were impressive achievements that were most positively received and did act to relieve some of the anxiety. We recall one athletic triumph over a very long sought goal and two architectural spectaculars. The first was the 1953 ascent of Mt. Everest by Edmund Hilary and Tenzing Norgay [12]. The new spirit was abundantly evident in the arts and architecture. The Guggenheim Museum (Fig. 3.2b) is a clear standout in not only New York but the entire world. This

was built in 1959 by the most famous of American architects, Frank Lloyd Wright [11]. The highly futuristic TWA terminal by the Finnish architect Eero Saarinen is most impressive, especially noting its construction date 1962, as presented in Fig. 3.2c [22]. Further, the general public was showered with a very broad array of highly prized technologies, viz., television, jet air travel, computers, air conditioning, etc.

The six developments with perhaps the biggest impact in science and technology in the years 1945–1961 were as follows: (1) the atomic bomb, August 1945; (2) the first electronic computer – 1946, the ENIAC[3] [6, 15]; (3) the discovery of the structure of the DNA molecule in (April 1953) [25]; (4) the first man-made object to orbit the earth, i.e., Sputnik on October 4, 1957 [18]; (5) the first human to orbit the earth was Y. Gagarin. This occurred on April 12, 1961 [8]; and (6) the first men on the moon, N. Armstrong and B. Aldrin in 1969 [2]. The new spirit was abundantly evident in the arts and architecture. See Fig. 3.3.

---

[3] The *E*lectrical *N*umerical *I*ntegrator *A*nd *C*alculator (ENIAC) was the first large general purpose electronic computer [15]. This was the result of the work by the team of J. Echert and J. Mauchly at University of Pennsylvania. This machine was commissioned to track trajectories of missiles. The machine was quite substantial, viz., 17,468 vacuum tubes, 70,000 resistors, 10,000 capacitors, and weighed 30 tons.

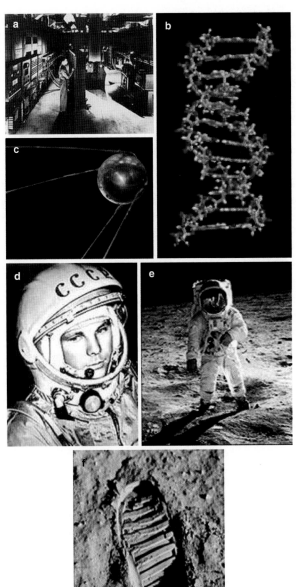

medicine and biology), financial activities, etc. The understanding of the double helix structure of DNA by Watson and Crick in 1953 [25] stimulated an exceedingly productive and dramatically expanding field of genetics with enormous impact on virtually all of biology and medicine. Fortunately, this is continuing and at an accelerating pace. It has extended broadly to oncology for genetic assessment of risk of development of tumor, diagnosis of tumor type and grade, the probability of a defined tumor and normal tissue response to the planned treatment, and risk of metastasis.

Two highly impressive firsts in space science were by Soviet scientists and engineers. This gave a vigorous, sustained, and positive stimulus to a sharp enhancement of the performance of US education in science and engineering. The response was strong and clearly effective in producing long-term benefits to US science. In July 20, 1969, Neil Armstrong and Buzz Aldrin were the first humans to walk on the moon. This event was quite widely celebrated. From that day, the USA has been the leader in space research and utilization of the new technologies for civilian and military functions. Now many countries have joined the USA and Russia in space programs. These diverse events have propelled the attitude of Americans into keen enthusiasm for science and expectation of a sustained stream of important advances. Fortunately, these high hopes have largely been met to this date.

In more general terms science, medicine, and technology have continued to advance into essentially every area of human knowledge and interest. In medicine, these have included: organ transplantation; vaccination programs resulting in near global eradication of several infectious diseases, e.g., poliomyelitis; antibiotics; chemotherapy for cancer patients; impressive gains in surgery; and the significant developments in radiation oncology.

Fig. 3.3 (**a**) Cpl. Herman Goldstein (foreground) sets the switches on one of the ENIAC's function tables at the Moore School of Electrical Engineering. (US Army photo) [6]; (**b**) model of the DNA molecule [5]; (**c**) The Soviet Sputnik launched in November 3, 1957, the first earth orbiting satellite [18]; (**d**) Y. Gagarin of the Soviet Union was the first human to orbit the earth, April 12, 1961 [8]; (**e, f**) Photograph of B. Aldrin taken by N. Armstrong, whose image is reflected in the visor, Footprint of B. Aldrin in the Sea of Tranquility on the moon. This is likely to persist for very many years [2]

3.2 General Status of Oncology in the Early Years After WWII

The "informed" opinion in many institutions in 1950–1960 was that eradication of death due to cancer was imminent due to the undeniably large gains in drug development and the intense cancer research programs in the USA and in many countries. There was the impressive regression of lymphomas by the available nitrogen mustard and alkylating agents, as used shortly after WWII [10]. An additional powerful contributor to that optimism was the demonstration by R. Hertz and associates at the NCI of a high frequency of remission of metastatic choriocarcinoma by treatment with methotrexate alone. Importantly, there were several well-documented long-term disease-free survivors [14]. The

Nuclear physics expanded dramatically after WWII in basic physics, industrial, and medical sciences and had a dramatic impact on radiation oncology. Computers are critical to operation of nearly all modern equipment, recording of events, mathematical modeling (extensively employed in

success of bone marrow transplantation to permit more aggressive chemotherapy was another positive development [20, 21].

There were extensive investigations employing basic chemistry and physics and radiation biology experiments based on in vitro and in vivo laboratory systems. There was a significant problem in the animal tumor models utilized. The experimental models were, with few exceptions, neither spontaneous autochthonous tumors nor even their very early generation transplants in syngeneic animals. Rather they were long serially transplanted chemically or viral-induced cancers. The observed responses were due in part to the immune rejection response against an antigenic tumor. A significant difficulty with such experiments is that in human oncology and in experimental animals, host immune reactions against their spontaneous tumors tend to be very weak.

An opinion commonly expressed and without equivocation during that period was "Why should talent, space and funds be used to develop radiation therapy centers, when the cancer problem is shortly to be eliminated by drugs in the 'pipeline'?" Thus, one could visit famous and very wealthy hospitals in 1970 and observe children under treatment for potentially curable diseases by 250 kVp x-ray beams. This was a quite distressing fact.

3.3 US Radiation Oncology in the 1945–1970 Period

This rather juvenile optimism regarding a certainty of eradication of cancer as a cause of death in the short term was only one factor in the comparatively slow development of radiation therapy in the USA. A perhaps puzzling aspect of American medicine during this period was that very few physicians specialized in any aspect of oncology. Surgeons, internists, and radiologists were practicing general surgery, medicine, or radiology. A consequence was that oncology was largely practiced as a single modality well into the 1960s, viz., little consideration of combined modality patient management. There was often the opposite of collaboration between surgery and radiation therapy. Chemotherapy was employed principally against the lymphomas and leukemias. By 1970, substantial changes were occurring in oncologic practice, especially the move toward a multi-disciplinary patient management. Medical students rarely had courses in oncology until ~1980. Their lectures on oncology were parts of more general courses in medicine and surgery, and even less commonly was a student exposed to patients being treated by radiation with a discussion of the basis for the use of radiation.

For approximately 1.5 decades after WWII, the USA was not the leader in radiation oncology. However, by 1950, there were three textbooks on radiation therapy in English, two were from the USA [13, 17] and one from the UK [16]. In addition, the very widely used book "Cancer" from the USA was written by pathologist L. Ackerman and radiation oncologist J. del Regato [1]. The gains in US radiation oncology in the late 1940s through the 1960s were enormously facilitated by the substantial "Brain Drain" to the USA. Mention is made of several of our early leaders who had been educated abroad: G. Fletcher (France), Simon Kramer (UK), Juan Del Regato (Cuba), Franz Buschke (Germany), and Fernando Bloedorn (Argentina) among many others [9]. By 1960–1965, the USA was abreast with Europe and ahead in some areas.

US radiation oncology community was markedly cautious in forming a professional society. Their first steps were quite timid, viz., formation of a club and not a proper society. The concern was to avoid an upset to the radiological organizations. The Club of Therapeutic Radiologists was created in 1958 largely by Juan del Regato. This event was during the annual meeting of the Radiological Society of North America (RSNA) in Chicago by a group of ~65 "radiation oncologists" from the total of ~100 in the USA. For several years, the club held its meetings during the annual meeting of RSNA. The site allocated to the club was in most years in a basement room of the Palmer House Hotel, adjacent to the kitchen. That provided a less than quiet background. Milford had been one of the main organizers and had been very active in pushing in both Boston and nationally for the separation of radiation oncology from general radiology over a long period. He served as the seventh president of the club, 1964–1965. Herman Suit, from the NCI, was one of the founding members of the club. Almost immediately Suit helped form the "Young Turk" group with Malcolm Bagshaw, Bill Powers, and Melvin Greim. They agitated, not in a very subtle manner, to transform the club to a society. The club responded to multiple pressures including the "Young Turks" and matured into a full professional society only in 1966. The name became the American Society of Therapeutic Radiology and Oncology. In 2009 the total membership was ~ 10,000.

Our club was preceded by the Radiation Research Society by 6 years, viz., established in 1952 and held its first meeting in 1953. The two societies have become quite close and have held combined meetings. This interactive relationship hopefully will continue. ASTRO's current programs have many parallel sessions covering combined modality treatment strategies, modification of radiation response, genetics applied to oncology, general radiation biology, physics, and history. In addition to the annual meeting, there is an impressive series of meetings directed to specific areas of interest.

Further, there are meeting times for the radiation therapists, nurses, and social workers. Similar professional societies for radiation oncology have been organized in many countries and regions, e.g., EORTC, the European organization, and JASTRO, the Japanese organization.

3.4 MGH Radiation Oncology in the 1945–1970 Period

To iterate earlier points, as of 1950, the MGH and Harvard had led in several radiation oncology areas. These included the following: the first radiology residency program in the USA was at the MGH (1916); the first US Tumor Clinic was at the MGH (1925); a leader in the use of ionization for measurement of radiation dose by Professor of Biophysics Duane and in the adoption of the Roentgen as the unit of dose in 1928 (Harvard Physics); the first clinical beam at 1.0 MeV, the Van de Graaff (VdG) in 1937 at the Huntington Memorial Hospital of Harvard, under the direction of a part-time MGH staff. The first clinical machine to operate at more than 1 MV was the 1.2 MV VdG at the MGH in 1939; the first (or very close to the first) to have a clinical 2 MeV beam (a second VdG) in 1948; and the important textbook by Homes and Schulz "Therapeutic Radiology" in 1950 [13].

MGH Röentgenology was only a component of the Department of Medicine until October 1944. At that point it became an independent department. In April 1945, the name was changed to the Department of Radiology. This was concurrent with the action of the Harvard Corporation to establish a separate Department for Radiology at the Harvard Medical School (HMS). Then in 1967, the MGH decided to separate the Department of Radiology into two departments, one for diagnosis and one for therapy. This was not realized until 1970. At the medical school, this separation of radiology into two departments did not occur until 1972. HMS was unique in American medicine with two departments – The JCRT led by Sam Hellman and the MGH Department of Radiation Medicine led by Herman Suit.

At the close of WWII, that the MGH had to have a great expansion of facilities and space had become evident to all observers. The results were these new buildings: Vincent Burnham, 1947; the Research, 1950; Warren, 1956; Pierce cardiopulmonary Laboratory, 1964; Gray Building Jackson and Bigelow Towers, 1968; parking garages on each side of North Grove Street, 1970. Not until 1975 was a Cancer Center established in the new Cox Building. Beyond activities "on campus" were the numerous community out-reach programs to West-End Beacon Hill, North End, Charlestown, East Boston, and Chelsea. These were definitely needed community services. One result was that cancer patients from

those populations strongly tended to come to the MGH. No new space was provided for radiation oncology between the move into the White building in 1939 and 1970. General references for this period are Castleman and Crockett [4] and Faxon [7].

In 1957, the hospital commenced an assessment of the need for a major expansion of radiation treatment facilities. This was later extended to a multi-disciplinary cancer center culminating in the Cox Cancer Center that opened in 1975. Milford Schulz was the only hospital staff who was near full time in the practice of radiation therapy during the 11-year period from 1942 to 1953 and is considered to have been a radiation oncologist. Milford was the first radiation oncologist in New England, one of the first in the USA. There were essentially no surgical or medical oncology sub-specialists in oncology at the MGH. During that period, Milford was one very busy man. In 1953, C.C. Wang, a fresh graduate from the MGH residency program, joined Milford.

Over the period 1945–1970, the staff slowly increased with growing patient numbers and related activities, see Table 3.1. In the 1960s, two additional staff were appointed and worked until the early 1970s. Melvin Tefft served for several years on the staff and then held positions as MSKCC, Brown University, and finally Chief at the Cleveland Clinic. George Zinninger was on the staff for a few years and then moved to Thomas Jefferson Hospital in Philadelphia. By 1970, there were ∼ 90 patients treated per day on a 6 days/week schedule. This steep increase in patient numbers was accompanied by no additional space or equipment.

The American Board of Radiology was established in 1934. Certification in Radiology was available until 1996 when all candidates for the examination had to choose between one of the sub-specialties. As of 1939, the minimum requirement for taking the examination in radiology was the satisfactory completion of a 3-year residency. The number of MGH radiology residents had increased from 1 in 1916 to 3 in 1939 to 6 in 1945 to 12 in 1957 and 30 in 1970. Twelve of the months were in radiation oncology. Although the Board did authorize training exclusively in therapy in 1939, the first MGH residents to select radiation therapy for their 3 years were Sidney Kadish, Susan Pittman, and Warren Sewall. They came into the specialty at the very end of the 1960s. Thus, by 1970 Milford and CC had three residents.

Table 3.1 Numbers of radiation treatments and radiation oncology staff, 1940–1969

Year	No. of treatments	Radiation oncologists
1940	3,781	0
1945	8,986	1
1955	17,226	2
1965	24,734	3
1969	32,180	4

3.5 Physics in Radiation Oncology

G. Brownell was recruited from MIT in 1949, as Director of the Physics Research Laboratory in the Research Building, Fig. 3.4a. In 1950 he proposed to William Sweet, Chief of Neurosurgery, the potential of improved imaging of CNS lesions by use of the annihilation radiation from positron-emitting isotopes. He promptly constructed a Mark I positron scanner using two sodium iodide detectors. This rapidly evolved into a PET scanner in 1952 and he was the first to use this system in medical diagnostic purposes for pathologies of the brain [3]. For his research, he had a cyclotron for production of radioisotopes for many MGH users. PET scanners have regularly been improved in resolution and now employ a spectrum of tracers. At present, PET scans are used in the assessment of the local extent, physiological characteristics of neoplasm, and presence of regional or distant metastasis. The PET scanner is a very significant contribution to medicine by the MGH.

A very important recruit in 1953 was Ted Webster from MIT. Milford was a major player in that recruitment. Ted was the first permanent full-time physicist in Radiology. He was appointed 13 years after the installation of the 1.2 MV and 5 years after the 2 MV Van de Graaff machines. He had the responsibility for all of the physics, diagnostic and therapeutic, radiation safety, and physics education of residents. He was responsible for the installation and commissioning of the ^{60}Co Theratron Junior in 1956. Webster appointed Rosemary Whipfelder, part-time M.Sc. physicist, to work with Milford and CC. In the early 1970s, Webster designed the shielding for the units to be installed in the new Cox Center.

Webster pursued a highly distinguished career in radiological physics. Figure 3.4b is a photograph of Ted Webster giving the William D. Coolidge Award of the American Association of Physicists in Medicine to Gordon Brownell in 1987. Ted Webster had received that award in 1983. Ted's contributions to MGH Radiation Oncology are considered further in Chapter 4.

3.6 Neurosurgery

William Sweet of the Department of Neurosurgery in the 1950s was one of the initiators of Boron Neutron Capture Therapy for patients with malignant brain tumors. This work was predominantly at the MIT facility [19]. The results were not judged to indicate a useful level of efficacy and the MGH program ceased. There have been several programs in Europe, the USA, and Japan investigating this therapeutic strategy. Sweet and Kjellberg with the team at the Harvard Cyclotron Laboratory initiated the third program in proton stereotactic radiosurgery in 1961. The first and second were the University of California, Berkeley, and University of Uppsala. The intent was to assess the efficacy of proton therapy to suppress pituitary function by single high-dose proton irradiation for hormonally active pituitary adenomas and later several other targets. This is covered in Chapter 6 on proton therapy.

3.7 C.C. Wang[4]

C.C. Wang (see Fig. 3.5) began his residency in radiology in 1950 and accepted the invitation to join the faculty in 1953. He continued in that position until 2002, viz., 52 years at MGH.

C.C. Wang was born in 1922 in Canton, China, and was the second son in the family of a preacher. In 1948, he graduated from the medical school in Kwei-Wang and

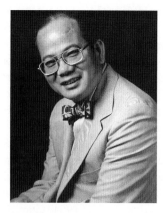

Fig. 3.5 C.C. Wang. MGH radiology resident 1960–1953 and staff radiation oncologist, 1953–2002

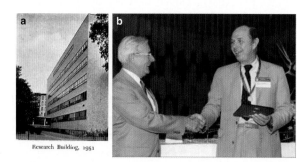

Fig. 3.4 (**a**) The Research Building that housed the physics research program. (**b**) Ted Webster presenting the William D. Coolidge Award of the American Association of Physicists in Medicine to Gordon Brownell in 1987

[4] This account is based on HDS working with and knowing CC over a very pleasant 35 years as a close friend and professional colleague. In addition, HDS interviewed CC for this book, read notes from CC, and other material.

was provided support by an aunt to come the USA for specialty training. CC often commented that he came on "a slow boat to San Francisco". CC had a 1-year general internship in Upstate Medical Center in Syracuse, New York (1949–1950), and then was admitted to the MGH radiology residency program in 1950. Larry Robbins had commented to CC's brother CA that "if CC is a fraction as good as you, we want him."

CC's older brother, CA, had been sent to the USA to attend Harvard College and Harvard Medical School. He then applied to the MGH residency program in surgery, was accepted, and on completion of the residency was appointed to the staff. This young man matured into an international star in the area of endocrine surgery (thyroid, parathyroid) and worked at MGH for his entire career.

C.C. Wang joined the faculty of the Department of Radiology in 1953 and was assigned to work with Milford Schulz in radiation therapy. He thus became the second radiation oncologist at the MGH. CC was put to the test shortly, as Milford had a 6-month sabbatical to assess the status of radiation therapy principally in Scandinavian and British centers. Milford wanted to have first-hand knowledge for his planned push for a separate department. During this 6-month period, CC was the one with the primary responsibility for the program but did have the active support of Larry Robbins, Department Chief.

In 1953, approximately 60–70 patients were being treated per day by the two clinicians. Additionally, CC and Milford were responsible for the operation of the program, supervising the therapists, nurses, secretarial, teaching residents, and the financial well-being of the department.

In his first year as staff, CC was the first author of a paper on the management at the MGH of 50 patients with Ewing's sarcoma published in the *New England Journal of Medicine*. CC's entire medical career was with the department, excepting for 2 years (1956–1958) duty in the US army and for the year 1961–1962 at the University of California at Berkeley to study particle beam therapy. That program was primarily a study of the effectiveness of helium ion irradiation to suppress pituitary gland function. This was the year, 1961, that W. Sweet and R. Kjellberg began their program of stereotactic radiosurgery based on the proton beam at the Harvard Cyclotron Laboratory (HCL) to ablate pituitary function and later to treat AVMs. Virtually all of the patients in this program were treated by Kjellberg. Milford and CC were not involved in any aspect of that phase of the MGH proton therapy program. CC rarely mentioned his year at Berkeley and that merely as a brief passing comment. He gave no hint of interest in participation in our planning to initiate fractionated dose proton therapy program or to participate in the treatment after it was started. The implication is of some severely hurt pride in not having been invited to participate in the start of the program in the early 1960s.

CC carried a very full clinical load over his 50 years as staff physician, namely he treated ∼ 25,000 patients. This was performed with high efficiency; his notes were always complete and up to date. He was extremely devoted to his patients, the residents, and the department. He rarely took his full vacation time. CC was characterized by a good sense of humor. His remarks to residents/fellows were peppered with well-targeted Chinese proverbs. To emphasize the necessity to avoid injury of normal tissues he often stated "you do not burn down a house to kill a mosquito"; "you cannot hit a home run if you do not see the ball." His attire was immaculate and invariably with a bow tie.

CC's skills and personal qualities resulted in his appointment as Clinical Director of the department in 1975. Also in 1975, he was promoted to the rank of Professor at Harvard Medical School in 1975. He held these titles until retirement in 2002, when Chris Willett became Clinical Director.

International fame came readily to CC for his quite significant contributions to radiation oncology. These include:

1. Initiation of the program of BID (two fractions per day) treatment for head/neck squamous cell cancers. Accelerated radiation treatment by one of several protocols is now commonly employed for the H/N squamous cell carcinomas.
2. Introduction of intra-oral cone (IOC) electron beam therapy as a boost dose for oral cavity lesions.
3. Development of interstitial therapy based on ^{192}Ir afterloading of angiocatheters.
4. Devised applicators for intracavitary therapy for a boost dose for nasopharyngeal cancer.
5. Author of two books: (a) *Radiation Therapy for Head/Neck Neoplasms* (three editions) and (b) author/editor of *Clinical Radiation Oncology* (two editions).
6. In addition, he published 180 papers.

He most enjoyed the opportunity to teach and work with the many residents and fellows that he helped educate. That affection was fully reciprocated. Also he was extremely well regarded by his colleagues, not only at MGH but in the medical community at large. Special honors to C.C. Wang include Gold Medals of ASTRO and the Chinese American Medical Society. Of quite special note is the endowed professorship at HMS, the C.C. Wang Professorship in Radiation Oncology. Dr. Nancy Tarbell is the first to hold that professorship. He was also an enthusiastic gardener and produced melons that would easily compete with the best of, say, Colorado.

CC and Pauline were a very devoted couple and extremely proud of their daughter, Janice. She is a graduate of Harvard Medical School and was an active anesthesiologist in Florida, but has now become an established architect.

C.C. Wang died on December 14, 2005.

3.8 Planning for the New Radiation Therapy Facility and Cancer Center

Milford was not alone among the hospital staff to recognize that the facilities for radiation therapy were rapidly becoming less than the state of the art and that the patient amenities were not meeting a reasonable standard. The need was manifestly obvious to any casual inspection, especially with appreciation that the treatments were for patients with a life-threatening disease.

Here is presented a brief chronological review of the diverse activities that led to the MGH comprehensive cancer center in the Cox building over the 18-year period of 1957–1975.

July 17, 1957. Committee on the Design and Location of Possible Facilities for Radiation Therapy and Research. This was the initial meeting of the first MGH committee to assess the needs for improvement of facilities for radiation therapy. The establishment of this committee was almost certainly the result, in part, of many conversations and letters between Larry Robbins, Milford Schulz, and the Administration.

Committee members were Drs. Earl Chapman, Chair, Dean Clark (Hospital General Director), Arthur K. Sullivan, and William Sweet. We note that there were no representatives from Radiology. K. Wright of MIT was an external consultant. He was a clinical physicist with the responsibility for the treatment planning and delivery at the Lahey Clinic radiation treatment program at the MIT Van de Graaff facility. He had developed some exceptionally elegant treatment techniques for cancers of the head/neck region. Suit visited MIT in 1953 while en route from Houston to Oxford and was extremely impressed by the creativity of the treatments. One technique was unique. This was for irradiation of targets of the base of skull, sinuses, and orbital regions. The strategy was (1) 360° rotation, (2) on-line imaging of the target by a modified fluoroscopic device, and (3) the fixation of two solid gold eye-shaped pieces to the head immobilization device so that as the patient was rotated, the gold pieces moved into the beam path and blocked irradiation of the eyes only for the segment of the 360° that the eye(s) were in the beam path. This was an early step in 4D image-guided radiation therapy. This is mentioned to note that they did obtain advice from outside talent.

The committee met multiple times and submitted a report to the Board of Trustees in July 17,1959, *vide infra*.

September 10, 1958. Report on the Radiologic Needs of the Massachusetts General Hospital prepared under the aegis of the Ambulatory Care Committee. Several pages were devoted to an assessment of the status of MGH radiation therapy. A recently completed survey of space available for radiation therapy in the 13 leading radiology departments of the country listed the MGH at next to the bottom. To meet the *average* space per procedure of the 13

institutions, the MGH program would need to increase space by a factor of 3. Further, emphasis was made of the fact that other institutions of New England now had acquired supervoltage equipment and had more adequate space than the MGH. Thus, in terms of facilities, the MGH was not in its accustomed position of clear leadership. Additionally, special emphasis was placed on the absolute necessity of allocation of adequate space for examination and consultation rooms in addition to actual treatment bays. This reflected the acute and daily frustration experienced by the staff and patients.

The need for facilities to conduct research into the biological effects of radiation was accepted by the administration as self evident and that the reality is that there is no area of medical practice at the MGH that can hold its position or advance unless it pursues research. This clearly obtains for radiation therapy, *viz* we must increase the understanding of the effects of radiation on tumor and normal tissues. Close proximity of the research space to the clinical areas contributes to the magnitude of success.

Regarding equipment, the request was for an additional 2 MeV unit and consideration was to be given for a linear accelerator or a Betatron.

July 17, 1959. The preliminary Report of the Committee on the Design and Location of Facilities for Radiation Research and Therapy was submitted to the Trustees. The members of the Committee had consulted with several persons in the USA and Europe.

The facility was proposed to be a collaborative effort between MGH, Harvard University, and MIT. The proposal for space at the MGH was (1) 30,000 ft^2 for clinical therapy and this include 3600 ft^2 for the tumor clinic (an important factor for Robbins and Schulz); (2) 15,000 ft^2 for physics research, to include a linear accelerator for research and clinical radiation therapy (G. Brownell and E. Webster); (3); the Thayer Building was suggested as the site for the new Radiation Center and (4) plans for later expansion.

Milford was quite aware that these points had been made earlier and that time was passing. He concluded that there was much talk but little movement toward an actual decision to commence planning the obviously needed new and greatly expanded facility. The impression in reading some of his notes was that his perception was rather that of one being politely listened to but not heard.

January, 1961. Celebration of the 150th Anniversary of the Authorization by the Legislature in 1811 to Build a General Hospital and an Asylum for the Insane. The hospital did not open until 1821 due to a several year delay resulting from the War of 1812. There had been plans to celebrate the 150th in 1971, viz., 150 years after the opening of the hospital. However, David Crockett judged that the MGH had to initiate its fund drive well before 1971 as a number of other Boston area institutions were planning major fund drives.

Hence, the decision to base the 150th year celebration on the date of the charter in 1811, i.e., 1961, not 1971.

At the celebration of the 150th Anniversary, Dean Clark, MGH General Director, presented plans for major new facilities. These included an ambulatory care center, a new facility with operating suites, a radiation therapy building, and new quarters for diagnostic radiology (presumably in that order of priority). Despite this nominal high priority, problems other than radiation therapy actually received the attention and funds over the subsequent several years.

In fact, the Trustees did appoint another committee to assess the status of radiation therapy at the MGH, again under the Chairmanship of Dr. Earl Chapman. Arthur Solomon of the Harvard Medical School and Dr. Henry Kaplan from Stanford University Medical School served as consultants. As part of this review, Dr. Chapman assessed the status of radiation therapy at centers in Sweden, Germany, and England. This spotlighted significant shortfalls in the program at MGH.

Clark retired shortly following the 1961 event and was replaced by the very young John Knowles. He moved forward with the Gray Building and surgical rooms. Significantly, he decided to initiate planning for the cancer center. A special committee of the Board of Trustees listed a new radiation therapy building as one of the three principal objectives from the 150th Anniversary program.

July 12, 1962. An MGH Committee met with representatives of the NCI and consultants to consider development of plans for the MGH Radiation Therapy program. Those in attendance included Francis O. Schmidt (trustee and MIT Professor), John Raker, Milford Schulz, C.C. Wang, Edward Webster, Adelbert Ames, Saul Aronow, and M. Potsaid. The guests included Drs. Faulkner Smith, Executive Secretary, Radiation Study Section, Division of Research Grants, NIH, M.M. Elkind, H.E. Johns, H. Vermund, and Nora Tapley. This clearly constituted a very prestigious team. Consideration was given to the strategy for development of the radiation therapy program at MGH and concluded that the MGH should apply to the NIH for funds to support development.

April 18, 1963. Milford Schulz's letter to John Knowles, General Director of the MGH.

This letter presents a lucid and compelling rationale for the MGH to continue as a leading center in radiation oncology. Also, the letter reflects a deep concern that progress had been far too slow and not certain of outcome.

Dear Dr Knowles,   April 18, 1963

The subject of your recent memorandum is one to which I have given many long hard thoughts-not only because it does represent my entire professional life and thus hopefully makes me somewhat of a qualified expert In these matters, but because I have a great affection for MGH and great concern for what goes on in it, how It develops and what the world outside thinks

of It and above all what we are doing and what we can do for the public sick with that disease we call cancer.

1. I am delighted that specific thought is being directed to the matter of what we are going to do about radiation therapy and its treatment at MGH. A decision as to the path we must take must be a deliberate one–right or wrong, and not occur by default.

2. I accept with enthusiasm the charge to explore with Dr. (David) Cogan or with anyone else the possibility of a joint effort directed toward the matter under consideration.

3. The idea of a cooperative venture in radiotherapy and related activities between the Massachusetts Eye and Ear Infirmary and MGH seems most attractive. Few know that the infirmary contributes about a third of our patients.

4. We must not get our thinking out of order. The thing we must first decide is not whether we want or can afford any particular piece of hardware, be it linear accelerator or what. Radiotherapeutic hardware is just a tool of the radiotherapist and though it is important and does have undoubted "front door" value, decisions about such matters are at about the third level of magnitude. The decision of first order is, "Shall MGH continue and grow in its position of eminence in cancer management?" This automatically implies the question, "Shall we make it possible at MGH to do the kind of radiotherapy which the present stage of development of the science requires?" That radiotherapy is pre-eminent among the presently available tools for dealing with this disease is, I fear sometimes not quite realized. Even if in the future some other means of dealing with this disease should occur, we still have the obligation to do presently the best we can with the means at hand. Then, having decided that we do indeed want to continue and to grow as a cancer center and not revert to the status of a community hospital, we then make decisions regarding the physical facility which will be required and then last of all the hardware we put into it.

5. Radiotherapy is not a matter of hardware. It is like all other medical activities a matter of men who use the hardware. The proposal that presently non-existent hardware in another non-existent facility be employed, even as a temporary expedient as a means of saving the cost of hardware, means in fact proposing that we bypass the existing staff and make it impossible for them to serve the institution and the patients in it.

6. MGH has been pre-eminent in the area of cancer control and I am fearful of an inversion of our thinking. This hospital is the center. This hospital has the experienced staff. This hospital has a going tumor clinic and an active program. This hospital has pioneered in super voltage radiation. We currently treat more than twice as many patients as the combined efforts of the other centers mentioned in the memorandum. The Children's Hospital treats 12 to 15 patients per day. The Deaconess treats about two dozen. The Beth Israel has a big day if it has ten. Even the Brigham, which is not currently under consideration in the program and which in fact just installed a 6 million volt linear accelerator, has a big day if it reaches 15 or 20 patients. We have a small day when we get down to 75, and 100 or more are not unusual. We give about 200 radium treatments per year. The Deaconess alone comes close to this, where about 40 such treatments are given per year and those by the surgeons and not by the radiotherapists and so for purposes of training and education are effectively lost. It is better they come to us than we go them.

7. The facility presently planned under the auspices of the medical school, to which you refer, is in fact not a clinical facility. It is a research and radiobiological facility under the direction of Henry Kohn, a friend of mine of many years. Dr. Kohn, though an M.D., is a biologist and not directly interested in the clinical problems of patient care. In fact, at San Francisco, where he now works, clinical radiotherapy is in an entirely separate department headed by Dr. Franz Buschke. Though we hope that our relations

with Dr. Kohn will be most cordial and intimate, he most of all does not expect to have any clinical responsibility. The clinical facility of which you speak, while it will come-and welcome-is still some way off.

8. This or any other hospital cannot maintain a strong cancer management service without an active and progressive program of radiotherapy supported in the strongest possible way by all internal sources. This is not to say that another parallel organization across town is not desirable. I believe it is, but certainly if we relinquish our position of eminence in this field, our tumor clinic which has served us so well and of which we are so proud will collapse and even soon the private activities in surgery will not be long in failing because of want of nourishment and reversion to habits of the past.

9. Radiotherapy is not just something, which can be done by referral to a machine or a facility. Modern radiotherapy, and I say this with some feeling, for radiotherapy today is much, much different than it was ten or fifteen years ago, requires a most intimate kind of teamwork involving not only the radiotherapist, who should be a good one, and his associated biologists and physicists (and hardware). But above all the cooperating surgeon and internist and such activity can serve the patient, best only when everyone works physically as well as philosophically together.

10. I don't believe we can afford to "procrastinate" or "experiment" in this matter. Certainly, once this Institution leaves this program to go to another, there will be no retrieving of it no matter how desirable we may think at a later date it might be to do so.

This brings me to my last thought for the moment. There are certain medical decisions in which a hospital such as ours has little or no choice of action. Money matters, important as they are, quite aside. Community hospital X can say, "No, we are not justified in spending the money which development of a first-class radiotherapy and cancer center would require. It is better for us to deal with these problems on a limited basis and send the more difficult, more exacting and expensive problems to the center" and in fact this is just what many community hospitals are doing-wisely. But we are the center. We are not a community hospital. We are a unique and in fact national institution and if we abandon any significant area of medical enterprise and do not provide the best available within our own internal framework, where is the patient to go? To provide such things is our obligation-our opportunity-yes, even our burden, and any decision to do otherwise requires of us an awfully good answer and this answer cannot be just dollars.

I am sorry that this has more to do with "feelings" than facts which you seek. I shall try to marshal them and give them to you soon, but I am off to Stockholm, Oslo and Copenhagen to renew old acquaintances at the Cancer Hospitals there. Perhaps I'll get some new facts there.

Sincerely,
Milford S. Schulz, M. D.

He copied this to Claude Welch, Laurence Robbins, David Cogan, Harold Schuknecht, and Paul Russell.

January 29, 1964. A request for 2500 ft^2 for research in radiation biology was submitted to the Massachusetts General Hospital Space Committee.

1965. Research Activity in Cancer. At the MGH, approximately \$2.25 M per year was devoted to cancer research. Basic research programs included biochemical characterization of tumors; hybridization of cells in vitro; origins of genetic variations of cell lines in vivo; cell surface properties;

patterns of simplification of normal antigenic make-up of cells; malignant transformation; new tumor-specific antigens; biochemical and biophysical properties of plasma membrane. There was discussion of the need for the radiation research laboratory and its location.

November 16, 1965. John Knowles emphasized the mutual interest of the MEEI and MGH in radiation therapy. Notation was made that the MGH would experience a net loss of patients were those patients referred to other centers. He also considered developing an arrangement for MGH to utilize facilities at MIT. However, there was recognition that Dr. J. Trump had already established a close and long-term working relationship with the Lahey Clinic that their patients were being treated at MIT. There was further discussion of the feasibility of use of the Thayer Building site for the new radiation therapy unit.

December 14, 1965. Oncology Planning Committee Meeting.

Attendees: Drs. Russell (Chair), Meader, Rita Kelley, Schulz, Sidel, Raker, McKhann, Zamecnik, Mr. Crockett, and Mr. Degen.

Dr. Sam Herman was the guest from the National Cancer Institute. There was a brief review of the plans for the cancer program at the MGH by Drs. Raker, Zamecnik for laboratory research, and Dr. McKhann for overall goals and research. Mr. Degen and Goff talked about a plan for a proposed new building showing different stages the construction could take. Dr. Herman emphasized the importance for being informed of all of the plans for radiation therapy in the Boston area. He reiterated three points that were made in a recent conversation between himself and Dr. Endicott of the NCI. First, medical schools will probably not go to the Cancer Institute for funds for their regional planning. But hospitals, such as the MGH, probably will do so. Second, Stanford University is interested in formulating a plan for cancer therapy built around radiotherapy with particular concern for instrumentation and development of hardware. Third, a committee on radiation therapy is going to convene in February, which includes Dr. Kaplan from Stanford and results from their Conference may be of value in MGH planning. He concluded by recommending that the MGH proceed to prepare and submit the application for funds from the NIH.

1966. Five years had elapsed since priorities for the MGH were specified at the 150th Anniversary of the MGH. John Knowles met with Sidney Farber at the Children's Hospital to discuss the planned expansion of the radiation therapy program and radiation research at MGH. He also explored with Dr. Ebert, Dean of Harvard Medical School, the use by the MGH of laboratory space in the Shields-Warren Building in the Longwood complex. These broad enquires by Knowles appear to have been a strategy to convince his diverse constituents that the MGH leadership had considered every conceivable option. We think that Knowles was not seriously considering "outsourcing" of the cancer program to the Longwood facilities but that these discussions were in fact only good "theater."

Knowles concluded that there was unanimity of our Staff, the other teaching hospitals, medical schools in Boston area, and the various community planning associations that a comprehensive cancer center at the MGH was needed. This was accepted as giving the MGH a green light to proceed. Although this appeared to be positive, the Board of Trustees decided that they had to delay a start of the new cancer facility due to the commitment to raise quite substantial funds for Surgical and Special Service Buildings. However, planning was started.

May 26, 1966. The Oncology Planning Committee. Attendees: Drs. Russell (Chair), Kelley, Castleman, McKhann, Raker, Robbins, Zamecnik, and Mr. Crockett. Dr. Robbins had gone ahead with the application to the American Cancer Society (ACS) for $400,000. Dr. Kelley, a member of the Board of Directors of the Mass Division of the ACS, commented that the ACS was not entirely happy with the MGH as relatively large amounts of money had been given previously as institutional grants but some of those funds had not been spent. She also noted that over the past years there was a continuing note of discord with some of our Trustees who are important figures in the United Fund and not sympathetic with the separate fund-raising by the ACS. The plan was for the application to be discussed with Drs. Daland, Robbins, and Schulz.

1967. The 154th Annual Report of the Trustees notes that Committees had been formed to search for new Chiefs of Anesthesiology, Radiology, Radiotherapy, and Urology. This meant that the decision had been taken to separate Radiology into two departments. This decision was 22 years after the decision was made to establish a separate and independent Department of Radiology, viz., 1945. Dr. Laurence Robbins requested that he be relieved of his administrative duties.

February 1, 1967. Report by Architects Rogers, Butler, and Burgun on the Radiation Therapy Facility. This firm had been charged to develop plans and budget for the Radiation Therapy facility on the site of the Thayer Building. The planning had not expanded to have a comprehensive Cancer Center.

The general plan was to construct the new radiation therapy building on a phased schedule with timing determined by availability of funds. Phase I was to be sited in the court between the Thayer and Warren buildings. This would provide 14,380 ft^2 for the radiation therapy division to accommodate three high-energy units, adequate exam rooms, and related clinic activities. For shielding purposes, this would be below ground level. Accordingly, radiation therapy would be divided between space in White II and the new building until Phase II is completed. Above the radiation area would be 5,400 ft^2 space for the tumor clinic. There would then be a two-level street entrance on Blossom Street to provide street access by elevator and stair to both the Radiation Therapy Department and the Tumor Clinic.

The Thayer Building was to be removed for Phase II, which would yield sufficient space for two additional treatment bays (a total of 5), the transfer of all radiation therapy from White II and for an expanded tumor clinic program. The foundation of the building would be specified so as to permit later expansion in height to equal that of the Baker building. The preliminary cost estimate was $3.427 M.

February 14, 1967. Meeting of Dr. J. Knowles with D. Crockett, J. Degen, S. Drury, and C. Wood. They accepted the plan of Rogers et al. as best probable plan for this project for radiation therapy. MEEI was to share in the project and pay 20%. The operation of the new department was suggested to be directed by the senior radiation therapist. Mention was made of the potential of a Steering Committee for overall guidance of the department and the submission of regular reports to a Joint Medical Planning Board. This was not a proposal for an independent department.

April 17, 1967. Radiation Therapy Planning Committee or the Oncology Planning Committee. John Knowles stated that there would not be a need to maintain a split department. He dismissed the idea of a Betatron, stating that it is not the best working machine. Further, he commented that the dosimetry is complicated and estimated that electron therapy is actually a fad, with applicability only to $\leq 10\%$ of the patients. In conclusion, the proposal by the committee was to construct a complete center and move all of White II at one time to the newly constructed space to be equipped with two linear accelerators, a cobalt unit) and the 250 keV machine. To assure continuous operation, one ^{60}Co unit was proposed as security from machine downtimes.

May 23, 1967. Oncology Meeting. Drs. Russell (Chair), Kelley, McKhann, Schulz, Meader, Knowles, Zamecnik, Raker, Castleman, Mr. Degen, and Mr. Crockett. Dr. Knowles indicated that from his visit to Stanford he did not think a Betatron was a good machine. Dr. Schulz indicated that there was a need for electrons of relatively high energy. He again articulated the pressing need for adequate space for examining rooms, dressing rooms, office space, and record space. He clearly voiced concern that the hospital be aware of the expanding capabilities for modern radiation therapy treatment at the Longwood hospitals and Boston City Hospital. The Committee concurred with Dr. Knowles that his selection of equipment was probably a good compromise at present and initial stage.

August 1967. The President of Harvard University appointed a committee to evaluate the status of Radiation Therapy at MGH and if appropriate to search for a Chief of the program. This is discussed further in Chapter 4.

1968. The firm Arthur D. Little submitted its report "A Report on the Administration and Organization of

Radiology." This document was another clear and strong support for greater space and modernization of equipment for radiation therapy and that facilities and space be provided for research in radiation biology. The 155th Annual report of the Trustees quotes the General Director saying "We look forward with increasing confidence to the future and have already started raising new capital for the next two pressing needs viz a modern radiotherapy facility with increasing facilities for radiobiology . . ."

February 2, 1968. The third meeting of the Committee on Radiotherapy. Present included Drs. J. Knowles, A. Leaf, P. Russell, H. Ulfelder, and D. Crockett. Invited guests were Dr. H. Abrams (Chief, Radiology, Brigham), Dr. F. Bloedorn (Tufts), M. Kligerman (Los Alamos), H. Kohn (Radiation Biology, Shields Warren Laboratory), and R. Walton (Manitoba Treatment and Research Foundation). The guests discussed the present difficulties and needs of the radiation therapy program with Dr. Schulz. Mr. Degen presented plans for the new facility at lunch. The discussion was taped and selected comments are given here:

F Bloedorn stated "it is not necessary to express one's horror with the facilities. We all agree that they are obsolete and far too small. . .. I think you have here one of the biggest radiotherapy loads in the country and only two or three departments in the country with more patients. You have to enlarge your staff, facility, and equipment in order to give proper care. Now why have things happened this way? Why hasn't an important hospital like this developed radiotherapy better? I think the main reason is that radiotherapy is responsible to radiology in general. When a man is not fighting his own battle, he doesn't fight with vigor and the same enthusiasm that you put into a fight of your own. My first impression is that you need an independent department of radiotherapy, not only to avoid dependence, but also to allow the department a proper training and research program. We all agree that Milford Schulz has achieved a great amount of work of good quality with very little facilities and is admired by all of his colleagues."

R. Walton: "I would agree with everything that Fernando has said. I am particularly struck by the size and excellence of the job that Milford has done under these extremely difficult conditions. Thus, I think he'd be first to admit, and in fact stated to us, that his dilemma is lack of space and lack of help. What this has meant is that his patients could not have the sophisticated quality of treatment that should be provided by the MGH. Secondly, I think that the patients have undoubtedly suffered from the crowding that exists. The clinical facilities and patient numbers in Winnipeg are comparable to that proposed for the MGH. In terms of space we occupy 65,000 square feet, of which about half can be related to clinical care patients." Walton also stressed the need to have radiation therapy separate from diagnostic radiology. Kligerman recommended a separate division or service for

Radiation Therapy and that the Radiation Service should have its own beds. All concurred that there could be four centers in Boston.

In consideration of candidates for the new position of Chief of Radiation Oncology M. Kligerman commented that it would be at least 5 years before the new MGH center would be physically available. He believed that Schulz should be kept in charge of Radiotherapy and given an independent department and then after the Unit is built select a bright young man at that time. This would be close to Schulz's retirement. All three consultants judged that Schulz is one of the best radiation therapists in the country and some strategy should be made to retain him. Dr. Bloedorn emphasized the importance of the good cooperation that Schulz has now with the other services and if one were to get a new and aggressive Chief, there would be a danger of losing Dr. Schulz. Dr. Kligerman suggested that a lay administrator attached to the department of radiotherapy might take care of many of the administrative details that Dr. Schulz must now manage. Although all members of the Committee agreed that Schulz is an excellent radiation therapist, some of the members opined that putting Schulz in a new environment with better equipment and a larger budget and giving him a separate department would not be likely to change reflexes that have been built up over the years. The group then listed possible candidates. All of these were judged to be well satisfied with their present position, and it was thought that none would be interested in the position were Dr. Schulz to remain as head of the department.

An undated letter (of approximately the same time) from Sam Hellman, Chief at the Joint Center for Radiation Therapy, strongly supported the development of a large program at the MGH.

May 9, 1968. Milford Schulz wrote an exceptionally strong letter to Dr. B. Castleman taking the position that as desirable as the separation of Radiology into Diagnostic and Therapeutic Departments was, there would be no relief from the extremely disadvantaged situation of the practice of radiation therapy in terms of space and equipment. The only immediate plus from the separation would be to make his voice heard by a larger fraction of the administration. Further, the MGH will shortly have to recruit young leaders. Unless changes are made and done so quickly, recruitment of top talent will be increasingly difficult. This letter indicates that Milford had been informed of the intent to make radiation therapy a separate department. Further, he also was aware of the plan to recruit a new and young Chief.

July 15, 1968. J.H. Knowles stated "facilities in our Tumor Clinic and in our radiotherapy area are essentially the same, with no improvement in equipment or space, since the White building was built in 1940." "One and all are agreed that we simply must expand and update our facilities for the care of the cancer patient." His position was supported by the rapid increase in number of radiation treatments administered per year as indicated in Table 3.1.

September 18, 1968. Letter from John Knowles to Howard Ulfelder, Chief of Gynecology and a leader of the group to have a new cancer facility. "Although it is most probable that the Trustees will allow us only to complete the first phase in moving the entire radiotherapy facility and tumor clinic to a location underground and one floor above ground abutted by the Thayer, Baker, and Warren Buildings, we would also like to show them a plan, which would remove the Thayer Building entirely with relocation of its occupants temporarily with ultimate location on unfinished floor or floors of the new building. I believe this will be prohibitively expensive in view of the present financial situation locally and nationally. But nonetheless, we should have the two alternatives available for discussion. I have discussed this with Mr. Goff, Mr. Crocket, and Dr. Castleman. Perhaps you should review it with them and with your committee. It has been suggested that Dr. Sohier would be an excellent one to do the actual writing and drawing together of material for application to such diverse sources such as the American Cancer Society, Mass Division, to say nothing of the development of a final brochure for our general public."

1969. The search committee for the new MGH Chief of Radiation Therapy began interviewing candidates.

3.9 Boston Radiation Therapy Programs Outside of the MGH ~1970

3.9.1 BU/BCH (Boston University/Boston City Hospital)

This information was obtained in part from the History of Boston City and Boston University Hospitals and from Dr. Kachnic, Chief at BUMC at this writing. Dr. Isamettin Aral was the radiation oncologist at BU/BCH. An important event in his tenure was the installation of a 42 MeV Siemens Betatron in November 1967. This unit had had an excellent performance record, an uptime of >95%. We arranged for treatment of select MGH patients at BU/BCH starting in 1971.

3.9.2 Tufts New England Medical Center

F. Bloedorn was recruited from the University of Maryland to develop a new and fully modern department of radiation oncology at Tufts. He came in 1967. At that time, Tufts had a single therapy machine, a 280 kVp unit at the Floating Hospital. The hospital instituted a major program of providing modern equipment for him. Bloedorn had a very well-established reputation for skills in brachytherapy and many referrals from well beyond New England. He oversaw the installation of two ^{60}Co units and in 1971 a 46 MeV Brown Boveri Betatron.

3.9.3 JCRT (Joint Center for Radiation Therapy)

Sam Hellman, young and clearly very talented, was recruited from Yale to head the JCRT in 1968. This was a consortium of the radiation therapy programs of five Harvard Hospitals: Brigham and Women's, Beth Israel, New England Deaconess, Boston Children's Hospital, and Boston Hospital for Women. The radiation treatment of patients of the Boston Children's Hospital and the Dana Farber Cancer Institute were given at the Brigham and Women's Hospital. By 1970, the supervoltage equipment at these four Hospitals was a 6 MeV Lin Acc , a 4 MeV Lin Acc, a 1 MeV resonant transformer, and a ^{60}Co unit, respectively. This Information was obtained from Bengt Bjarngard, former Head of Physics at the JCRT (personal communication 2007). The total number of new patients per year was ~1200.

This summary demonstrates a rapidly changing Boston radiation therapy community. None of the MGH staff interviewed nor material examined in the archives by HDS was there a statement(s) indicating concern by the MGH regarding the substantial upgrading of the other Boston facilities.

An exceptional indicator of the comprehensive nature and quality of the care provided by the Boston academic centers is that to this date no radiation oncology facility has opened that has not been a part of one of the academic centers in Greater Boston.

References

1. Ackerman LA, del Regato JA. Cancer: diagnosis, treatment, and prognosis. St Louis: Mosby; 1947.
2. Armstrong N, Aldrin B. NASA. Photographs in http://en.wikipedia.org/wiki/Apollo_11. Accessed on 2010.
3. Brownell GL, Sweet WH. Localization of brain tumors with positron emitters. Nucleonics. 1953;11:40–45.
4. Castleman B, Crockett DC, Sutton SB. The Massachusetts General Hospital, 1955–1980. Boston, MA: Little, Brown and Company; 1983.
5. DNA molecule. http://en.wikipedia.org/wiki/DNA. Accessed on 2010.
6. ENIAC the first electronic computer. http://en.wikipedia.org/wiki/ENIAC. Accessed on 2010.
7. Faxon, N. The Massachusetts General Hospital, 1935–1955. Cambridge, MA: Harvard University Press; 1959.

8. Gagarin, Yuri. http://en.wikipedia.org/wiki/Yuri_Gagarin. Accessed on 2010.
9. Gagliardi RA, Wilson JF, eds. A history of the radiological sciences: radiation oncology. Reston, VA: Radiology Centennial; 1996.
10. Gilman A, Phillips FS. The biological actions and therapeutic applications of B-chloroethyl amines and sulfides. Science. 1946;103(2675):409–15.
11. Guggenheim Museum. Guggenheim website. Scott Gilchrist/stock.archivision.com. With permission. Accessed on 2010.
12. Hilary E, Norgay T. Summit of Mt Everest. 1953. http://en.wikipedia.org/wiki/Tenzing_Norgay#cite_note-0. Accessed on 2010.
13. Holmes G, Schulz M. Therapeutic radiology. Philadelphia, PA: Lea and Febiger; 1950.
14. Li M, Hertz R, Spencer DB. Effect of methotrexate on choriocarcinoma and chorioadenoma. Proc Soc Exp Biol Med. 1956;93(2):361–6.
15. McCartney. ENIAC: the triumphs and tragedies of the world's first computer. New York, NY: Berkley Books; 1999.
16. Paterson R. The treatment of malignant disease by radium and x rays. London, UK: Edward Arnold and Company; 1948.
17. Portman, U. Clinical therapeutic radiology. New York, NY: Thomas Nelson and Sons; 1950.
18. Sputnik 1, the first earth orbiting satellite. Launched in Nov. 3 1957. Wikipedia website. Available at http://en.wikipedia.org/w/index.php?title=Sputnik_1&printable=yes. Accessed on 2010.
19. Sweet WH, Javid M. The possible use of neutron-capturing isotopes such as boron 10 in the treatment of neoplasms. I. Intracranial tumors. J Neurosurg. 1952;9(2):200–9.
20. Thomas ED, Storb R, Clift RA, et al. Bone-marrow transplantation (first of two parts). New Engl J Med. 1975;292(16):832–43.
21. Thomas ED, Storb R, Clift RA, et al. Bone marrow transplantation (second of two parts). New Engl J Med. 1975;292(17):895–902.
22. TWA Terminal of 1962 by E Saarinen. With permission. http://www.greatbuildings.com/buildings/TWA_at_New_York.html. Accessed on 2010.
23. United Nations Building, © Copyright Lee W Nelson, www.inetours.com. Accessed on 2010.
24. General Assembly of the United Nations. Declaration of Human Rights, 1948. United Nations website. Available at http://www.un.org/Overview/rights.html. Accessed on 2010.
25. Watson JD, Crick FH. Molecular structure of nucleic acids: a structure for deoxyribose nucleic acid. Nature. 1953;171(4356):737–8.

Chapter 4

The New Department of Radiation Oncology 1970–1975

4.1 Establishment of the MGH Department of Radiation Oncology[1]

The Department of Radiation Oncology was established effective June 1, 1970, with separation of radiology into imaging radiology and therapeutic radiology. Accordingly, the Chief of Radiation Oncology would report directly to the General Director of the hospital, John Knowles, and serve as a member of the General Executive Committee. An interesting point is that then and for many years, the Chief of Radiation Oncology was the only oncologist on the General Executive Committee.

4.2 Recruitment of the First Chief of Radiation Oncology at MGH

The MGH had decided to (1) build a Cancer Center on the site of the Thayer Building for the radiation, medical, and surgical oncology programs; (2) recruit a Chief for the new department of radiation oncology, and (3) develop a laboratory and clinical radiation research program.

In early 1967, the hospital requested Harvard Medical School to conduct a national search for the Chief of Radiotherapy at the MGH. This process is described by the December 22, 2004, letter to HDS from Jack Eckert, Rare Books Librarian, Countway Library:

In August 1967, Harvard's President, Nathan Pusey, appointed an ad hoc committee to consider the present and future status of radiotherapy at MGH and, if warranted, to search for and nominate a candidate to a tenured position in that field. The physicians asked to serve on the ad hoc committee were Drs. Benjamin Castleman[2], Chairman, Herbert L. Abrams[3],

Sidney Farber[4], John H. Knowles[5] (ex officio), Henry I. Kohn[6], Alexander Leaf[7], Paul S. Russell[8], and Paul C. Zamecnik[9]. It appears that Samuel Hellman and Howard Ulfelder were subsequently added, or at least were part of the committee at the time it submitted its report in July 1970. There were also three external consultants – Drs. Fernando G. Bloedorn, Morton M. Kligerman, and R. J. Walton – who had made a site visit and recommendations concerning the radiation therapy program. Deliberations of the ad hoc committee were suspended for a year due to a funding problem in 1968. You were one of four candidates interviewed. According to the information I have at hand, you were serving as the Alvan T. and Viola D. Fuller-American Cancer Society Visiting Professor of Radiology at Harvard in 1968–1969 academic year, and was subsequently appointed as the Professor of Radiation Therapy and chief of the Department of Radiation Medicine at MGH in January 1971 (retroactive to July 1970).

The following section is a personal account of the recruitment by HDS:

For the 1969 spring term, I was invited by Sam Hellman to give a course in radiation biology and to participate in several departmental activities at the Joint Center of Radiation Therapy as the Alvin T. and Viola D. Fuller Visiting Professor of Radiology. I accepted and enjoyed a wonderful 4 months in Boston. In May, the Search Committee at the MGH invited me for an interview. Fortunately for me, the available talent pool in radiation therapy was small, in the USA and in Europe.

I had just had my 40th birthday and had been Chief of the Section of Experimental Radiation Therapy at the University of Texas M.D. Anderson Cancer Center (MDACC) in Houston for 10 years. My educational and professional background was BA in Biology, University of Houston, 1948; MD, Baylor University College of Medicine, 1952; M.Sc., Biochemistry, Baylor University, 1952; D.Phil., Oxford University, 1956; staff of the Radiation Division of the NCI (Bethesda), 1957–1959; and British and American Boards in radiation therapy.

---

[1] The initial name of the department was Radiation Medicine but later changed to Radiation Oncology and will be so designated in the sequel.

[2] Chief of Pathology at MGH.

[3] Chief of Radiology at Peter Bent Brigham Hospital.

[4] Director of the Dana Farber Cancer Institute.

[5] General Director, viz., President of the MGH.

[6] Senior Biologist at the Joint Center for Radiation Therapy.

[7] Chief of Medicine at MGH.

[8] Chief of Surgery at MGH.

[9] Senior Biologist at MGH.

H.D. Suit, J.S. Loeffler, *Evolution of Radiation Oncology at Massachusetts General Hospital*, DOI 10.1007/978-1-4419-6744-2_4, © Springer Science+Business Media, LLC 2011

I was recruited in 1959 to the M.D. Anderson Cancer Center (MDACC) to develop the Section of Experimental Radiotherapy and to work in the laboratory and in the clinic on a 50:50 time basis. Laboratory research at MDACC commenced immediately on the radiation biology of spontaneous and early generation syngeneic transplanted murine tumor systems and of murine normal tissues. Importantly, during a visit to the Texas Inbred Mouse Co. to consider buying mice for experimental studies, I met and discussed experimental animals with Robert Sedlacek, an employee. He described his concept for a defined flora and pathogen free (DFPF) mouse colony. I judged that his concept had highly important potential and was entirely feasible. Dame fortune smiled and I succeeded in short order to obtain a new position and recruited him. He accomplished our goals of providing exceptional quality mice in large numbers for experimentation. Several of his developments were patented and are in wide use to this day. Our colony was the only DFPF in an academic center in the USA and one of very few even today. Some of research talent recruited were H. Rodney Withers, Luka Milas, Ian Tannock, Vlatko Silobrcic, and others. Further, I had the great fortune of serving as the supervisor for two graduate students, Larry Thomson and Helen Stone. They received their Ph.D. degrees from the University of Texas (MDACC was a component of their graduate program). This laboratory program was supported by a NCI RO 1 grant, a NCI Research Career Development Award, and $100 K per year institutional support.

Several of my clinical and research contributions are mentioned here. At MDACC I worked for the 11 years primarily as a sub-specialist in connective tissue oncology. The clinically significant gain was to appreciate that recent studies, especially of T. Puck, strongly indicated that cells of sarcomas were not inherently more radiation resistant than epithelial tumor cells. The combination of moderate dose radiation and less than radical surgery for extremity soft tissue sarcomas was soon demonstrated to be effective. This strategy became known as limb salvage treatment. In addition, I had proposed, organized, and conducted with the Gilbert Fletcher one of the first phase III trials of radiation and chemotherapy, viz., radiation alone vs radiation combined with 5 FU for pharyngeal carcinomas. There was faster tumor regression but no gain in long-term local control in the radiation + 5FU group. Further, I worked with the machinist Bailey Moore and modified the Fletcher applicator for the intracavitary treatment of patients with carcinoma of the uterine cervix for afterloading, i.e., sharply reducing radiation exposure to hospital personnel.

Selected laboratory research findings were

1. Dose–response curve for local control of tumor is a straight line on a Logit response frequency vs Log dose grid for early generation syngeneic transplants of spontaneous tumor systems, i.e., any change in dose alters response probability.
2. Introduced the term TCD_{50}, i.e., the dose that would on average control half of tumors.
3. TCD_{50} increased linearly with log tumor volume.
4. The murine solid tumors investigated had large hypoxic fractions. In fractionated irradiation, "re-oxygenation" was a large response modifier.
5. Quantitative transplant studies yielded no evidence of host immune reaction to spontaneous mammary carcinomas of the C_3H mouse.
6. Ph.D. student L. Thomson studied L 59 cells in vitro. He demonstrated that cells killed by low radiation doses often proliferated through 3–6 post-radiation divisions before undergoing pyknosis or apoptosis. Lethal sectoring was frequent among surviving cells.
7. S. Gallagher, MDAH breast cancer pathologist, was not able to identify residual tumors at 3 weeks post single doses corresponding to TCD_1 or TCD_{95}, i.e., no morphological features to distinguish between tumor cells that were cytologically intact but reproductively dead or viable.

In administrative functions, I had served 2 years as Chair of the Hospital Research Committee and as a member of the President's Advisory Committee.

At the MGH interview in May 1969, MGH plans and intentions for a multidisciplinary cancer program and a new building were convincing and certainly attractive. Strengths of the new position included the exceptional reputation of the hospital and medical school combined with the commitment to a major expansion in oncology and a completely new department of radiation therapy. In addition, there were comments by Search Committee members on the long leadership in oncology and radiotherapy by the MGH. There was no ambiguity in their wish for the MGH to be a leader in radiation therapy and broadly in oncology.

I presented a general summary of goals for the department were I to be the Chief. These included (1) faculty to work assiduously to improve continuously the effectiveness of patient care; (2) we would work as sub-specialists for tumors at specific sites or age, viz., pediatric patients; and (3) our staff would be effective members of the multidisciplinary oncology teams/clinics. There would be a resident program with designated time for research for each resident. Further, I stated that in my department there would be no house cases, i.e., every patient would be the formal responsibility of a staff radiation oncologist with residents participating in all aspects of the patient's care. This was in contrast with the tradition in some MGH major departments.

The new department would include a Division of Radiation Physics assigned to build and then sustain a front line physics and technology program. That division would operate a departmental machine shop. There would be a laboratory research program in the broad area of radiation biology of tumor and normal tissues. This would require the transfer of the defined flora mouse colony to the MGH.

I had known and greatly respected Milford and CC and discussed with them their view of future needs of the department. Additionally, I met with Dr. L. Robbins (Chief of Radiology) and several of the hospital staff. All appeared to agree with the stated goals.

In June, I was pleased to receive a letter inviting me to accept the MGH position. However, the letter was severely disappointing in that there was no mention of institutional support for the biology research program. My response was that despite the extremely attractive clinical opportunities, I had to decline the offer due to the absence of specific hospital support for a research program. Later that summer at a meeting in Tokyo, a young radiation oncologist friend mentioned that he had just declined an invitation from the MGH to be the new Chief.

David Crockett, Director of Development, was requested by J. Knowles, General Director,[10] to generate the required institutional support for the radiation biology program. I was invited to come back to Boston in February 1970, for discussions with Knowles, the committee, and Mr. Crockett. David readily arranged the required institutional support for the laboratory program. He and I rapidly developed a close personal friendship that continued to his recent death.

---

[10] The title of the CEO of the MGH is now President.

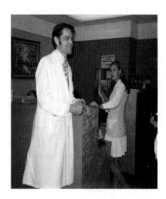

Fig. 4.1 Herman Suit in the Sarcoma Clinic at MDACC near the time that he accepted the invitation to come the MGH. This photograph was taken by one of his patients

On April 14, I met again with John Knowles and accepted the position as Chief of the new department and Professor at the Harvard Medical School. Knowles indicated that the name Radiotherapy was not attractive in its implication that radio equipment would be employed. I proposed Radiation Medicine to reflect the increasing use of radiation in the treatment of patients with non-malignant diseases in addition to the central focus on malignant tumors. Agreement was reached. The plan was for me to be appointed as of June 1, 1970, on a half-time basis until September 1, 1971 (see Fig. 4.1). Dr. Fletcher agreed with this plan and that H.R. Withers would become the Chief of the Section at MDAH in September, 1971.

4.3   Start-Up Activities of the New Department

In 1970, the medical staff had four full-time radiation oncologists, viz., Milford Schulz, C.C. Wang, Melvin Tefft, and George Zinninger. Both Melvin and George moved to other centers in the early 1970s. There was one part-time treatment planner, Rosemary Whipfelder, with back-up by Ted Webster, Head of Physics for Radiology. There were three residents: Sidney Kadish (1968), Susan Pittman (1970), and Warren Sewall (1970) who had joined Schulz and Wang. Vincent Chang came with HDS for his residency. A dedicated team of radiation therapists and nurses effectively performed their functions in the seriously overcrowded and highly stressed space on White 2. Also a small secretarial and a very pleasant but rather ineffectual billing staff was in place.[11] There were also offices for M. Schulz and C.C. Wang. Our treatment equipment comprised a 2 MV Van de Graaff, a ^{60}Co Theratron Junior (55 cm SSD), a 280 kVp orthovoltage machine, and a good supply of radium. The

actual space available for the three machines, an examining room, secretarial area, patient waiting room, staff offices, and record storage was along one short corridor on White 2. This team was treating ~90 patients per day. We were provided substantial space in the Temporary Building II (Temp II), a remnant from WW I in front of the Bulfinch. This would house the animal colony, research laboratory, office space for the new staff, and the machine shop.

4.4   New Staff, 1971–1974

Clinicians appointed were Ann Chu (1971) from MDACC, Rita Linggood (1973) from St. Bartholomew's Hospital, London, and Noah Choi (1973) from Tufts. New physicists were Miriam Gitterman (1971) from Memorial Sloan Kettering, Art Boyer (1971) from MDACC, Michael Goitein (1972) from UC Berkeley, Karen Doppke (1973) from U Wisconsin, Ed Epp (April, 1974) as Head Radiation Biophysics Division (20% time until 1975), and Clift Ling (1974) from Memorial Sloan Kettering. Biology staff were Robert Sedlacek and Jan Vaage (1971) from MDACC. Claire Hunt was the new secretary and in effect the general manager. All of the new staff were housed in Temp and were close to the new animal colony and the resulting "bouquet," not appreciated by all.

4.5   Clinical Program

This team was fully confident that we would contribute to advancing the care of cancer patients. We were quite aware that there had been substantial gains in the fight against the infamous crab (Fig. 4.2) and we were to make further and important gains. Here we present an image of the crab under sustained attack from numerous sources. These include the NCI, radiation, genetics, chemicals, and surgery among the many participating in the productive work to reduce progressively the impact of cancer. Our intent was to make several central hits by intense effort by the entire team of clinicians, physicists, biologists, biomathematicians, radiation therapists, nurses, medical records, secretaries, social workers, administration, dieticians, receptionists, and others.

There was a prompt effort to engage fully in the Tumor Clinic and to augment our interactions with the medical oncologists and surgeons.[12] This was an important aid in

---

[11] Several patients at follow-up examination asked HDS if the treatments were free as they had not received a bill. This was corrected as soon as some of the pressing medical care needs had been achieved.

[12] None of the surgeons limited their practice to oncology at that time.

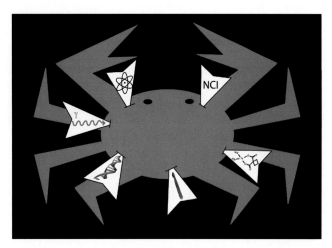

Fig. 4.2. The crab (Cancer) under serious attack by many medical and scientific teams (Wolfgang J. and Suit H.)

the development of multi-disciplinary planning and care of the MGH cancer patients. Milford concentrated on thoracic, breast, and pelvic tumors; CC devoted most of his time to H/N and pelvic tumors; Ann Chu worked primarily on breast and pelvic tumors; Rita Linggood treated the CNS and pediatric patients; Noah Choi specialized on thoracic tumors; and HDS worked predominantly with the mesenchymal tumor patients and managed a spectrum of other tumor categories.

One of the first accomplishments for the White II space was the improvement of the small and unattractive patient waiting area. Almost immediately after his appointment, HDS requested that the patient waiting area be updated with new furnishings, etc. Quite fortunately, almost simultaneously with that request, a well-known patron of the hospital complained in a letter to Dr. Knowles that the waiting area was comparable to that in a train stop in a village in a remote area of Czechoslovakia. With this jolt, there was a prompt response and no further mention that these aspects of patient care could "do" until the move to the Cox.

Concurrent with the swirl of activity to upgrade steeply our technical facility by the physicists and clinicians, several clinical papers were produced. Most notable was the M. Schulz Janeway Lecture of the American Radium Society of 1974 entitled "The Supervoltage Story" [9]. This is discussed in Chapter 2. He was a member of the group that revised the staging system for laryngeal cancer [11]. A technical development was scleral plaques for irradiation of conjunctival lesions [10]. Hatfield and Schulz [7] presented the case histories of five patients who developed radiation sarcoma following radiation treatment for breast carcinoma. Wang and Schulz with Oliver Cope published a paper with their surgical colleagues on the use of limited surgical resection

of breast carcinoma [3]. They also wrote on combined radiation and surgery for carcinoma of the supraglottis [16]. CC developed an applicator for intracavitary irradiation of the nasopharynx [15]. The risk of osteoradionecrosis of the temporal bone was another subject of interest [14].

With W. Russell and R. Martin, Suit completed the analyses of the clinical and pathological characteristics of their series of 100 sarcoma of the soft tissue patients managed by moderate dose radiation and less than radical surgery at MDACC. They reported positive results [12, 13]. These data formed the basis for the staging system of soft tissue sarcomas. That experience was the starting point for the MGH program on limb sparing management of soft tissue sarcoma of the extremities.

4.6　Residency Program, 1970–1974

In 1970 the program of residency in radiation oncology was formalized and expansion begun. In addition to S. Kadish, S. Pittman, and W. Sewall, the residents starting in the 1971–1974 period were Vincent Chang, Arthur Elman, Luiz Fagundes, Bob Heller, Gerry Sokol, Joel Tepper, Gene Kopelson, Stuart Gilbert, and Tim Russell. Fellows included Bruce Walz and Joel Busse. Lecture series on radiation oncology and on physics were initiated. The residents rotated between the clinical staff members, participated in all phases of the patient evaluation, tumor clinic, simulation, treatment, and follow-up examinations. They also were active in Tumor Clinic sessions.

4.7　Special Clinical Initiatives

4.7.1　Lease of Boston University Betatron for Treatment of MGH Patients

There was a clear need to have x-ray beams of energy higher than 2 MV and electron beams of useful energy. HDS learned in 1971 that the betatron at Boston University was utilized lightly and that there was an opportunity to have access to high-energy x-ray and electron beam. He soon made arrangements to commence treating some MGH patients there. This was later formalized (October 1972) in a leasing arrangement for the machine from 1:30–4:30 each afternoon, Monday–Friday. Ann Chu went to BU three afternoons a week and HDS went two afternoons. The betatron was used principally in the treatment of our Gyn, GU, pelvic sarcoma, and a few H/N (for electrons) patients.

4.7.2 Proton Therapy Program for Fractionated Irradiation of Cancer Patients

The planning and developmental work on this program commenced early in 1972 and the first patient was planned and treatment commenced in late December 1973. This program was based on a 4 day/week schedule as a joint effort between the Harvard Cyclotron Laboratory and MGH radiation oncology. Turn to Chapter 6 on Proton Therapy for a detailed discussion of this program.

4.7.3 Radiation Therapy at the Waltham and the Mt. Auburn Hospitals

C.C. Wang attended tumor rounds at the Waltham Hospital and Milford Schulz participated in tumor rounds at the Mt. Auburn Hospital. Soon after his appointment, Noah Choi spent approximately half-time at the Mt. Auburn Hospital supervising the radiation treatment there.

4.8 Clinical Physics

For several years, clinical physics had been provided by Rosemary Whipfelder, a part-time dosimetrist and treatment planner. Thus, in June 1970, clinical physics was exceedingly thin for a patient load of ~90 patients treated/day.

The first full-time dosimetrist-treatment planner in the hospital was Miriam Gitterman, M.Sc. who was recruited from Memorial Sloan Kettering (MSK) by Ted Webster, Ph.D., Head of Physics of the Department of Radiology. She started work on January 1, 1971. Webster was very important in aiding her to commence the long overdue changes in clinical physics. For example all calculations had been done on slide rules. Hand-held calculators were purchased. A perhaps interesting note is that the cost in 1970 dollars was $125 for a unit, the equivalent of one available today in a drugstore for ~$10 (2009 dollars). She made an arrangement with Memorial Sloan Kettering to perform computer dose distribution calculations on information that she sent by a venerable teletype machine. This was a certainly modest but definite start toward modern treatment planning.

A radiation therapy machine shop was established in Temp II in 1971 with Bill Niepert as the head. He and two assistants are pictured in Fig. 4.3. With the later departure of Niepert, Leo Codere became the Head.

Our physics capabilities were dramatically enhanced with the arrival of Art Boyer in September 1971 from MDACC.

Fig. 4.3 The departmental machine shop in Temp II in 1971

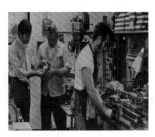

Major gains in space and equipment commenced immediately. These included a much improved ionization chamber, a digital electrometer, and a Farmer chamber, with triax cables. Art assumed responsibility for the operation of the Van de Graaff, the ^{60}Co Theratron junior, and the orthovoltage machine. A large project for Art was the purchase, installation, and commencement of operation of the simulator. The hospital was arranging the purchase of a substantial number of Picker units and we were able to tag a Picker simulator onto that order with virtually no delay. The second room was the clinical physics work area. Art was one of the first (certainly ahead of commercial providers) to design and bring into clinical use, laser systems to align patient position on a daily basis using surface markers [1]. He also supervised the modification of the Fletcher-Suit afterloading applicators to use ^{137}Cs rather than radium sources, shown in Fig. 4.4. These were made in the machine shop of the new department. Boyer and Gitterman started a physics lecture series for the residents.

An extremely important addition to the faculty was Michael Goitein from UC Berkeley in early 1972; see Chapter 6 for description of his contributions. Merriam, Art, and Michael formed a very effective team of three. They arranged the purchase of an Artronix computer system,[13] for treatment planning. This resulted in a huge change in the accuracy and precision of treatment planning and the frequency of treatment planning.

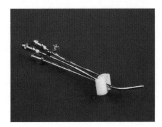

Fig. 4.4 The Fletcher-Suit applicators were modified for afterloading with ^{137}Cs sources. This was organized by A. Boyer

---

[13] The small Artronix PC-12 computer had been designed as a student project by the first computer science class at Washington University in collaboration with the Radiotherapy Department.

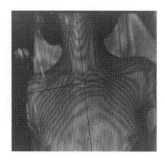

Fig. 4.5 A Moiré camera view of an anterior chest wall

Arthur and Michael developed a Moiré camera system for use in design of compensator systems to correct for patient surface irregularities [2]. Figure 4.5 illustrates the changes in the grid when projected onto an irregular surface and that those changes could be employed to reconstruct the 3D contour of that surface and employ that information in treatment planning.

Michael reported investigations on techniques for flexible beam shaping [4], mathematical modeling of unusual dose fractionation [5], and errors in immobilization [6].

Another most valuable recruit was Karen Doppke, from the U Wisconsin (1973). She accepted a heavy responsibility for treatment planning and dose measurements and, following Merriam's move to New Hampshire in 1986 to be a high school physics teacher, became Head of the Treatment Planning Team and has continued to the present with great effectiveness. She was the co-author of a paper describing a wedge filter interlock system for 4 MV linear accelerators [8].

4.9 Planning the Move to the Cox Building

A major and clearly important responsibility was the design of the space for radiation oncology in the new Cox building and the selection, purchase, and monitoring the construction and installation of the linear accelerators. The physicists and several of the clinicians began planning the radiation therapy space and equipment for the Cox building.

Art and Michael began planning with the clinicians for the equipment to be in the new department in the Cox building. The hospital trustees had decided that the machines were to be manufactured in North America in order to reduce the risk of prolonged down-time in the event of a war, e.g., we had to avoid the risk of a problem in trans-oceanic transportation of parts in the event of another war. This reflected the impact of WWII on certain aspects of hospital function. The departmental and hospital decision was Varian machines: a Clinac 35 with a 25 MV x-ray beam and two Clinac 18s with 6 and 10 MV x-ray beams. Electron beams were available from 6 to

32 MeV. They had several work sessions at Varian facilities in California in testing the linear accelerators prior to shipping. Art designed a scanner to measure beam flatness and symmetry at all gantry angles. This was built in our machine shop and was of great value in commissioning the new linear accelerators.

Art had also raised concern regarding the neutron dose for the high-energy x-ray beams, as they had not been adequately allowed for in planning the shielding for the new machine rooms. Detectors were obtained and the finding was an unacceptable high neutron dose. This problem was corrected by adding borated polyethylene to the inside of the door. Also, Boyer was a very active participant in the commissioning of the new linear accelerators.

On Cox ground floor there were to be rooms for three linear accelerators and two new ^{60}Co units. Additionally, there would be a generous work area for the residents and a separate work area for the physicists and treatment planners. Further, there was to be a nurse's office area, space for a social worker, and a staff lounge. A clearly important space was that for a pleasant and ample patient/family waiting area. The floor plan for Cox ground was presented in the Introduction.

The animal colony and research labs would be on Cox 7 and part of Cox 6. The engineer's work area and the machine shop would be in Cox 4. Office space for the clinical and physics staff and the secretarial teams were to be on Cox 3.

The first project in the actual construction of the Cox building was demolition of the Thayer Building, see Fig. 4.6.

Dr. Edward Epp was appointed as Head of the Division of Radiation Biophysics early in 1974. He commenced work, 20% time, in ~ April 1974 and was here full time as of January 1975. He was heavily involved in all of the activities from April forward. Then, there was the process of conducting performance testing in the factory, installation at the MGH, and then the commissioning of each machine

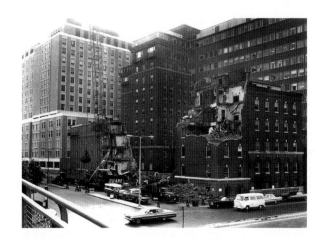

Fig. 4.6 Demolition of the Thayer building

according to an exhaustive and detailed protocol. Epp's role is discussed fully in Chapters 5 and 8 on clinical physics and on biological research, respectively.

4.10 Administrative Support

This was principally performed by Claire Hunt, Executive Secretary for the department. Claire dealt readily with the substantial paper work for each new appointment to the medical, physics, and biology staff in addition to the many more appointments to the various support staff. In addition there were the residents and the entire array of educational efforts that involved Claire to some extent. Additionally, residents, research fellows, and staff at all levels benefited from her TLC.[14] She managed the paper work for equipment purchases (treatment planning computer, simulator, calculators) and modification of Temporary Building II (Temp II) to accommodate the special mouse colony to meet Sedlacek's specifications, and many other items. Claire helped get the proton therapy program going in December 1973 and participated in the preparation of the application to the NCI for support for the clinical evaluation of proton therapy. Further, she assisted in preparation of the application for renewal of the NCI RO 1 of HDS. In addition to these efforts, there were numerous tasks as part of the oversight of the building and equipment for the new department in the Cox building. There was a major shift in scale and style of the departmental operations with the move into the Cox building in 1975.

Claire was a highly important part of the team that managed these: (1) arrange for the lease of the BU betatron; (2) move of Ed Epp and Clift Ling from Memorial Sloan Kettering to the MGH and then immediate recruitment of biologists and physicists; (3) transfer of Rakesh Jain and team from Carnegie Mellon to the MGH; (4) work with Susan Woods in the administrative aspects of the proton therapy program; (5) participation in the quite protracted negations to get the IOEBT (intraoperative electron beam therapy) unit installed in OR 43; (6) communication with the JCRT; (7) interactions with HMS regarding appointments and teaching; (8) arrangements with community hospitals and a vast array of other activities. Each of these diverse responsibilities grew and not slowly.

The departmental staff continued growth as patient numbers increased and new activities initiated. A group photograph of the staff at ~1976 is shown as Fig. 4.7.

A person of central importance in realization of the Cox Cancer Center and much of the MGH radiation oncology

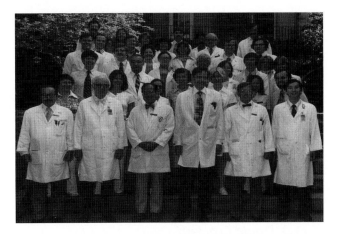

Fig. 4.7 Staff of the department of radiation oncology at ~1976

program was David Crockett. The biographical sketch on Crockett definitely merits a read.

4.11 Biographical Sketches of the Participants, 1970–1974 (Presented in Alphabetical Order)

4.11.1 Art Boyer and His Wife at the Time of Their Move to MGH

In September 1971, Art Boyer and his wife Suzanne (Fig. 4.8) moved from the MDACC to the MGH as the first full-time Ph.D. physicist in radiation oncology. Arthur arrived on this planet in September 1945 in El Paso, TX. For undergraduate studies, he earned the BA in 1966, University of Dallas, and then his Ph.D. in physics in 1971, Rice University. During his graduate studies he was part time in medical physics at MDACC. Art worked very successfully at MGH for 15 years, 1971–1986 as described above.

In 1986, Art returned to the MDACC. There he obtained an NCI RO 1 to develop the software for IMRT. He arranged for Thomas Bortfeld to come from Heidelberg to collaborate on this project who had developed the concept for part of his

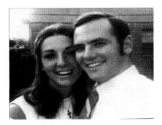

Fig. 4.8 Art and Suzanne Boyer

---

[14] TLC is an abbreviation of Tender Loving Care.

Ph.D. thesis (see Chapter 5). They had a major success and IMRT is now a very commonly used technique for radiation planning and delivery. After just a few years, Boyer moved to Stanford as Professor and Director of their radiation physics program. Wishing to be closer to his homeland, he recently accepted the position as Head of Radiation Physics at Texas A and M Medical School. Arthur has had many awards of distinction. Interestingly, in 2000, Bortfeld was recruited to the MGH as Director of Physics Research and in 2009 as Head of the Radiation Biophysics Division.

4.11.2 David Crockett

David Crockett (Fig. 4.9) was the Director of the Development Office. He was the crucial person in generating the funds for partial support of the department's laboratory research, the Cox building, the seventh floor research laboratory, and the A. Werk Cook and the Andreas Soriano endowed professorships. David proposed the establishment of a Visiting Committee for the department. At that time there were only a few departments with their own Visiting Committees. David was an active member of our committee and attended all of its meetings.

David Crockett was born in Ipswich, MA, in 1909 to a medical family. His father was a Chief of Staff of the MEEI. David attended the Milton Academy and Harvard College, graduating in 1932. Prior to the start of WWII, in 1939, David was made Executive Secretary of the precursor of the Voice of America. During World War II, he had several important assignments behind the enemy lines in military Intelligence in the North Africa and European theatres, see Fig. 4.9. Quite fascinating in his history is that he met Marion in the military intelligence corps and they later married. David in his military uniform is shown in the figure. David and Marion were of Boston Brahmin families and were known among the financially prominent Boston area families. They had the good fortune to have had a wonderful family and a long and happy marriage. They lived in Ipswich, less than a mile from Crane's beach.

In 1946 he was engaged by the MGH to organize the 1951 celebration of the 150th anniversary of the creation

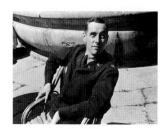

Fig. 4.9 David Crockett

of the MGH in 1811. That event was a clear success and David stayed at the MGH for a long and exceptionally productive career yielding numerous major benefits to the hospital. Crockett was extremely knowledgeable and careful. These characteristics were combined with an excellent and wry sense of humor. He was a master raconteur. Buildings for which his fund raising was extremely important include Edwards, Gray, Jackson, and Cox and a long list of smaller but important projects. David was the person responsible for discussing the need for a cancer building with Jessie Cox. He recalled "I had that famous luncheon which produced the unexpected result. I asked Jessie Cox to come to lunch at the Trustees Room with John Knowles, Howard Ulfelder and myself." David had to leave the luncheon to deal with an unexpected death of a patron of the MGH. Upon his return he continued, "So, Mrs. Cox said to me, as I came back looking rather shattered, you were just about to tell me how I could do this. I said, well I need 9 million dollars and I'm hoping that if you give me 50% of it so that the Trustees will allow us to go forward and raise the balance. Oh, she said I'll give the whole thing." The result was that she paid for the building, i.e., $9 M.

Subsequently, he talked with her sister, Jane Cook, and she funded the laboratory on Cox 7 and had it named the Edwin Steel Laboratory in honor of her first husband. Then she endowed the A. Werk Cook Professorship of Tumor Biology at HMS to be used in our department. This was in honor of her second husband. These two women were the heirs of the Hugh Bancroft fortune (*Wall Street Journal*, Barron's weekly and Dow Jones Industrials). Later, David was the responsible person for arranging the Andres Soriano Professorship in Radiation Oncology at the MGH. This was funded by Jose Soriano, a son of Andreas Soriano, to honor his father, a former MGH patient from the Philippine Islands.

In response to a question about the decision to establish a separate department of Radiation Oncology and to have a Cancer Center he commented, "Well, the most important fellow as I recall was Milford Schulz. Milford had acted in the most diplomatic and farsighted way. He was absolutely splendid." C.C. Wang "was a great fellow. He was always urging me on – in a huge way." Robbins wasn't going to support it with enthusiasm. The proposal to have a Cancer Center and a "full scale radiation therapy department did not have the support of either Churchill or Bauer. Bauer was the Chief of Medicine and Churchill the Chief of Surgery. Bauer's opposition as Chief of Medicine was that he felt and stated publicly that there was no point in spending so much money on equipment to treat cancer because cancer would be solved before the equipment would be built. Churchill opposed the center proposal because he didn't believe in spending money for anything except surgery." "Ben Castleman (Chief of Pathology), Howard Ulfelder (Chief of Gynecology) and Rita Kelly (medical oncologist) were terribly important in this whole thing." "There was really no serious push for the new Cancer Center until Howard Ulfelder got into the act. He got into the act because he had a son who had died of a cancer. That was the motivation behind Howard's tremendous drive. He really did a great job for you – a great fellow. He was Chief of Gynecology and Chief of Vincent Memorial Hospital, a component of the MGH."

Bob Buchanan was very involved in the proton program. That was very important. Buchanan was concerned because of the magnitude and cost of the project and we didn't have the money to build it.

The message was that Radiation Oncology had been well provided to perform the expected developments and achievements.

4.11.3 Karen Doppke

Karen Doppke (Fig. 4.10) decided on physics for her career and entered Dr. Cameron's Radiological Physics program at the University of Wisconsin. There she received a B.Sc. and M.Sc. in physics and in math. She performed extremely well and received an appointment as instructor. One early responsibility was the organization of a laboratory course for training in Radiological Physics. In addition, she conducted research on radiation damage to thermoluminescence material.

Karen moved to Boston in 1973 with her husband who had been appointed as Head of Physics at Brigham and Women's hospital. She was recruited to the MGH staff in 1973.

Karen quite quickly became a very active participant in the Boyer, Goitein, Gitterman, and Biggs team for the installation and commissioning of the three new linear accelerators and two ^{60}Co units in the Cox building. Later, she was involved in interface dosimetry, e.g., solid tissue–air cavity studies, with Epp and Boyer. Another important effort was that with Goitein in getting the 3D treatment-planning system into clinical service. This has matured into the CMS treatment-planning system. Additionally, she did substantial work on treatment planning for individual patients. Karen

has served with great effect as the Director of the treatment-planning unit. Her teaching activities included many lectures in the physics series for residents and fellows plus special teaching of treatment planners, and young staff fresh from their Ph.D. in physics.

She has combined this with work in the ACR, including Radiation Oncology Accreditation for clinical physicists-treatment planners. Karen has been a highly effective and very much respected staff member for 35 years, serving as the mainstay of the treatment-planning unit. In 2007 she was given the "Alumni of the Year" award by her college for undergraduate studies.

4.11.4 Miriam Gitterman

Miriam (Fig. 4.11) graduated from the Philadelphia High School for Girls and then the University of Pennsylvania with a major in physics. She became interested in the potential of medical physics and earned M.Sc. in Radiological Physics from Cornell University Graduate School of Medical Sciences, Sloan Kettering Division.

Miriam was the first full-time physicist in radiation therapy at the MGH, starting work in January 1971. In addition to participating in the start of computer-based treatment planning and developing plans for the Cox building, she played a substantial role in the brachytherapy program. She designed and oversaw the brachytherapy laboratory. In addition, she participated in teaching biologic effects of ionizing radiation to nurses and technologists.

After 17 years in radiation therapy at the MGH, she relocated to southern New Hampshire and taught high school physics and chemistry in public schools and at Phillips Exeter Academy. Currently she consults in the New England area, teaches yoga in her home studio, and sails the coast of Maine with her husband in their 42 ft sail boat.

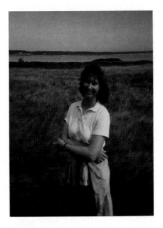

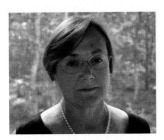

Fig. 4.10 Karen Doppke

Fig. 4.11 Miriam Gitterman

4.11.5 Claire Hunt

Claire (Fig. 4.12) accepted the position of Executive
Secretary in the new department in 1971. Previously she had
worked as a secretary in the laboratory of Michael Young.
She had three Executive Secretary positions offered. She
was, however, particularly keen to learn about and participate
in the oncology program and accepted our offer. For an office
she had space in Temp II adjacent to the office of HDS. Her
office was immediately opposite the entrance to the mouse
colony readily identified by a slight but characteristic odor.

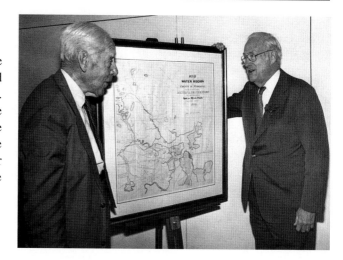

Fig. 4.13 Lawrence E. Martin with David Crockett

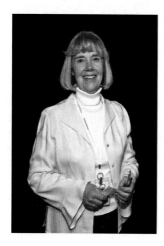

Fig. 4.12 Claire Hunt

Claire dealt readily with the substantial paper work for
each new appointment. She evidenced no difficulty in coping
with a continuously enlarging job description. The various
departmental social functions were organized and managed
by Claire, e.g., the Christmas party, Science Festivity day,
various receptions, and other functions. Also great fun for the
entire department was the summer lobster gala at the south
shore home of Agnes Fiore who hosted the event and was
supported administratively by Claire.

Her work included direct supervision of the expanding
secretarial staff. Claire was extremely effective in performance of the secretarial work not only for HDS but for one
or two additional staff. Claire retired to Marblehead in March
2004 and became intensely and happily involved in the large
and important art world there.

4.11.6 Lawrence E. Martin

Larry Martin (Fig. 4.13) worked in finance at the MGH from
1951 to 1972 and for many yeas served as the CFO and
Associate General Director of MGH. In discussing the decision to have a cancer center and a new and greatly expanded
department of radiation therapy, Larry commented, "I don't

think there was any one event or factor that precipitated
the decision to have a Cancer Center. There was a ground
swell of discussions over a number of years." Key players in
the decision to separate Radiation Medicine from Radiology
and the consolidation of cancer activities in the Cox building were several. Highly important was the push by Howard
Ulfelder, Chief of Gynecology. "Milford Schulz was a prime
mover in getting the hospital to recognize the fact that there
should be a separate department of radiation medicine. As a
matter of fact, he organized a letter campaign. Schulz wrote
letters to the General Executive Committee. Milford was a
very direct individual and very enthusiastic. Sometimes he
was a bit over enthusiastic, but he made his point." "I don't
think Larry Robbins was particularly adverse to the separation of the department and was quite helpful on that."

Martin commented that John Raker, a surgeon, who ran
the hospital Tumor Clinic, was a big pusher for creating a Cancer Center for the MGH. Rita Kelley, a medical
oncologist, helped a great deal to focus on the development
of a cancer center. Ben Castleman, Chief of Pathology, was a
major ally in the effort to get the new Cancer Center. "I don't
recall anyone who was against the development of a cancer
center, even though it took money and space."

"When it came to money, David Crockett was the prime
mover. He along with Jane Claflin convinced Ms. Cox to fund
the building and then Ms. Cook to finance the research laboratories for Radiation Medicine and subsequently endow the
A. Werk Cook Professorship in Tumor Biology."

Larry did not judge that the activities at BU (a new betatron), Tufts (recruitment of F. Bloedorn and obtaining a
betatron), or the JCRT (the new young Sam Hellman as the
Chief of that program) were important factors in the decision
to build the MGH cancer center.

As CFO, Larry Martin was a critical player in our negotiations with the central administration for the continuously

expanding need for staff, space, and equipment. HDS enjoyed working with him and considered him to be genuinely interested in the well-being of our patients.

References

1. Boyer AL. Laser "cross-hair" sidelight. Med Phys. 1978;5(1): 58–60.
2. Boyer AL, Goitein M. Simulator mounted Moiré topography camera for constructing compensating filters. Med Phys. 1980;7(1):19–26.
3. Cope O, Wang CA, Chu A, et al. Limited surgical excision as the basis of a comprehensive therapy for cancer of the breast. Am J Surg. 1976;131(4):400–7.
4. Goitein M. Flexible beam-shaping device. Radiology. 1974;110(3):734–5.
5. Goitein M. The computation of time, dose and fractionation factors for irregular treatment schedules. Br J Radiol. 1974;47(562): 665–9.
6. Goitein M, Busse J. Immobilization error: some theoretical considerations. Radiology. 1975;117(2):407–12.
7. Hatfield PM, Schulz MD. Postirradiation sarcoma. Including 5 cases after x-ray therapy of breast carcinoma. Radiology. 1970;96(3):593–602.
8. Lane RG, Doppke KP. A wedge filter interlock system for 4 MV linear accelerators. Radiology. 1975;116(02):452.
9. Schulz MD. The supervoltage story. Janeway Lecture, 1974. Am J Roentgenol Radium Ther Nucl Med. 1975;124(4):541–59.
10. Schulz M, Weist F, Gemählich M, et al. Radioactive scleral shells in the treatment of conjunctival tumors. Am J Ophthalmol. 1970;70(5):783–6.
11. Smith RR, Caulk R, Frazell E, et al. Revision of the clinical staging system for cancer of the larynx. Cancer. 1973;31:72–80.
12. Suit HD, Russell WO. Radiation therapy of soft tissue sarcomas. Cancer. 1975;36(2):759–64.
13. Suit HD, Russell WO, Martin RG. Sarcoma of soft tissue: clinical and histopathologic parameters and response to treatment. Cancer. 1975;35(5):1478–83.
14. Wang CC, Doppke K. Osteoradionecrosis of the temporal bone – consideration of Nominal Standard Dose. Int J Radiat Oncol Biol Phys. 1976;1(9–10):881–3.
15. Wang CC, Busse J, Gitterman M. A simple afterloading applicator for intracavitary irradiation of carcinoma of the nasopharynx. Radiology. 1975;115(3):737–8.
16. Wang CC, Schulz MD, Miller D. Combined radiation therapy and surgery for carcinoma of the supraglottis and pyriform sinus. Laryngoscope. 1972;82(10):1883–90.

Chapter 5

Photon and Electron Physics at MGH 1975–2008

5.1 General Strategy for the Photon and Electron Physics Program of MGH Radiation Oncology

One certain strategy to increase therapeutic efficacy of radiation therapy is to advance radiation physics and the associated technology including improvements in distribution of radiation dose and radiation safety. This includes an increased accuracy of (1) definition of the target contours in 4D; (2) intra-fraction target position in 4D; (3) planning of radiation dose distribution to the defined target, including Monte Carlo dose calculations where appropriate; (4) delivery of the planned dose; (5) access to the complete array of radiation modalities; (6) maintenance of a detailed record of each patient; (7) rigorous adherence to quality assurance (QA) procedures; and (8) working effectively as members of the oncology team.

5.2 Radiation Biophysics 1974–1997. The Edward Epp Era

5.2.1 Appointment of the First Head of Radiation Biophysics

After an intensive search procedure, a Harvard Search Committee recommended Edward R. Epp (Fig. 5.1) of the Memorial Sloan-Kettering Cancer Center (MSK) for the newly created position of Head of the Radiation Biophysics Division at the MGH and Professor of Radiation Oncology (Biophysics) at HMS. He accepted and began work part time in April 1974 (1 day/week) and then full time on January 1, 1975. Ed continued in this role until retirement in 1997, after 22 years of valuable and productive leadership in physics at the MGH.

Clift Ling came with Ed from MSK to work in medical physics and in the radiation biophysics laboratory. Ed also

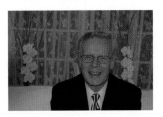

Fig. 5.1 Edward Epp

appointed Peter Biggs, Dale Kubo, and Joe Leong as full-time clinical physicists in this early phase of the division.

Ed was intensively involved in the details of planning the testing of the linear accelerators (linacs) at the Varian factory, installing and commissioning of the three new linear accelerators and two ^{60}Co units at MGH. Then Ed and team commenced and sustained clinical operation of these machines at a very low down-time. While Ed took direct responsibility for the photon section, M. Goitein was given the responsibility for the physics component of the proton program. Michael additionally had the responsibility for the computer group (IT). Peter Biggs had additional responsibility for the engineers and the machine shop. Importantly, Ed directed the education in physics of residents and post-doctoral fellows.

5.3 Installation and Commissioning of the New Equipment for the Cox Center

The departmental plan was to have a comprehensive array of "state-of-the-art" equipment to provide external photon and electron beam therapy and brachytherapy based on the highest technology feasible. The daunting challenge in 1974 was the installation, commissioning, and start of clinical use of the four new treatment machines, viz., three Varian linear accelerators: a Clinic 35 (25 MV x-ray and 6–29 MeV electrons), two Clinac 18s (10 MV x-rays and 4–18 MeV electrons) plus two AECL ^{60}Co units, a Theratron 780 gantry unit, and an Eldorado-78 non-gantry unit (insufficient space for a gantry). None of the machines on White 2 were transferred to the Cox Center.

H.D. Suit, J.S. Loeffler, *Evolution of Radiation Oncology at Massachusetts General Hospital*,
DOI 10.1007/978-1-4419-6744-2_5, © Springer Science+Business Media, LLC 2011

For the acceptance procedures, physicists and engineers tested the linacs at the factory in Palo Alto, CA. Physicists active in this testing program and in the commissioning of the machines after installation at the MGH included Peter Biggs, Art Boyer, Karen Doppke, Michael Goitein, Miriam Gitterman, and Clift Ling. The engineers participating in this project were Robert Johnson, Al Kennedy, and Dennis Mento; they were experienced and had been recruited from the Harvard Cambridge Accelerator Laboratory. The protocol for the commissioning of each of the machines was exceptionally thorough, detailed, and meticulous. This process was especially tense for the physicists due to their own anxiety and those of the clinicians to commence use of these radiation beams and for all of the machines to work as planned. Much work at nights and weekends was required in performing the complex array of measurements on each machine. Quite happily, this complex and labor-intensive process went well and achieved the desired end result.

Table 5.1 lists the major radiation treatment machines in the department from 1970 to present. One linear accelerator and the two ^{60}Co units were brought into clinical operation in 1975. Two additional linear accelerators later went into service, one each in 1976 and 1977. This effort for the x-ray and electron beams was largely completed in 1978. One quite special linear accelerator was the Siemens unit that provides 6–18 MeV electrons for intraoperative electron beam therapy (IOERT). This was installed in the new OR 43 in 1996.

The mean life span of the linear accelerators in our department has been 17 years. This short life span was due to the aging of mechanical components and the manufacturers regularly introducing new technical features, e.g., independent jaws, multiple leaf collimators (needed for IMXT), portal imaging systems, and many more.

As noted in Chapter 4 we began computer-based treatment planning in 1972. This was quite an early system and we regularly upgraded to new systems or to modification of the system in use. The progressive upgrades have been TP 11–34, 1980; ROCS, 1984; an in-house RX system was used for select cases, 1994–1997; CMS, 1997. This system has been upgraded, almost yearly to the present; Corvus, 1999. IMXT is planned on both CMS and CORVUS.

Clinical Advances. Epp et al. determined that prominent air cavities in the sinuses and in the upper respiratory track cause under-dosing on the far side of the cavity in the beam path of a 10 MV x-ray beam, due to loss of electron equilibrium in transiting the cavity [16].

Peter Biggs was heavily involved in the intraoperative electron beam therapy (IOERT) program from the initial planning to the first clinical treatment in 1978 to the present. The clinical start was based on the Clinac 35 on Cox ground floor. Ultimately a total of 342 patients were irradiated in Cox ground floor over a period of 18 years (1978–1996). Peter organized the purchase, installation, and commissioning of

Table 5.1 Time line of MGH treatment machines. This table was prepared by Peter Biggs

Machine name	Room #	Photons (MV)	Electrons (MeV)	Date in	Date out
Van de Graaff	White 2	2	–	1948	1975
Picker 280 kVp	White 2	0.28	–	Uncertain	1977[a]
Cobalt Jr	White 2/Cox LL	1.25	–	1956	1978[b]
Contact Unit	Cox LL	50 kVp	–	1973	2010
Theratron 78	Cox LL	1.25	–	1975	1989[c]
Theratron 780	Cox LL	1.25	–	1975	1996
Clinac 18	Linac 1	10	4–18	1975	1995
Clinac EX	Linac 1	6, 15	6–20	2003	–
Clinac 18	Linac 2	10	4–18	1977	1992[d]
Clinac 2100C	Linac 2	6, 10	6–20	1993	2006[e]
Clinac iX	Linac 2	6, 10	6–20	2006	–
Clinac 35	Linac 3	8, 25	6–29	1976	1989
Siemens KD2	Linac 3	6, 23	6–21	1990	2001[f]
Clinac EX	Linac 3	6, 18	6–20	2001	–
Clinac 4/100	Linac 4	4	–	1984	2002
Clinac 600C	Linac 5	4	–	1990	2007
Clinac iX	Linac 5	6	6–20	2008	–
Clinac 2100C	Linac 6	6, 10	6–20	1996	–
Siemens ME	OR 43	–	6–18	1996	–

[a]Transferred to Cox 7 laboratory for radiation biology research.
[b]Transferred to Cox LL for 1975–1978.
[c]Theratron 780 was moved into this room when the linac 5 was installed.
[d]Installed x-ray tube on this machine; first use of IGRT at MGH.
[e]Cone beam CT.
[f]Electron energies never used.

the new linac (electron beams of 6–18 MeV) for IOERT in OR 43. This entered clinical operation in 1996. He and his team published evidence for low-level production of photon/neutrons in the new IOERT facility that required correction [2, 20]. Biggs and group designed and supervised the fabrication of the cones in our shop and then determined dose distributions for the IOERT cones in 1981 [2, 5, 6].

Figure 7.1 is a photograph of an array of cones that were in use near the start of the program. They similarly prepared the cones for electron intra-oral cone therapy used by C.C. Wang [4].

J. Leong made an important contribution to our field, viz., the first system (1986) for digital processing of high-energy x-ray portal films to be of value in rapidly determining the position of the target in patient treatment and digital fluoroscopy [22, 23]. Rabinowitz and Broomberg, medical students, working with Leong and Goitein in 1985 were among the first to measure the variation in the interfraction target position [27]. Another early contribution of Leong and Shimm in 1987 was a method for assessing target motion during treatment [24].

Kubo and Shipley, in 1982, designed and introduced lead shielding systems for protection of the testes during irradiation of pelvic tumors [21]. In 1986, Biggs and Shipley developed a device for improving beam flatness and width [3].

5.4 Special Units for Which Biggs Had Responsibility

5.4.1 External X-Ray and Electron Beam Treatment Planning

Photon/electron external beam treatment-planning activities have increased steadily over the period 1970–2009 with the increasing number of patients and the rapid growth in technical complexity. These included 3D conformal treatment, IMXT, 4D CT, and 4D IGRT. As treatment plans have regularly become more complex, there is often more than one plan per patient to provide for decreasing treatment volume, viz., boost dose and, recently, dose painting. Further, QA has become progressively more stringent. (See Chapter 4 for discussion of the physics from 1970 to 1975.)

Karen Doppke joined the group in 1973 and has worked with impressive effectiveness as Head of the treatment-planning unit since 1986. She and her team of 9 plan the photon/electron treatment of the ~ 210 patients treated/day. Karen and her group interact closely with clinicians in defining margins of target and organs at risk (OAR), then preparing treatment plans, and working on the QA program. The planning of the proton treatment for the ~ 50 patients under proton treatment is performed by a separate group, managed by Judy Adams, see Chapter 6.

5.4.2 Brachytherapy (BRT) and Radionuclides

In 1970, all BRT was based on radium and that was stored in a safe in the small record room on White 2. Preparation of the radium tubes or needles for clinical use was done under conditions of only modest protection of the physicians and physicists. A constant goal has been to have the lowest practicable exposure dose to all hospital personnel. To this end,

there was a prompt change to afterloading for intracavitary treatment of uterine tumors and replacement of radium with ^{137}Cs due to its much lower photon energy. Later, in 1976, Wang et al. replaced radium by ^{192}Ir for interstitial therapy [33]. ^{125}I was the isotope for the BRT treatment of patients with prostate cancer and for selected other sites. ^{125}I emitted the very easily shielded 27 keV photons and was employed for special patient problems.

T. Mauceri manages the clinical physics of our intracavitary and interstitial program, viz., the isotope laboratories, preparation of the isotopes for each BRT patient, and calculations of dose distributions. The radioisotope laboratory has been quite restless as evident by the high frequency of change in its location. This laboratory was moved to a newly designed and equipped laboratory in Baker basement in 1977. When the Baker building was demolished in 1992 for the construction of the Blake building, the laboratory was transplanted to the basement of the Vincent Burnham building. In 2007, the laboratory moved to the Bulfinch building when the Vincent was to be demolished and the site cleared for the Third Century building. This new lab provides an exceptionally fine work space, even with windows, and all needed modern equipment.

All of our BRT procedures (intracavitary and interstitial) were low dose rate until 1991 when we purchased a Nucletron MicroSelectron Unit for high dose rate and remote control afterloading, featuring one 10.0 Curie ^{192}Ir source for the Gyn procedures. The short half-life of ^{192}Ir requires four "change-outs" of the source per year. Advantages included easily planned special dose distributions, low-energy photons, and minimum feasible exposure to all staff. There is no handling of radioactive sources. This technique has been employed in virtually all Gyn brachytherapy procedures after Tim Russell joined the staff in 2002 as Head of the Gyn unit. In 2006, he obtained a new high dose-rate unit with several advanced features. Most of the interstitial BRT procedures now utilize the high dose-rate unit. In part this is due to the ease of sharply improving dose distribution due to capability of selection of dwell times at each point in the implant.

The total numbers of BRT procedures were 259, 334, and 442 in 1998, 2002, and 2007, respectively. In 2007, of the total, 372 were high dose rate. There were 59 implants as treatment for prostate cancer patients (permanent low dose rate) and 11 low dose-rate applications at other sites.

5.4.3 Engineering

The unit has had three full-time engineers for the photon program. Their effectiveness is evidenced by a very high "up-time," viz., 98% for our linacs. In 1975, the Engineering staff was Bob Johnson and Al Kennedy who had transferred from the high-energy physics lab at Harvard's CEA. Shortly, Dennis Mento joined the group and later became the Head of the unit. Staff during Mento's time included Ken Rice, Wayne Philips, John Glidden, Jamie Urribarri, and Jim Wilson. Tony Hou replaced Dennis Mento as Head of the unit when he had to take disability leave. Tony had a long experience with medical accelerators at the Universities of Michigan and Tufts. Recent recruits to his team are Troy Gayle (from Wentworth Institute) and Jeffrey Sullivan (IBA and FHBPTC); these three are presented in Fig. 5.2a.

The work of these engineers extends beyond maintenance of linear accelerators to the ^{60}Co units, the 50 kVp machine, simulators, the radioisotope laboratory, the radiation machines on Cox 7 (the Steele Laboratory) and CNY (Dr. Held), mechanical service on the Overly doors on Linac 1 and 2 rooms. (Currently this is provided by an outside vendor.) There is a separate engineering team of 10 at the F.H. Burr Proton Center, managed by Steve Bradley (see Chapter 6).

5.4.4 Machine Shop

A machine shop was established in 1971 at the start of the department. This was directed by Bill Niepert (Chapter 4 for photo). Leo Codere succeeded Niepert and continued in that role until he retired in 1985. The shop was transplanted to

Cox 4 in April 1977. Lenny Wasileski was the next Head of the shop and has remained in that position to this date. Our shop is very well equipped and is regularly upgraded. The present equipment includes specialized lathes, milling machines, and a block cutter. Several of the major construction projects are given in the footnote.[1] The shop functions as a source of design and fabrication of new devices/instruments (not commercially available) for patient treatment, physics and biology research programs. Additionally, the shop system is of major value in repair and maintenance of the department's diverse and complex technical and mechanical devices.

The machine shop functions at the HCL were transferred to the new FHBPTC at its opening in the MGH campus. This provided a shop and machinists immediately adjacent to the cyclotron, gantries, and other complex gear. The FHBPTC machinists are a component of the department's shop systems and work under the supervision of Lenny.

Beyond projects for the department, our machine shop has made a variety of items for radiology, anesthesia, engineering, and the Shriners Burn Institute. Staff in August 2008 include L. Wasileski, A. Brown, and D. Yves at the Cox 4 shop and J. MacDonald and Y. Delva at the proton center shop. The Cox 4 team is shown in Fig. 5.2b.

---

[1] Major items built by the machine shop:

a.   Intraoral cone system for linear accelerators.

b.   Intraoperative cone system for linear accelerators.

c.   All brachytherapy applicators (GYN, head and neck, etc.). Built CT guided brachytherapy device for HDS.

d.   Diagnostic x-ray system on the old Linac 2 (Clinac 18) in ~1981– 1982. First use of IGRT.

e.   Harvard cyclotron: x-ray tube holders and attachments for patient support assembly FHBPTC: STAR: rebuilt all parts for new system.

f.   FHBPTC: all parts for retractable floors in gantry 1 and 2.

g.   FHBPTC: Designed and produced all brass aperture and range compensator blanks used for proton therapy.

h.   Beam spoilers, x-ray graticules, side paddles, safety devices, wedges, standard chest tissue compensators.

i.   "Coffee tables" for extra patient shielding for pregnant patients. Also built stand with lead to interpose between linac head and patient for same purpose.

j.   Adapted scissor lift for treatment of heavy (>400 lbs) patients.

k.   Built large number of pieces of equipment for physics research and development on the linear accelerators. Fabricated all the devices used for daily QA by the therapists and monthly/annual QA by the physicists.

l.   Stand-mounted cassette holder for port films.

m.   Applicators for 50 kVp unit, including IORT still devices, still in use as of this month.

n.   Various items for the research programs at Cox 8 and Charlestown labs of Drs. Jain, Held, and Gerweck.

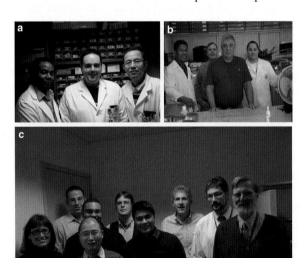

Fig. 5.2 (**a**) Tony Hou (*right*), Troy Grayle (*left*), and Jeffrey Sullivan (*center*) are the engineers for the Cox building radiation equipment. (**b**) D. Yves, A. Brown, L. Waslieski, and M. Aris in the Cox 4 machine shop. (**c**) Greg Moulton, Head of the Computer and Information Technology Unit, and members of his team

5.5 Computer and Technology Unit

This unit evolved in the 1980s. Initially, the computer needs were provided principally by Michael Goitein and Art Boyer. They arranged the purchase of our first computer-based treatment-planning system, Artronix in 1972. Goitein was the principal physicist involved in the progressive upgrading and expanding of our computer equipment and staff and served as director of the IT unit until 1997. He engaged Greg Moulton as Site Manager/Programmer Analyst in 1982, Ken Paiva in 1988 as a programmer for treatment-planning software at MGH, and Andrew Meglis in 1989 for the 3D treatment planning for treatment of eye tumors. Later, Meglis was a participant in bringing IMPAC Record + Verify into regular service. Long-term employees who started in the mid-1990s in addition to Greg are Phil Graceffa and Michael Russell. Shashidhar ("Sashi") Kollipara was a long-term employee but left with Skip Rosenthal to join Ken Gall and the Stillwater Company. Hanne Kooy, Ph.D., joined the Radiation Biophysics Division in 1997 and became Director of IT for the department.

Current IT computer staff as of December 10, 2007, are presented in Fig. 5.2c.

Greg Moulton	Systems Manager and Supervisor
Andrew Kaplan	Systems Manager
Michael Russell	Systems Manager
Philip Graceffa	Senior Project Manager
Daniel Griffin	Senior Systems Analyst
Tom Madden	Senior Programmer Analyst
Jian Pu	Senior Programmer Analyst
Brinda Paramasivam	Programmer Analyst III
Khai Le	Computer Systems Coordinator I
Tim Lehane	Systems Support Special

5.6 Radiation Biophysics 1998–2008. George Chen Era

A Harvard Search Committee performed an international search for the Head of the Biophysics Division. Their unanimous recommendation was that George Chen (Fig. 5.3) from the University of Chicago be invited to succeed E. Epp as the Head of the Division of Radiation Biophysics at the MGH and Professor of Radiation Oncology (Radiation Biophysics) at the Harvard Medical School. Fortunately, he accepted and commenced work at the MGH early in 1999 and continued through 2008.

5.6.1 Major Advances

The major advances in medical physics to be considered are 4D CT imaging, 4D IGRT, IMXT,[2] Iris, and the dural plaque.

5.6.2 4D CT Imaging. First Clinical Use Was at MGH

In 1986, Joe Leong commenced use of on-line digital fluoroscopic imaging to assess movement of the target during delivery of an individual fraction [23]. Bortfeld et al. in 2002 assessed the impact of intra-fraction motion on dose delivery by IMXT [9, 10]. At that time, there was an increasing awareness that the standard CT scanning yielded significant errors in imaging of moving targets, despite the major increase in speed of CT scanning. Jong Kung questioned the ability of even the new and faster helical scanning (tube rotation of 0.5 s) to assess accurately the geometrical shape of tumors that moved during respiration. To quantify the extent of distortions in standard CT imaging, Chen, Kung, and others developed an experimental method to investigate this question. They employed a mechanical stage that provided 1 cm uniform "superior to inferior" motion of a 6 cm ball (a simulated lung tumor), i.e., a total of 2 cm for each respiratory cycle. Thus, at 15 cycles/min the motion of the ball is $\sim$ 2 cm in 4 s or $\sim$5 mm/s, Fig. 5.4a. Chen et al. in 2004 [12, 13] then completed several computer simulation analyses of the scan and motion parameters that would affect the imaging of a moving object. Variables studied included the speed of scanning, number of slices, slice thickness, motion amplitude, etc. The resulting images are well illustrated in Fig. 5.4b by experimental imaging using the system in Fig. 5.4a. The upper row of images are by standard helical scanning and the lower row are images from the 4D scanning technique. These confirmed the predicted major distortion in size and contour of the moving ball using conventional helical CT scanning. Clearly, 4D scanning eliminates nearly all of the distortions. The clinical relevance is convincingly shown by the standard

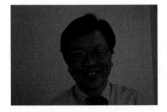

Fig. 5.3 George T.Y.C. Chen

---

[2] IMXT is used in this department to designate intensity-modulated x-ray therapy and IMPT for intensity-modulated proton therapy.

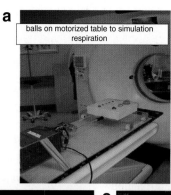

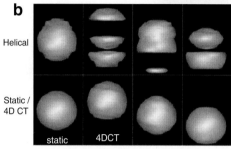
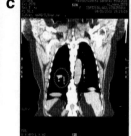
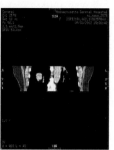

Fig. 5.4 (**a**) Photograph of the experimental set up for CT scanning of a moving 6 cm ball, 10 mm from superior to inferior or 20 mm per complete cycle. (**b**) Comparison of images by standard helical scan and by 4D CT of 6 cm ball that moved over a 1 cm range and 15 respiratory cycles/min to simulate normal respiration. The *upper row* is by standard helical scanning and the *lower* images from 4D scanning. The latter exhibits only very slight distortion. (**c**) Standard and 4D CT images of a lung tumor

and the 4D CT of a tumor in a lung in Fig. 5.4c. These studies have resulted in 4D CT being adopted as standard imaging for mobile targets in this department.

Proof of principle (2003) for 4D CT was established by E.C. Ford at Memorial Sloan Kettering and S.S. Vedam at Medical College of Virginia with helical CT scanning technique. One of the limitations of this early implementation was the long scan time. Then in 2004, G. Chen and E. Rietzel began work with GE and their physicist T. Pan on an evaluation of their prototype 4D CT method utilizing a multi-slice CT scanner [26]. The technique differed from earlier work in that it used a modified cardiac scanning algorithm developed at General Electric Research Laboratories by T. Pan. They completed several theoretical analyses of the potential and the constraints of its clinical use, viz., the speed of taking individual slice(s), interpretation of the data taken over the entire field of interest, the number of passes. Chen and his team began clinical studies with Noah Choi on patients with lung tumors. This 4D CT technique was commissioned and employed in the first ever 4D CT on a patient for treatment planning. This is now our standard imaging technique in patients planned for treatment of mobile lesions at MGH, viz., principally thoracic-pelvic tumors. This is being employed in an increasing number of centers in several countries.

One important detail is the necessity of use of patient-specific characterization of the target motion throughout the

respiratory cycle as demonstrated by Rietzel et al. in 2006 [29]. Another complicating aspect of the move to progressively smaller PTVs considered by Rietzel et al. in 2006 is that the 3D contour frequently becomes distorted, viz., an inconstant shape throughout a respiratory cycle [28]. Additionally, the tumor often shrinks with irradiation. This importance of target motion on image quality continues under investigation.

Evidence of the rapid enhancement of image quality is demonstrated by the work being conducted by the imaging research unit in Radiology at the MGH. This powerfully demonstrated the extremely high resolution of the imaging of the middle ear, Fig. 5.5a. The 4D CT image of the human lung in Fig. 5.5b was produced by 256 thin slice scans at the Cancer Center in Chiba, Japan, and is provided by S. Mori, He was a fellow with G. Chen and team on several high-technology projects. George predicts that we will have imaging at least with as high resolution in the near future.

5.6.3 4D Image Guided Radiation Therapy (4D IGRT)

Chen et al. [13] have been leaders in 4D IGRT. Participants in this program have included T. Bortfeld, M. Engelsman,

Middle Ear Comparison

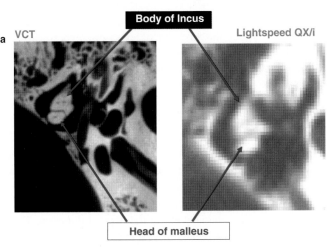

a VCT   Lightspeed QX/i

Body of Incus

Head of malleus

256 Slice Scanner 4D CT

b

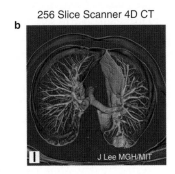

J Lee MGH/MIT

Fig. 5.5 (**a**) Extremely high resolution of the human middle ear taken at the MGH Radiology Imaging Research unit. (**b**) 256 thin slice 4D CT of lung taken at Chiba and provided by S. Mori, a fellow with G. Chen

D. Gierga, H. Kooy, H.-M. Lu, G. Sharp, and J. Wolfgang. An impressive group of very talented post-doctoral fellows have contributed quite importantly to our rapid gains in correcting for target motion during the actual irradiation. This progress by MGH is well documented by extensive publications, viz., [1, 7, 8, 15, 17–19, 25, 30–32].

There has been a long-term concern regarding the large volumes of radiographically normal lung necessarily included in the PTV throughout each respiratory cycle to assure that the target is in the beam for the duration of irradiation of each field of each treatment session. This fact has been the main stimulus in the intense effort to generate clinically useful 4D imaging and 4D dose delivery capabilities. The greatest motion for nearly all pulmonary tumors is in the superior–inferior planes, but for some there is clinically significant motion in the other two planes. There is appreciation of the reality that even after determining the size and configuration of the target in 3D at a point in time and the extent and pattern of movement of the tumor in the superior–inferior, anterior–posterior, and lateral planes throughout the respiratory cycle, there must be correction for distortion of the anatomic shape and size of the target during these motions.

The three most actively studied strategies to maintain the target in the beam throughout each treatment session are: (1) gating of beam-on time to a defined segment of the respiratory cycle; (2) breath hold; and (3) tracking. For each, the patient is made as comfortable as feasible and after a brief period of quiet breathing treatment can start. The points of minimal target motion are at maximum expiration and at maximum inspiration. Limiting beam-on to maximum inspiration is attractive due to a minimal volume of normal lung in the PTV. However, there is much greater variability at that point in the respiratory cycle resulting in higher error frequency and longer treatment sessions. The most commonly employed technique for lung and hepatic lesions is gating, i.e., beam-on is confined to just before, at, and following maximum expiration, viz., a beam-on time of ∼30% of the respiratory cycle. For patients who are able to manage a useful breath-hold time at maximum expiration, use of respiratory gating yields decrement in PTV. The third option is tracking of the target during the complete respiratory cycle. For this, fiducial markers are implanted in the target and the multileaf collimators are adjusted $\sim \leq 0.4$ s during irradiation of each field. This allows correction for motion and changes in contour of the tumor. There has to be determination of the target position at a defined point in the respiratory cycle before the start of each fraction. The patient breathes quietly and the respiration is monitored by RPM or other system. Planning and delivery of irradiation of moving targets is complex and carries increased risk of errors.

Engelsman et al. [15] estimated that gating or breath-holding would permit field margins lateral to the edge of the defined CTV to be reduced by 7–12 mm for maximum range of peak-to-peak target motion of 20–30 mm (10–15 mm Sup-Inf). Were target motion to be ≤ 10 mm, the gain would be marginal at 1–2 mm. The vast majority of patients at quiet respiration, 89%, have a breathing motion of ≤ 10 mm. The clinical gain from the technical effort to achieve a PTV of 1 or even 2 mm is likely to be modest and perhaps not outweigh the required effort and time combined with an increased risk of error. The exception probably would be for tumors near abutment of CTV on a sensitive critical structure and the total dose planned.

4D IGRT is being extended into the proton therapy program, especially with the move into intensity-modulated proton therapy (IMPT). This move is in progress by a large team of physicists and engineers.

An additional direction of improvement is the move to Monte Carlo method for dose calculation of selected patient characteristics. Harold Paganetti is leading this component of the project, see Chapter 6. Each advance in these technologies requires additional time and staff combined with more demanding QA systems. These strategies are under critical evaluation at the MGH.

5.6.4 Intensity-Modulated X-Ray Therapy (IMXT)

This new treatment delivery system is considered in some detail in that it is manifestly of high importance and was developed by T. Bortfeld, currently a member of our faculty since 2000 and Head of the Radiation Biophysics Division starting in January 2009. Bortfeld developed IMXT at Heidelberg and M.D. Anderson Cancer Center with A. Boyer, our first Ph.D. physics staff member.

Thomas Bortfeld's early contribution to the field of radiation oncology was development of the concept of intensity-modulated x-ray therapy (IMXT) and bringing this into clinical practice. This contribution is described in his papers [9, 11]. IMXT allows the radiation oncologist to confine the high radiation dose much more closely to the PTV and thereby reduce risk of injury to non-target tissues for a specified dose to the target. This permits a higher dose to the target and thus a predicted higher probability of tumor control. A concern that is not quantified at present is the clinical impact of the low dose "bath" to the large volumes of normal tissues, a consequence of the use of more fields than for 3D conformal x-ray therapy, viz., $\sim$ 6–10 vs 2–4.

The physics of IMXT is summarized here. Because of the much higher number of degrees of freedom of beam direction in IMXT, treatment planning for IMXT is a mathematical and computational challenge. This requires solution of an optimization problem with about 104 variables and 106 constraints. Bortfeld developed the first fully functional 3D IMXT treatment-planning system around 1990 as a Ph.D. student and post-doctoral fellow (with Professor Wolfgang Schlegel) at the German Cancer Research Center in Heidelberg, Germany.

Bortfeld employed fast "scaled gradient projection" algorithms for the solution of the IMXT treatment-planning problem. This approach has been adopted by many researchers in the field. Today his method is implemented, albeit in modified form, in many commercial IMXT planning systems. Thomas was the first to show that very attractive spatial dose distributions are achievable with a relatively small number (<10) of intensity-modulated beams, i.e., many fewer beams then generally predicted to be necessary. This reduced number of beams made clinical implementation of IMXT on multileaf collimator (MLC) equipped machines practical. In 1992–1993 Bortfeld pioneered IMXT delivery with MLCs while a visiting fellow with Arthur Boyer at the MDACC in Houston.[3] Bortfeld devised a method to translate an IMXT treatment plan into specific MLC positions for each beam,

making the delivery of IMXT readily feasible on the available treatment machines. This method has become a standard reference method, known as the Bortfeld–Boyer technique. They performed the first IMXT phantom experiment on an MLC treatment machine. The phantom was stacked with radiographic film to measure the 3D distribution of dose.

In 1993, on his return to Heidelberg, Bortfeld visited Memorial Hospital in New York and assisted in the installation of his IMXT system. There it was used in 1995, in modified form, to perform the world's first MLC-based intensity-modulated x-ray treatment of a patient. Thomas and his team were the first to recognize the importance of interactive IMXT planning capabilities, viz., the treatment planner to steer the plan interactively in the desired direction. They developed and implemented interactive features in their planning system. Further, this interactivity was combined with a new capability to maintain dose to selected organs at or less than defined levels and the dose distribution throughout specific organs, viz., a dose-volume histogram. This observation led to the integration of dose-volume parameters in IMXT planning. Bortfeld first presented the concept and implementation of interactive dose-volume IMXT planning at the ICCR (International Conference in the use of Computers in Radiotherapy) in 1997, where it was fully embraced. Once again, these concepts have been adopted in all commercial IMXT planning systems today. More recently, Bortfeld has started a collaboration with mathematicians at Fraunhofer in Germany and MIT in Cambridge, where the idea of interactive multi-objective plan optimization is being further developed.

A significant question for IMXT has been the accuracy of planned dose delivery to a moving target. Bortfeld showed that the motion problem is not worse for IMXT than 3D conformal therapy. This team generated estimates of the indications for correction of patient position errors. Bortfeld and team were among the first to generalize the basic concept of IMXT to other treatment modalities, most notably proton therapy. They developed a planning system for intensity modulated proton therapy (IMPT) and demonstrated the potential of IMPT relative to conventional proton therapy and to IMXT.

In October 1999, MGH became the beta test site for Varian's HELIOS system for IMXT. Testing of the system was begun by Hanna Kooy, Piotr Zygmanski, and Jong H. Kung. Then in March 2000, the clinical version of HELIOS was released for general use. Very shortly, in June 2000, MGH treated its first patient using HELIOS IMXT, a sarcoma patient. In 2000, Thomas Bortfeld was recruited to our faculty and was quite active in the clinical implementation of IMXT at MGH. In July 2002, MGH switched to the CORVUS IMXT system in early 2007; we upgraded to CMS IMXT system.

---

[3] Boyer was the first Ph.D. physicist in our department (1971), see Chapter 4.

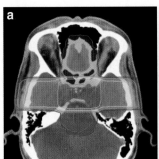
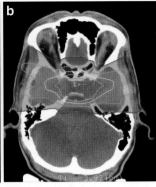

Fig. 5.6 (**a**) 3D conformal vs (**b**) IMXT treatment plans for a patient with a tumor of the pituitary gland

Comparison of 3D conformal and IMXT treatment plans is given in Fig. 5.6a, b for treatment of a patient with a pituitary gland tumor. The dose distribution is clearly delivering lower doses to non-target tissues by the IMXT plan. There is, however, a large volume of normal tissues receiving low doses due to the increased number of fields. This is likely to increase the risk of low dose in very late injury.

IMXT is employed in a steeply increasing fraction of patients treated with intent to cure. Currently, ∼ 30–40% of such patients at the MGH are treated by IMXT methods. Despite the improved conformation of the high dose volume to the defined CTV, there is concern regarding the risk of late injury or secondary radiation cancer in tissues beyond the PTV due to the large number of fields employed. This results in a "bath effect" with a much increased volume of normal tissues receiving a low radiation dose.

5.6.5 Integrated Radiation Therapy Imaging System (IRIS)

As an important step toward providing intra-fractional near fluoroscopic imaging of the target or selected fiducial markers, Barbeco, Jiang, and Sharp developed the IRIS system [1]. This is further developed for tracking special markers [31, 32]. Figure 5.7 is a linear accelerator with diagnostic

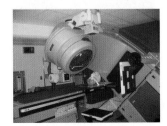

Fig. 5.7 The IRIS on a linear accelerator

x-ray units (80–125 kVp) mounted on each side of the head at 45° to the central axis of the beam. Thus, the system can take bi-planar images at 90°, e.g., there can be orthogonal images simultaneously available to the operators during irradiation of each field. The detectors are flat panel digital units with the image visible in <1 s. This constitutes a major advance over the system employed earlier that required development of a film. Importantly, there is no necessity for the images to be AP and lateral. The treatment-planning program can generate digital reconstructed radiographs (DRR) to show the image that should be seen at the planned angle and thus no time spent in rotation of the machine head.

5.6.6 Stereophotogrammetric Video

Another technical development in which MGH has led, including clinical implementation, is the use of stereophotogrammetric video for patient positioning and monitoring [19]. MGH had been approached by a small company focused on using 3D video technology for patient positioning (VisionRT, London). They were familiar with 2D video-guided patient-positioning studies done at the University of Chicago by Chen et al., and were interested in having MGH evaluate their technology. S. Powell and A. Taghian were beginning to use partial breast irradiation (PBI) with hypofractionation and were keen to assess the new breast-positioning methods. The AlignRT system was installed at MGH and applied to PBI to evaluate its accuracy. Students and fellows involved in this project included R. Berbeco, C. Bert, a graduate student from GSI, Darmstadt, and M. Riboldi, a fellow from Milan. Faculty participating include David Gierga and Hsiao-Ming Lu. The system consists of two camera pods suspended from the ceiling that map the patient's surface very accurately by projecting a pattern and visualizing this with stereo cameras. The system can capture the surface in both single flash and continuous video. Initial experiments established that the inherent accuracy of this system is better than 0.4 mm and 0.5°. The system was then tested against various options to set up breast: lasers, chest wall alignment, or clip alignment (using DIPS[4]/developed at MGH). A critical study was to measure quantitatively the target registration error (TRE) of these various methods of breast set-up. In TRE, the alignment modality under test is compared to "ground truth," which was chosen to be clip-based alignment (clips are registered at treatment time to the reference digitally reconstructed radiographs [DRRs]). Riboldi found that average alignment accuracy from lasers or

---

[4] Digital Imaging for Patient Set-up.

chest wall was ~6–8 mm, with variations as large as 1.4 cm (due to skin elasticity). Statistically there was little difference between the two conventional methods. Surface imaging was found to be accurate to ~3 mm, and clips were "accurate" to 2 mm. Since the clips were ground truth, theoretically its TRE should be zero. The figure of 2 mm was determined to be the practical limit, because after radiographic capture of the clip positions, and digitization by DIPS, it determined a specific move to align the clips perfectly with the reference image. This move was made during patient treatment, but a confirmatory radiograph post move showed that on the average, in a real patient, the moves were good to only ~2 mm.

Riboldi et al. are extending the formalism of TRE to 4D, viz., proposing a methodology that characterizes the ability to irradiate with high accuracy a moving target using a very narrow PTV. In principle, this would advance our development in IGRT by providing a quantitative metric to evaluate and quantify the accuracy of various IGRT schemes.

5.6.7 Dural Plaque Project

Sarcoma abutting the dura present a major problem for radiation therapy, viz., only 0–4 mm from dura to the cord surface, the minimum being tumor abutting dura and pressing dura against the radiation-sensitive spinal cord. In our chordoma/chondrosarcoma patients, the not infrequent story was that tumor had been peeled off dura. The technical problem was delivery of a high boost dose to the dura while respecting cord tolerance. This project has progressed through several phases.

For the first two patients Suit used 20 kVp x-ray beams. By the time of the third patient, T. Mauceri and G. Chen had a β-ray plaque system ready. This had a steeper dose "fall-off," viz., a superior dose distribution. This was developed in conjunction with John Munro of Implant Sciences, a small business that developed, among other devices, radioactive sources for brachytherapy. The first was the use of ^{90}Y in solution. This was not attractive due to a real risk of spillage.

T. Delaney carried this forward to an effective and convenient method [14]. Currently, a plaque is made that matches the involved segment of the dura, based on measurements on the MRI. A non-radioactive sheet of ^{89}Y is bonded to a substrate. This device is then activated in a nuclear reactor to transmute the metal to ^{90}Y, a β-emitter with a maximum energy of 2.3 MeV and a depth dose profile of 100, 52, 28, and 14% at 0, 1, 2, and 3 mm depth. For 2 mm of CSF, the dose on the cord surface is ≤ 3 Gy for a dural dose of 12 Gy and only <0.1 Gy at cord center. The plaque is then applied directly to the exposed dura for a few minutes to deliver a dose of ~12 Gy. There is almost no dose to any of the OR personnel. This is discussed in more detail in Chapter 10 with photographs of an exposed section of the dura after resection of the vertebral body and the plaque applied to the affected segment of the dura. Tom Delaney has obtained a very high local control rate of the sub-clinical disease on the dura with his new technology.

Radiation oncologists from several centers have approached Tom regarding this technique. A potential problem is that the technique is quite specialized and applicable to a rather limited number of patients. The company Implant Sciences has moved to other projects and the availability of the device from a commercial vendor is uncertain in the autumn of 2008.

5.7 Radiation Biophysics. Thomas Bortfeld Era 2010-Present

Thomas Bortfeld (Fig. 5.8) was appointed to succeed George Chen on January 1, 2009. A major goal is to achieve effective integration of the photon and proton components of the clinical physics units. He has initiated a series of changes and the prospects for success are high. Another goal is to provide biological model estimates of the TCP and NTCP to the clinicians for each radical treatment plan with the option of the physician to ask for calculations to be repeated with different values for parameters of concern. This is to be combined with uncertainty bands shown for critical isodose contours. Additionally, there is expected that dose distributions will be computed using Monte Carlo math for complex heterogeneity of densities.

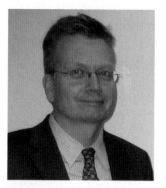

Fig. 5.8 Thomas Bortfeld

5.8 Education Program

This is presented in Chapter 10 on Education.

5.9 Affiliated Hospitals

The physics division is responsible for the clinical physics at BMC, Emerson Hospital, North Shore Cancer Center, and the Newton Wellesley Hospital. The physicists at these hospitals are appointed by the MGH and have appointments in our department and we are responsible for the quality of the clinical physics service. The MGH is responsible for the medical staff at Jordan Hospital radiation oncology department but not for the physics.

Over the past 35 years, our physics unit has, at variable times, had responsibility for radiation physics at Mt. Auburn and Waltham hospitals. This continued until the hospitals were purchased by the Beth Israel-Deaconess (BID) hospital system. Additionally there were periods of involvement in the physics at Cape Cod Hospital and the South Suburban Radiation Center.

5.10 Biographical Sketches (Arranged Alphabetically)

5.10.1 Peter Biggs (Fig. 5.9)

As a London grammar school (our high school) student, Peter concentrated in physics, chemistry, and math and was at or extremely close to the top of his class. His favorite was physics with the "hands-on experiments." He described his student days as being greatly influenced by a spectacularly engaging science teacher. Peter's family was not in science or medicine. His other interest was language and he took classes in French, Latin, Greek, German, and Spanish. He majored in physics at the Imperial College, London, with no little success. He was admitted into the Ph.D. program and received a fellowship for 2 years of experimental work at nuclear physics research center near Frascati, Italy. After completing his thesis, he had a profitable fellowship at the new high-energy physics laboratory at Daresbury, Lancashire. He then accepted an invitation of Sam Ting to join his group, based at MIT. Ting conducted a major experiment at the Brookhaven National Laboratory (BNL). Peter was part of the Ting research team that worked long and hard at BNL. As such Peter was an important participant in the work that discovered the J particle. This was rewarded by a Nobel Prize for Ting. Although he did not receive the big prize, Peter was a co-author on several of the primary articles dealing with that work.

While at BNL, he learned of scientists investigating the biological effects of radiation and the biomathematical modeling of those effects. This stimulated interest in the medical uses of radiation. He spent 1.5 years at the Joint Center for Radiation Therapy (JCRT) learning of clinical radiation physics and then was recruited to the radiation biophysics program at MGH.

For many years Peter has been responsible for clinical photon physics. This has included heavy involvement in the commissioning of the new linear accelerators for the Cox Center 1974–1977, subsequent machine replacements, the Lin Acc installation in OR 43 for IOERT, establishing quality assurance programs, and bringing IMXT into regular clinical use. Further, he has been responsible for several technical units described above.

Presently, he is involved in the design of the new facility in the Third Century that is to house most of the department, see Fig. 1.1 for the architects' drawing of this new building.

5.10.2 George Chen

George Chen (Fig. 5.10) is a first generation American whose parents were from China. He was born and went to high school in a suburb of New York City. A strong influence on George's interest in physics was his high school physics teacher, a graduate of MIT. That physics course included significant laboratory work. For university, George went to MIT and was startled to find that all of the students had been in the top $\geq 10\%$ of their class. For the first time he had to study reasonably hard to perform well relative to this new

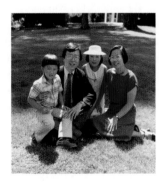

Fig. 5.10 This is a fine photograph of the young George Chen with his family

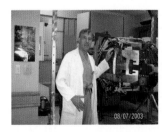

Fig. 5.9 Peter Biggs

class of competitors. This he did and then entered the physics Ph.D. program at Brown University. His thesis work was on high-energy spark chamber phenomena at the Brookhaven laboratory. His impression was that he was a "cog" in a very big wheel which definitely was not his career goal. This provoked a sharp change in plans to a career that provides more personal involvement and also might benefit other humans. He saw a notice in the Brown newspaper from the Harvard School of Public Health regarding an M.Sc. program in medical physics. He signed up to learn in depth this new specialty in physics. This led to work in the Bengt Bjarngard group at the JCRT. He volunteered to work on edge scattering effects of proton irradiation with Michael Goitein, for a 6-month period. Perhaps affected by this exposure to particle beam radiation therapy, he went to Lawrence Berkeley Laboratory of UC Berkeley and worked for 9 years with J. Lyman and C. Tobias in physics and with J. Castro and T. Phillips in radiation oncology.

Subsequently, he was recruited by Ralph Weichselbaum to be the Head of their Physics program at the University of Chicago. There he worked with success in his aim to achieve clinical applicability of co-registration of PET, CT, and MRI images. He arranged collaboration with several physicists on this large project. Chen's new appointees include Thomas Bortfeld, Steven Jiang, Greg Sharp Jong Kung, John Wolfgang, and David Gierga. His principal interest was development of 4D CT and 4D IGRT in collaboration with Thomas Bortfeld and several staff and post-doctoral fellows. The latter include Shinichiro Mori, Eike Rietzel, Christoph Bert, Marco Riboldi, among others.

George has enjoyed success in developing productive collaboration with physicists at the CENSSIS Center at Northeastern University, Boston University, Rensselaer Polytechnic Institute, and other centers in the USA and abroad.

5.10.3 Edward R. Epp

As a young man, Ed (Fig. 5.11) became fascinated with the intellectual challenge of chess. He played regularly and with ever more intensity. His performance regularly advanced. Ed was a regular competitor at regional and then national meets. In 1989 he won the New England Open by beating three National Masters. Then in 1991, Ed was made a National Master by the United Stated Chess Federation. He still carries the title of Expert Class. One evening in the 1980s he invited nine physics and math faculty and fellows from around the medical centers to his home for a competition. He and each of the nine had their own chess board. Ed moved from one board to the next with alacrity. These nine games were spirited with a high level of attention and within a mere few

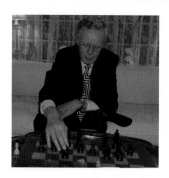

Fig. 5.11 Edward R. Epp

hours, Ed had politely and with no apparent anxiety cleared the deck. His reputation as a worthy chess opponent was clearly established.

Ed was a native of the plains of western Canada. As a youth he became interested in science and this matured into physics. He was a student at the University of Saskatchewan and earned the B.Sc. and the M.Sc. in physics. For the M.Sc. his mentor was Harold Johns, the world's most highly regarded physicist in medicine in the 1960s and 1970s. Johns was the second to install a ^{60}Co unit and one of the earliest to install a betatron. He moved to Toronto and was the Head of Physics at the Ontario Cancer Institute and Princess Margaret Hospital and continued leading many advances. Johns was the author of the famous text on physics for radiation oncology. Thus, Ed had an early exposure to world-class medical physics and this was an important factor in his career path.

Epp next had a year working in the Department of Electrical Engineering at the National Research Council in Ottawa. However, Ed decided that his goal was in physics. For this, he moved to McGill University in Montreal, and received the Ph.D. in nuclear physics in 1955 under John Foster. Due to his experience with ^{60}Co units under H. Johns, he was offered a clinical physics position at the Montreal General Hospital. While there he met and married Shirley, the head nurse on the 14th floor. The next change was his recruitment to Memorial Sloan Kettering Institute as Head of the Division of Physical Biology and Professor of Radiation Biophysics at Cornell University. There his research was primarily in biological effects of radiation at extremely short pulses and high dose rates in an investigation of the mechanism of the oxygen effect on radiation response using cell survival curves of bacterial systems. For further discussion of this research, go to Chapter 7 on Radiation Biology. Ed brought Clift Ling, a nuclear physicist, from Sloan Kettering to MGH to work on clinical physics and on Ed's lab research projects.

Ed was responsible for defining the procedures for testing of the linear accelerators at the Varian factory and the commissioning of the machines at the MGH. These were as rigorous as any applied to clinical machines at any facility. Ed was responsible for the appointment to the photon/electron staff of Peter Biggs, Clift Ling, Joe Leong, and Dale Kubo. He established the engineer group, the radionuclide laboratories, the information technology/computer group, and the much expanded machine shop.

5.10.4 David Gierga

David (Fig. 5.12) decided to major in nuclear engineering as an undergraduate physics student at Rensselaer Polytechnic Institute, in Troy, NY. His studies at MIT in nuclear engineering involved much time on the design of nuclear reactors or atomic weapons. He decided to change direction to medical applications of radiation. His Ph.D. thesis involved the design of a neutron delivery system for a radiation treatment for rheumatoid arthritis.

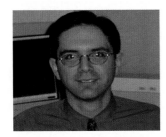

Fig. 5.12 David Gierga

David came to the MGH as a post-doctoral fellow in 2001 to learn clinical physics and conduct research. He was promoted to a staff position in 2003. His principal research effort has been on the 4D treatment-planning project. Additionally, David works on 3D imaging of the surface of the breast. He also is investigating Monte Carlo dose calculations for use in designing radiation shielding and for radioactive plaque design. Additionally, David works on the clinical use of IMXT. Further, his clinical efforts include image-guided therapy, stereotactic radiosurgery, high dose rate brachytherapy, and quality assurance.

5.10.5 Jong Kung

Jong Kung (Fig. 5.13) moved from Seoul Korea to New York City as a 12-year-old lad with his parents. For high school he attended Brooklyn Technical High School and was quite interested in physics and math. This was to some extent because of the interaction he had with the physics teacher. Also, in his high school, there were physics lab studies. For university, he went to New York University as a physics/math major. He made top grades in all physics and math courses

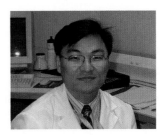

Fig. 5.13 Jong Kung

and graduated Magna Cum Laude. Then he went immediately into graduate school for physics at Brown University. He studied for 5 years and produced several papers on the Inflationary Universe and Cosmic String Theory.

For his post-doctoral fellowship, he went to the Harvard-Smithsonian Astrophysics Institute in Cambridge, 1990–1993. He then decided to become a physics teacher and worked in that capacity at Bates College in Maine to 1995. During this time he learned about careers in medical physics. For this, he entered the M.Sc. program at Columbia university. At this point he was recruited by George Chen to the University of Chicago. There he performed at a very high level for ~ 1.5 years and accepted the invitation to move to the MGH with George in 1998.

Important activities of Jong at the MGH include start of the 4D CT imaging on patients; analysis of dose distributions in IMXT of pulmonary tumors; study of ultrasound imaging for direct imaging during gated treatment; development of the physical basis for the use of Lamour frequency of ^{17}O (non-radioactive) for imaging of hypoxic zones in tumors, and other researches.

5.10.6 Joe Leong

Joe Leong (Fig. 5.14) came from Hong Kong to study physics at MIT. He ranked in the top 30 of 6500 high school students in a city-wide examination. He had been attracted into physics after Sputnik in 1957 and the subsequent space programs in the USA and USSR. He performed

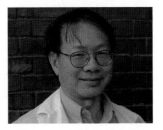

Fig. 5.14 Joe Leong

well and was invited to do his Ph.D. work at MIT. This was a very positive time. For his thesis project much of his work was at Brookhaven National Laboratory working on the search for "Charm" particles. His group did have success. There he met and talked with scientists studying radiation effects on biological systems, and their use of mathematical models. He became interest in medical application and then spent 1.5 years as a fellow at the Joint Center and then accepted an appointment at the MGH. Here his major interests have been improving imaging systems for target positioning before and during each treatment session. On a personal note, his one child is a graduate of Harvard. After spending 2 years as a Fulbright scholar at the Max Planck Institut für Neurobiologie in Germany, he is now in an M.D., Ph.D. program at Stanford with concentration on neuroscience.

5.10.7 T. Mauceri

Tom's (Fig. 5.15) interest in physics comes from an interest in music. He was active in drum music and rock bands from 12 to 30 years of age. From Northeastern University he graduated with a B.Sc. in Physics in 1978 with a determination to learn the physical basis for the design and operation of stereo equipment and loudspeakers. His plan was to go to graduate school to study acoustical engineering.

Plans do change and his did with the invitation combined with a fellowship to study Medical Physics at Boston University for 1 year. He accepted and stayed there for 3 years under Jacob Spira and studied the physics of diagnostic and therapeutic radiology. He was next at Lynn Hospital. He

did graduate study and received the M.Sc. at the University of Lowell in 1987. His thesis was on the effects of the materials used in ionization chamber construction on the measured dose in heterogeneous material.

In September of that year he joined the MGH clinical physics program and was assigned the responsibility for oversight of the brachytherapy program. In the intervening 20 years he has participated in the commissioning of seven linear accelerators (at MGH and at affiliated hospitals) and two HDR remote afterloaders. In addition he designed a facility for total body pig for the surgical transplant unit irradiation and he was the principal designer of new isotope labs. He has also been responsible for developing new brachytherapy programs and techniques for HDR, prostate, endovascular, and dural brachytherapy. In addition, he has been able to pursue clinical research in various areas of medical physics. These have led to several publications.

5.10.8 Greg Sharp

Greg (Fig. 5.16) was born and educated in Racine, WI. His early ambition was to become a creative writer, viz., novels. In addition he was quite attracted to math and science. Greg had an excellent time in high school biology labs, particularly the hands-on aspects. He was admitted to the University of Wisconsin with a scholarship in engineering, and majored in electrical engineering. As part of the course, he spent 1 year in an IBM laboratory, where he developed a writable CD-ROM, and then 1 year as an exchange student in Japan. His time in Japan was quite a happy period. After graduation, he returned to Japan for a 4-year period working for Intergraph Corporation. There he participated in the development of several products that were put on the market, a very satisfying experience. While in Japan, he also married Tomomi. Further he learned the Japanese language. He is still able to read and converse in Japanese.

After the 4 years Greg and Tomomi returned to the USA. Tomomi attended a medical residency and Greg entered graduate school at the University of Michigan in electrical engineering. His thesis title was *Robust and Stable Multi-view 3D Surface Registration.*

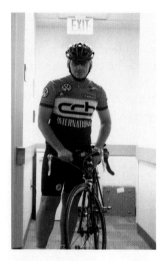

Fig. 5.15 Thomas Mauceri. Thomas is a serious cross country cyclist and has been into competition. Currently, he cycles with groups for intense but fun rides

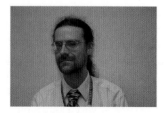

Fig. 5.16 Greg Sharp

Immediately after graduation, Greg came to the MGH on a post-doctoral fellowship to work with S. Jiang and G. Chen on image-guided radiation therapy (IGRT). He made major contributions to the IRIS project, which has been brought into clinical operation. He is now intensively into the 4D IGRT development project. In addition, his current projects include fluoroscopic guidance in patient positioning for photon and proton treatments and deformable image registration.

5.10.9   John Wolfgang

John (Fig. 5.17) comes strong science family, viz., his father is a Ph.D. in electrical engineering (Duke) and had served in a Navy electronics units in WWII and then proceeded to electrical engineering school. Young John was the youngest of four children, having a brother and two sisters. Although born in Indiana, he had his childhood and youth in Arizona. He attended the University of Arizona with a major in physics. John did some work in chemistry but decided on a career in physics and entered East Texas State University located in the relatively small town of Commerce, TX (presently, it is Texas A and M in Commerce, TX). He became strongly motivated by his supervisor for the Masters degree. Their work resulted in several published papers. By this time his interest in physics was "on high" and he moved to the more competitive Rice University for the Ph.D. degree in applied physics. The thesis study was on condensed matter theory; this included nanoscale work. During this time he met the young woman who was to be his wife. For his first 1.5 years post-graduation, he worked for America Online but then responded to a notice of post-doctoral fellowships at MGH and applied for one. He was accepted for a position with T. Bortfeld. There he concentrated on IGRT and the uncertainty secondary to target motion. This proved to be an extremely fruitful experience for John. After a period, he decided that he should become much better informed on straight clinical physics. He then transferred to the group with Peter Biggs, Jong Kung, David Gierga, Karen Doppke, Tom Mauceri, and others. His performance was assessed as being of high quality and he was appointed to the staff in 2002.

John is clearly one very happy man with his wife and a young son, born in 2007. A touching photograph of the baby's hand in the palm of John's hand is included here (Fig. 5.18).

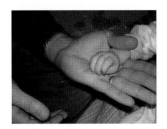

Fig. 5.18 A touching photograph of his son's hand in the palm of John's hand

5.11   Faculty Who Have Moved to Other Institutions

Steve Jiang (2000–2006) Steve joined MGH in September 2000. His research was focused on image-guided radiation therapy. In 2006, Steve moved to the University of California San Diego. Steve's description of his research projects:

1. Real-time tumor tracking. With strong support from George, as well as funding and hardware from Varian, we have built a unique on-board x-ray imaging system, which is called Integrated Radiotherapy Imaging System (IRIS). This system has served as the hardware platform for real-time tumor tracking. In terms of software development, we have developed algorithms for (a) tracking multiple implanted fiducial markers, (b) tracking lung tumor mass without implanted fiducial markers, (c) predicting tumor motion, (d) identifying tracking failure, (e) modeling tumor trajectory, etc.
2. Image-guided respiratory gated radiotherapy. Based on Varian RPM system, we have developed an image-guided gating procedure, including key technologies like 4D CT patient simulation, breath coaching, gating patient set-up, cine mode EPID for treatment verification. This procedure has been implemented at MGH.
3. Tracking tumor motion using dynamic MLC. We have developed algorithms for tracking tumor with dynamic MLC.

I have supervised 6 student internships, 4 post-doctoral fellows and co-supervised 7 Ph.D. students.

Clift Ling. Clift was active in the general clinical physics program, but with special attention to the BRT program using ^{125}I for treatment of prostate cancer patients. Clift left to become Chief of Radiation Physics at Georgetown in 1979, the University California at San Francisco in 1985, and then to Memorial Sloan Kettering in 1989.

Hideo Kubo. Kubo was recruited from Sloan-Kettering Institute. Kubo developed new aspects of absolute dosimetry by special methods in calorimetry. He moved from the MGH to the University of Rochester as the Chief of Physics. From

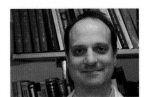

Fig. 5.17   John Wolfgang

there he was recruited to be the Professor and Head of Physics in the Department of Radiation Oncology at the University of California at Irvine.

References

1. Berbeco RI, Jiang SB, Sharp GC, et al. Integrated radiotherapy imaging system (IRIS): design considerations of tumour tracking with linac gantry-mounted diagnostic x-ray systems with flat-panel detectors. Phys Med Biol. 2004;49(2):243–55.

2. Biggs PJ. Evidence for photoneutron production in the lead shielding of a dedicated intra-operative electron only facility. Health Phys. 1998;74(1):96–8.

3. Biggs PJ, Shipley WU. A beam width improving device for a 25 MV X ray beam. Int J Radiat Oncol Biol Phys. 1986;12(1):131–5.

4. Biggs PJ, Wang CC. An intra-oral cone for an 18 MeV linear accelerator. Int J Radiat Oncol Biol Phys. 1982;8(7):1251–6.

5. Biggs PJ, Noyes RD, Willett CG. Clinical physics, applicator choice, technique, and equipment for electron intraoperative radiation therapy. Surg Oncol Clin N Am. 2003;12(4):899–924.

6. Biggs PJ, Epp ER, Ling CC, et al. Dosimetry, field shaping and other considerations for intra-operative electron therapy. Int J Radiat Oncol Biol Phys. 1981;7(7):875–84.

7. Boldea V, Sharp GC, Jiang SB, et al. 4D-CT lung motion estimation with deformable registration: quantification of motion nonlinearity and hysteresis. Med Phys. 2008;35(3):1008–18.

8. Bortfeld T, Boyer AL, Schlegel W, et al. Realization and verification of three-dimensional conformal radiotherapy with modulated fields. Int J Radiat Oncol Biol Phys. 1994;30(4):899–908.

9. Bortfeld T, Jokivarsi K, Goitein M, et al. Effects of intra-fraction motion on IMRT dose delivery: statistical analysis and simulation. Phys Med Biol. 2002;47(13):2203–20.

10. Bortfeld T, van Herk M, Jiang SB. When should systematic patient positioning errors in radiotherapy be corrected? Phys Med Biol. 2002;47(23):N297–302.

11. Bortfeld TR, Kahler DL, Waldron TJ, et al. X-ray field compensation with multileaf collimators. Int J Radiat Oncol Biol Phys. 1994;28(3):723–30.

12. Chen GT, Kung JH, Beaudette KP. Artifacts in computed tomography scanning of moving objects. Semin Radiat Oncol. 2004;14(1):19–26.

13. Chen GT, Kung JH, Rietzel E. Four-dimensional imaging and treatment planning of moving targets. Front Radiat Ther Oncol. 2007;40:59–71.

14. DeLaney TF, Chen GT, Mauceri TC, et al. Intraoperative dural irradiation by customized 192iridium and 90Yttrium brachytherapy plaques. Int J Radiat Oncol Biol Phys. 2003;57(1):239–45.

15. Engelsman M, Sharp GC, Bortfeld T, et al. How much margin reduction is possible through gating or breath hold? Phys Med Biol. 2005;50(3):477–90.

16. Epp ER, Boyer AL, Doppke KP. Underdosing of lesions resulting from lack of electronic equilibrium in upper respiratory air cavities irradiated by 10MV x-ray beams. Int J Radiat Oncol Biol Phys. 1977;2(7–8):613–9.

17. Flampouri S, Jiang SB, Sharp GC, et al. Estimation of the delivered patient dose in lung IMRT treatment based on deformable registration of 4D-CT data and Monte Carlo simulations. Phys Med Biol. 2006;51(11): 2763–79.

18. Gierga DP, Chen GT, Kung JH, et al. Quantification of respiration-induced abdominal tumor motion and its impact on IMRT dose distributions. Int J Radiat Oncol Biol Phys. 2004;58(5):1584–95.

19. Gierga DP, Riboldi M, Turcotte JC, et al. Comparison of target registration errors for multiple image-guided techniques in accelerated partial breast irradiation. Int J Radiat Oncol Biol Phys. 2008;70(4):1239–46.

20. Jaradat AK, Biggs PJ. Measurement of the neutron leakage from a dedicated intraoperative radiation therapy electron linear accelerator and a conventional linear accelerator for 9, 12, 15(16), and 18(20) MeV electron energies. Med Phys. 2008;35(5):1711–7.

21. Kubo H, Shipley WU. Reduction of the scatter dose to the testicle outside the radiation treatment fields. Int J Radiat Oncol Biol Phys. 1982;8(10):1741–5.

22. Leong J. Use of digital fluoroscopy as an on-line verification device in radiation therapy. Phys Med Biol. 1986;31(9):985–92.

23. Leong J. Implementation of random positioning error in computerised radiation treatment planning systems as a result of fractionation. Phys Med Biol. 1987;32(3):327–34.

24. Leong J, Shimm D. A method for consistent precision radiation therapy. Radiother Oncol. 1985;3(1):89–92.

25. Neicu T, Berbeco R, Wolfgang J, et al. Synchronized moving aperture radiation therapy (SMART): improvement of breathing pattern reproducibility using respiratory coaching. Phys Med Biol. 2006;51(3):617–36.

26. Pan T, Lee TY, Rietzel E, et al. 4D-CT imaging of a volume influenced by respiratory motion on multi-slice CT. Med Phys. 2004;31(2):333–40.

27. Rabinowitz I, Broomberg J, Goitein M, et al. Accuracy of radiation field alignment in clinical practice. Int J Radiat Oncol Biol Phys. 1985;11(10):1857–67.

28. Rietzel E, Chen GT. Deformable registration of 4D computed tomography data. Med Phys. 2006;33(11):4423–30.

29. Rietzel E, Liu AK, Doppke KP, et al. Design of 4D treatment planning target volumes. Int J Radiat Oncol Biol Phys. 2006;66(1):287–95.

30. Seco J, Sharp GC, Wu Z, et al. Dosimetric impact of motion in free-breathing and gated lung radiotherapy: a 4D Monte Carlo study of intrafraction and interfraction effects. Med Phys. 2008;35(1):356–66.

31. Sharp GC, Jiang SB, Shimizu S, et al. Prediction of respiratory tumour motion for real-time image-guided radiotherapy. Phys Med Biol. 2004;49(3):425–40.

32. Tang X, Sharp GC, Jiang SB. Fluoroscopic tracking of multiple implanted fiducial markers using multiple object tracking. Phys Med Biol. 2007;52(14):4081–98.

33. Wang CC, Boyer A, Mendiondo O. Afterloading interstitial radiation therapy. Int J Radiat Oncol Biol Phys. 1976;1(3–4):365–8.

Chapter 6

Proton Therapy Program

6.1 Textbook on Proton and Charged Particle Radiotherapy

An important contribution to this discipline is the book *Proton and Charged Particle Radiotherapy* written and edited by Thomas Delaney and Hanne Kooy (2008) (Fig. 6.1) [4]. This book is a comprehensive and current presentation of the history, present status, and probable future of particle beam therapy. DeLaney and Kooy's book is one of the first books in this field and clearly constitutes an important contribution to the understanding of the rationale, details of planning, and delivery of radiation dose by proton beams combined with substantial data on treatment outcomes.

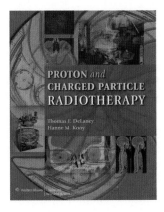

Fig. 6.1 The book on proton and charged particle radiotherapy by T. Delaney and H. Kooy [4]

6.2 Rationale for Proton Radiation Therapy

Protons, neutrons, and electrons are the three clinically studied constituents of an atom. The proton is positively charged and is defined as having a mass of 1 and a positive charge of 1. The actual mass is 1.67×10^{-30} g. Neutrons have no charge and a mass just very slightly greater than that of the proton. Electrons have a mass of $\sim 1/1850$ of the proton but a negative charge of 1. For clinical proton beams, the protons are accelerated by injection of hydrogen ions into a rapidly changing and intense magnetic field.

The entire rationale for use of proton beams in radiation therapy is that for nearly all treatment situations the yield is a superior distribution of the biologically effective dose relative to that by the highest technology photon beam therapy. A superior dose distribution is one that for a specified dose and dose distribution to the target delivers less dose to non-target tissues.

This superior dose distribution is based on the physical fact that protons have a finite range in a defined tissue and that range is determined by the proton energy and the tissue density and atomic composition along the beam path. The consequence is that by proper selection of the distribution of proton energies, a beam can be designed that achieves a uniform dose across the tissue volume of interest (spread-out Bragg peak or SOBP) with near-zero dose deep to the target and a reduced dose proximal to the target. This is illustrated in Fig. 6.2a by the display of the depth dose curve of a high-energy x-ray beam and a clinical proton beam. The tissue depths that receive higher dose by the photon beam to the uninvolved normal tissue deep to and proximal to the target are shown in stippled black. The superficial few mm receive a lower dose by the x ray beam (this region is colored gray). This is the basis for combining protons and x rays in the treatment of certain superficial sites, viz., reduced dose to skin.

In 1946, during his 6 months on the faculty of the Harvard Physics department after World War II, Robert Wilson (Fig. 6.2b) published a powerful and convincing comprehensive rationale for the use of protons and heavier charged particles in clinical radiation therapy [41]. This paper has been seminal for the field of particle beam radiation therapy. He had quite recently returned from World War II duty at Los Alamos on the Manhattan Project. Wilson stated that he needed to make "atonement for involvement in the development of the bomb at Los Alamos," viz., make a contribution from nuclear physics to benefit humanity [40].

These gains by protons relative to photons pertain for every beam path. Proton beams may be applied in as

H.D. Suit, J.S. Loeffler, *Evolution of Radiation Oncology at Massachusetts General Hospital*, DOI 10.1007/978-1-4419-6744-2_6, © Springer Science+Business Media, LLC 2011

Fig. 6.2 (**a**) Depth dose curves for a high-energy x-ray and an energy-modulated proton beam. (**b**) The young Robert Wilson and his bride

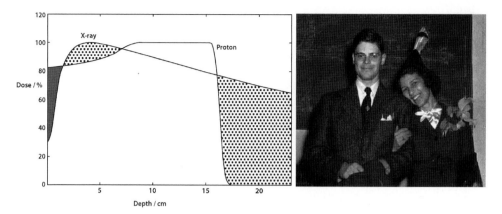

many ways as can x-ray beams, viz., number, direction, co-planar, non-co-planar, intensity modulation, 4D IGRT (four-dimensional image-guided radiation therapy). The result is a lesser dose by proton therapy to tissues not suspected of involvement by tumor for virtually all anatomic sites.[1] This yields an increase in the patient's tolerance. Hence, dose to the target tissues may be increased and result in a higher tumor control probability (TCP), and minimal increase in normal tissue complication probability (NTCP). Where the TCP by the standard of care x-ray treatment acceptable, the target dose would not be changed but the lesser dose to normal tissues would yield a lower NTCP.

For an easy appreciation of the dose sparing by proton therapy examine Fig. 6.3a,b that displays the dose distribution for irradiation of a superior pubic ramus chondrosarcoma by IMXT and proton beams. Similarly, there is a dramatic difference in dose to the thoracic–abdominal–pelvic structures in a patient with medulloblastoma treated by irradiation of the thecal sac by protons in contrast to that by x-rays due simply to the finite range of the proton beam achieving virtually no dose anterior to the vertebral column. This contrasts with the substantial dose exiting the contents of the thorax, abdomen, and pelvis anterior to the vertebral column by x-ray beams.

An important question is, does a higher target dose yield a higher tumor control probability (TCP)? The answer is a clear "yes." That opinion is based on extensive data from dose–response assays of long-term local control of spontaneous cancers studied as early generation transplants in syngenic mice and irradiated uniformly at a defined volume and observed for times sufficient to score virtually all local regrowths. The dose–response curves, logit TCP vs log dose,

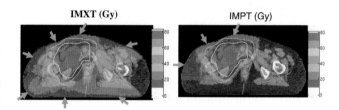

Fig. 6.3 (**a**) Dose distribution for irradiation of a superior pubic ramus chondrosarcoma by IMXT and (**b**) by proton beams

are steep, straight, and independent of fractionation, i.e., any change in dose for a defined fractionated schedule results in a change in response probability. The clear implication is that any change in dose to a tissue results in a change in response probability, either TCP or NTCP. The change might be too small for clinical demonstration, but nonetheless be real.

Widely accepted as a clinical truism with very wide applicability is that the dose to elicit a specified level of normal tissue injury decreases with area/volume irradiated to a specified dose and increases with dose fractionation. This was shown early for human skin [25].

There has been concern by some clinicians that the dose–response curves for human tumors are not steep and that increases in dose will achieve little gain in TCP but will augment NTCP. Such opinions are judged to reflect the considerable heterogeneity among patients included in outcome analyses with respect to tumor volume, dose and dose distribution, the quality and duration of follow-up examinations, and pathological type/grade. Such heterogeneity results in a flattening of the dose–response curve. The slope of the dose–response curve for tumor or normal tissue of an individual patient is almost certainly to be of comparable steepness to that of tissues (tumor or normal) in an inbred animal population and irradiated to a specified volume and dose fractionation schedule. Indeed,

---

[1] For superficial lesions, electron beams provide similar benefits, except that there is a substantially wider penumbra and much less steep decrease in distal fall off.

Terahara et al. in 1999 [35] determined the γ_{50}^2 for chordoma of the skull base to be 3.7 by correcting for dose heterogeneity by use of the equivalent uniform dose for each voxel. This value differs only slightly from that for tissues of inbred animal systems, viz., minimal genetic heterogeneity.

There was and is concern of an increased risk of marginal failures due to the employment of progressively decreasing treatment planning margins (PTV) around the defined target to increase tolerated dose to the target and/or decrease dose to normal tissues. The goal of virtually every technical advance since 1895 has been to decrease treatment volumes. Consider the improvements since 1920 to the present in beam energy, i.e., 140 kVp $\rightarrow$ 250 kVp $\rightarrow$ ^{60}Co gamma rays $\rightarrow$ linear accelerator 4–30 MeV x-ray beams combined with portal films, simulators, computer-based treatment planning systems, CT, MRI, PET, US, MRS, PET-CT,[3] and others. Additionally, 4D image-guided external beam therapy is currently being introduced by George Chen and team [2]. Local control probability has increased progressively over this period. A pertinent fact is that local failures are predominantly central, i.e., within the clinical treatment volume (CTV).

These predicted gains for proton therapy are being investigated by comparative treatment planning studies, biomathematical models, and analysis of clinical results vs dose and specific fractionation protocols. Based on superior dose distributions, proton therapy is likely to replace x-ray therapy for radical dose irradiation of most sites within two decades at most major medical centers [31]. Further, as proton beams are low LET, phase III clinical trials of x-ray vs proton beams are not warranted for those sites that comparative treatment planning demonstrates a superior dose distribution. That is, there is no rationale to use phase III trials to assess the magnitude of the gain from a lesser dose of low LET radiation. Rather our energies, time, and resources should be directed to assessing the most effective dose for specified dose fractionation schedules, proton vs carbon ions, and the dose modification needed for combining proton radiation with chemical and biological agents and surgery, etc. [32].

6.3 Radiobiological Studies

The initial relative biological effectiveness (RBE) studies on the Harvard Cyclotron Laboratory (HCL) proton beam using a ^{60}Co beam at the MGH as the reference radiation began with the experiments by J. Robertson, Harvard School of Public Health, and published in 1975 [27]. He employed the H4 hepatoma cell line with colony formation as the endpoint for cell survival. RBE was essentially constant at 1.00 from the plateau, across the 5 cm SOBP to the mid-point of the distal peak, at 10.5 cm. Just beyond that point, the RBE increased to ~1.4 along the declining edge of that distal peak. The effect was to produce a biological "hot spot" of ~8% for a few millimeters just at and beyond the distal Bragg peak. This increasing RBE along the declining distal edge increased the effective beam penetration by 1–2 mm. Further, the RBE was independent of dose down to 1 Gy. Thus, we had access to RBE values for the HCL beam very early.

Joel Tepper, as a resident, led the team in determining in vivo RBE values of our 160 MeV proton beams, employing jejunal crypt cell survival, acute and late skin reactions at the mid-portion of a 10 cm SOBP [34]. Proton radiation was given in single doses or in 20 fractions, 3 h between fractions (~1.1–1.6 Gy/fraction). The results for jejunal crypt cell survival are presented in Fig. 6.4a. For this series of RBE determinations, the values were in the range of 1.13–1.23. Importantly, RBE was nearly independent of dose per fraction over the range ~1.1–15 Gy.

These experiments were complimented by extensive studies on seven normal tissues and two tumors by M. Urano and his team in our department [38, 39]. The RBE values from these diverse in vivo experiments ranged between 0.73 and 1.33.

For our clinical study, an intermediate value of 1.10 was selected and employed as a generic value, i.e., independent of dose, dose per fraction, and tissue for the plateau and SOBP with recognition that there was a small "hot spot" of $\leq$10% over the few millimeters of the distal most portion of the SOBP.

In 2002, Paganetti et al. reviewed the extant published values from in vivo systems and concluded that the available evidence indicates that the best estimate of the mean RBE is 1.10 [23]. The scattergram of these RBE values is shown in Fig. 6.4b. These results provide no support for the expected increase in RBE with decrease in dose down to ~1 Gy. The RBE value of 1.10 has been adopted by the International Commission of Radiological Units (ICRU). In their Report 78 on prescribing, recording, and reporting proton-beam therapy the recommendation is that the RBE value of 1.10 be used as a generic value [11].

---

[2] The γ_{50} is a measure of the slope of the dose–response curve at the 50% point and is the percent point increment in response probability for a 1% increase in dose.

[3] These abbreviations represent the following: CT for computerized tomography; MRI for magnetic resonance imaging; PET for positive emission tomography; US for ultrasound imaging; MRS for magnetic resonance spectroscopy; and PET-CT for an integrated CT and PET imaging system.

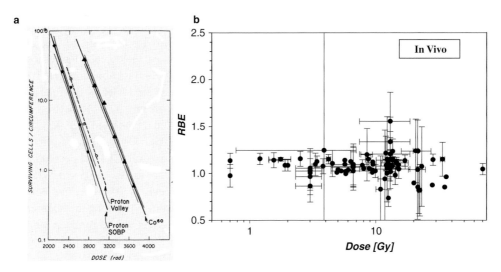

Fig. 6.4 (**a**) Jejunal crypt cell survival for radiation administered in 20 equal fractions by spread-out Bragg peak 160 MeV proton beams vs ^{60}Co beams [34]. (**b**) The published proton RBE values for in vivo systems are presented in this figure. The mean value is 1.1 [23]

6.4 Commencement of the MGH-HCL Proton Therapy Program

6.4.1 The Harvard Cyclotron Laboratory

The first Harvard cyclotron was built in 1937 and generated a beam of 12 MeV protons. Professors K. Bainbridge and K. Street were the physicists involved in building this unit. A Nobel Prize was awarded to E. Purcell for his research on this cyclotron: "The Focusing of Charged Particles by a Spherical Condenser." When needed by the Manhattan project in WW II young Robert Wilson was sent to make arrangements for the transfer of the cyclotron to the government in 1943. The sale price was $1. The agreement was that after the war, the cyclotron would be returned or replaced. This is described in *"Brief History of the Harvard University Cyclotrons, 2004"* by Richard Wilson [40].

After the war, K. Bainbridge was again the lead person in obtaining approval for a new physics building and a new and a much more powerful cyclotron. The new cyclotron was funded principally by the Office of Naval Research. Those participating in the planning and construction of the new machine during 1945–1949 included K. Bainbridge, J.C. Street, E. Purcell, Robert Wilson, and R. Wickman.

Considering this clear rationale from straightforward physics, the potential positive impact of proton treatments on the probability of success rate was not difficult to appreciate. Importantly, time moves forward with zero pause and that the potential of this new beam needs assessing and to be made available widely.

The first beam from the new Harvard cyclotron was in June 1949 and was ~90 MeV. There was an obvious need

for higher energy to conduct the planned physics experiments. Definitive work on the redesign was completed in April 1956 and produced a 160 MeV beam. The machine was massive by hospital standards then or now; see Fig. 6.5. The proton therapy program was conducted in the Harvard Cyclotron Laboratory. This was modified to provide examining rooms, patient waiting area, office space, and sizeable machine shop.

This proton beam was employed for an array of experiments and the treatment of 9116 patients over the 41 years of its clinical use: proton stereotactic radiosurgery from 1961 to 2002 and fractionated irradiation of malignant and benign lesions from 1973 to 2002 (Janet Sisterson. Personal Communication, 2006). The HCL physics team responsible for the HCL operation and continued improvements were A. Koehler, W. Preston, Richard Wilson, Bernard Gottschalk, Janet Sisterson, Kris Johnson, Miles Wagner, plus many others. Andreas Koehler, Richard Wilson, Bernie Gottschalk,

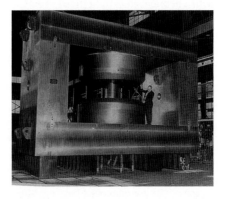

Fig. 6.5 The Harvard cyclotron being installed. The scale of the machine is appreciated by its size relative to one of the physicists

Fig. 6.6 (**a–e**) Photographs of
Andy Koehler, Richard Wilson,
William Preston, Bernie
Gottschalk, and Janet Sisterson

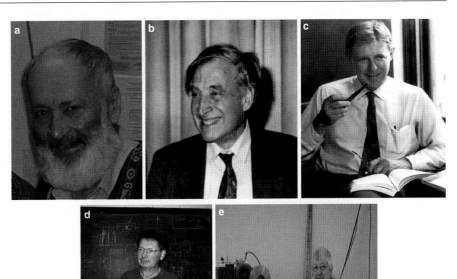

and Janet Sisterson are shown in Fig. 6.6a–e. The Harvard cyclotron was closed in 2002 [40].

Proton radiation biology was initiated in 1952 at the E O Lawrence Berkeley Laboratory by Tobias et al. using the laboratory rat [36, 37]. In 1957 and 1958, Lawrence et al. reported on the initial University of California Berkeley experience in proton irradiation of the pituitary to suppress hormone production in patients with breast tumors [16, 17]. Protons were next used in radiation therapy by the group at the Uppsala, Sweden, in 1957, reported by Falkmer et al. in 1962 [5]. The third center was the MGH-HCL program that opened in 1961 by neurosurgeons Kjellberg and Sweet [13]. For each center, treatment was almost entirely single fraction and in several patients a few fractions.

6.4.2 The Initial Efforts to Implement Proton Therapy in Our Department

Suit's account of the start of the department's proton program is given here. Starting June 1970, my job description essentially was to develop the department, including a physics and radiation biology program. There was no mention of proton therapy. However, I was seriously interested in the potential of proton therapy and visited the Harvard Cyclotron Laboratory (HCL) and had discussions with Andy Koehler, Bill Preston, and Dick Wilson. I was warmly received and informed that a program of 4 treatment days per week for fractionated therapy would be welcome. There was serious interest in proton therapy with curative intent for cancer

patients. They judged that Kjellberg's stereotactic radio-surgery (single fraction) treatments could be readily accommodated on a 1 day per week schedule. The medical annex to the HCL had been built from funds provided by a NASA grant to W. Sweet, Chief of Neurosurgery, for proton treatment of neurosurgical patients. He had also obtained a NASA research grant for the start of clinical studies.

This highly positive situation was a clear signal to commence working toward prompt implementation of a proton therapy program. I had been unaware that several letters had been sent to Dean Ford urging that the cyclotron be closed by December 31, 1967, and the space used by physics. Indeed, there had been a party at the HCL in December 1967 to celebrate the many successes of the cyclotron over nearly 20 years of operation and to salute the next users.[4] The closure obviously did not occur as MGH increased its contributions to the HCL. The HCL was evidently keen to provide time for the fractionated dose proton treatment program and thus increase utilization and income.

Harvard Medical School wished to establish guidelines for the study of proton therapy of cancer patients. A meeting was convened at the HCL in 1971[5] to assess the roles of the MGH and the Joint Center for Radiation Therapy (JCRT) in the Harvard proton program. Those in attendance included (1) J. Adelstein, Dean of Faculty Affairs, at the Harvard Medical

---

[4] A Koehler. Personal Communication Nov 16, 2007, by phone.

[5] No records of the meeting have been located. The listed attendees are according to my recollection.

School; (2) Dick Wilson and A. Koehler, the Harvard Physics Department; (3) S. Hellman, Chair of the JCRT; and (4) H. Suit, MGH. The conclusion was that (1) the JCRT group would concentrate on high technology photon therapy and (2) the MGH team, in collaboration with the HCL team, would be responsible for an assessment of clinical efficacy of proton beam therapy. This arrangement continued until the closure of the HCL in 2002. The JCRT group has enjoyed many important successes in advancing photon therapy.

Michael Goitein was recruited in December 1971 and started work in early 1972. He initially wished to learn the basics of radiation therapy and worked with the photon physicists. Michael did have a large and relevant knowledge base from his many years of work in nuclear physics. After several months, he became actively involved in the proton effort while continuing to contribute importantly to the photon program. In the late spring of 1972, he organized a 1 day "mini-symposium" at the MGH on the feasibility and rationale for radical dose proton therapy by conventional dose fractionation on the Harvard Cyclotron Laboratory (HCL). Namely, the clinical plan would be one variable, viz., dose distribution. This was attended by several nuclear physicists from Harvard, MIT, Ken Robinson of the CEA,[6] and a senior physicist from Princeton Particle Accelerator Laboratory, in addition to the MGH staff. This provided the forum for a highly useful exchange of information and thoughts re technical requirements and medical rationale for the clinical use of protons. To no surprise, the recommendation was that we move energetically to develop a beam line for large fields, dosimetric systems, and various pieces of equipment needed for patient positioning, etc. In parallel, there was agreement that radiobiological evaluation of the HCL proton beam should commence.

Quite importantly, Koehler and Preston had designed, tested, and described in July 1972 a relatively straightforward system for generating a flat dose across the volume of interest, the spread-out Bragg peak (SOBP) [14].

6.5 Clinical Experience of Proton Therapy 1973–2008

6.5.1 Policy of Proton Therapy Program 1973–2008

The policy of the program has been to accept patients for proton treatment for whom an important increase in dose to target was judged feasible and, hence, a predicted increase in TCP. Additionally, for several sites proton therapy has been employed primarily to deliver lesser dose to normal tissue, viz., no change in TCP but a reduction in NTCP.

The basic strategy for this evaluation of the superior dose distribution of proton beams in radiation therapy was as follows:

(1) Obtain NCI funding for clinical study and development of proton therapy
(2) Change only one variable, viz., dose distribution of low LET radiation
(3) Employ standard dose fractionation, except for uveal melanoma
(4) Develop computer-based treatment planning systems for proton therapy
(5) Concentrate resources on curable patients
(6) Generate long-term follow-up data to assess TCP and NTCP
(7) Develop closely interacting physician–physicist teams
(8) Be intensively involved in multi-disciplinary clinics
(9) Conduct clinical trials, viz., dose escalation

6.6 Initial Treatment of MGH Cancer Patients by Fractionated Proton Therapy

J. Knowles, General Director of the MGH, provided funds for the treatment of the initial several patients, with the proviso that we apply to the NCI to fund this clinical study. This was no problem as we were already at work on an application to the NCI.

Late in 1973, the new beam line was ready and we began to select our first patients. Treatment at the HCL was constrained by three major factors: (1) the energy of 160 MeV, i.e., a range in water of 159 mm; (2) fixed horizontal beam, i.e., no gantry and no feasibility of one; and (3) the several miles distance from the MGH campus. Many patients were treated in the lateral decubitis, the sitting or the standing position and a small proportion were in the supine position for lateral fields. Due to the intent to utilize the minimum achievable PTV,[7] the policy was that prior to irradiation of each field on each day, a bi-planar set of radiographs were obtained to check target position, viz., alignment according to the position of anatomic fiducial points, viz., physician inserted gold seeds or well-defined anatomical marks. The patient support system was moved as indicated and the filming repeated. This procedure was iterated until the planned alignment of beam on the target was achieved.

---

[6] Cambridge Electron Accelerator. Robinson made preliminary plans for using the CEA for patient treatments.

[7] The PTV is the planning treatment volume or the volume to receive the planned dose; this is larger than the CTV to ensure that all of the CTV, in fact, receives the intended dose despite patient movement and setup errors.

The world's first patient treated by protons using low dose per fraction is shown in the treatment position (Fig. 6.7a). This patient was a 4-year-old boy with a posterior pelvic rhabdomyosarcoma and no detected metastatic tumor. The aim was to deliver a much reduced dose to the pelvic contents, viz., GI structures. This patient did not require anesthesia. Treatment was started in December 1973. Treatment was by combined posterior 42 MV x-ray (low skin doses and near uniform dose across the target) and 160 MeV proton beams. In addition he received chemotherapy. His treatment was well tolerated as predicted. Michael Goitein, H. Suit, and Joel Tepper are reviewing the treatment setup portal films in Fig. 6.7b. The primary lesion regressed completely and there were minimal GI symptoms. He later developed metastatic disease and succumbed.

The second patient was a 31-year-old woman with a locally recurrent chondrosarcoma of the left petrous ridge at 2 years post-partial resection. The CT scanner was bulky and could not examine as far down as the skull base. Treatment planning was based on detailed analysis of standard radiographs and tomographic series. She was also treated by a combination of 42 MV x-rays and 160 MeV protons in the seated position. This patient is alive but with a local recurrence. The third patient was a 54-year-old man status post simple excision of a 10 × 5 cm Grade II myxoid liposarcoma sarcoma of his posterior thigh. Post-treatment, this patient committed suicide as he became convinced that pain in the treatment volume meant that the sarcoma was recurring, despite being informed that examinations indicated no evident tumor, but cause of pain undetermined.[8]

When the proton treatments were restarted in 1975, technology had advanced such that CT imaging was available for most body sites. The large-field fractionated dose treatments were performed in the same room as was the stereotactic radiosurgery until the second room for the large-field treatments became available in 1977.

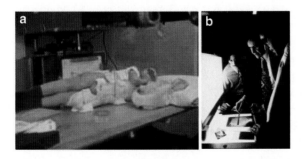

Fig. 6.7 (**a**) The world's first patient treated by low dose per fraction proton therapy. (**b**) Review of the position confirmation films by M. Goitein, H. Suit, and J. Tepper

---

[8] A distinct possibility is that the pain was secondary to injury to the sciatic nerve by the radiation and surgery.

6.7 New Concepts and Method for Treatment Planning

Michael Goitein displayed a high level of ingenuity and originality in creating these systems: first, computer-based treatment planning system used clinically; design proton beams that allow for density heterogeneity along the beams path; beams eye view; dose volume histogram; and calculation of dose uncertainty [6–9]. This is a formidable record of creativity and industry and all directed to improve care of patients. These methods are employed worldwide for treatment planning for photon and proton beam therapy. These developments by Goitein made a valuable contribution to medical physics that has had a clearly positive impact on the care of many patients.

6.8 NCI Funding of Our Study of Proton Beam Radiation Therapy

Substantial time and effort were directed to writing our first application for NCI support for the clinical evaluation of proton treatment and physics developmental work. This was funded in 1976 for 3 years. This support by the NCI has continued through to the present. The grant changed from an RO 1 to a PO 1 in 1979. M. Goitein served as co-principal investigator of these P 01 grants. J. Loeffler became the PI in 1996 and T. DeLaney in 2005. Without this NCI support, our program to assess the clinical efficacy of proton therapy could not have been performed. The current PO-1 is a collaborative effort with the proton group at MD Anderson Cancer Center. Throughout this period of 37 years, the effective and sustained support of the MGH staff in our department, colleagues in other departments, and the administration has been critical to any successes we have enjoyed.

6.9 Clinical Treatment of Cancer Patients by Proton Beams

A critical feature of our treatment methodology from the first patient to the present has been to assess target position by biplanar diagnostic quality films or other imaging techniques prior to treatment of each field on each day with adjustment of patient position until the target is correctly positioned. This does increase the time per dose fraction. The gain has been employment of quite narrow PTVs. Target alignment for mobile structures currently employs 4D imaging.

Patients in the early phase of the program had skull base and spine sarcomas (chondrosarcoma and chordoma), uveal melanoma, paranasal carcinoma, prostate cancer, and

Table 6.1 Local control results by proton radiation therapy

Tumor	No. patients	Dose Gy (RBE)	Dose/fraction Gy(RBE)	Local control	Reference
Chordoma of skull base	115	69	1.8	59 at 5 years	[35]
Chondrosarcoma of skull base	200	72	~1.9	95% at 15 years	[28]
Chordoma of sacrum	9	74	~1.9	8/9 at 5 years	DeLaney 2010, unpublished
Uveal melanoma	2069	70	14	95% at 15 years	[10]
H/N adenocystic carcinoma	23	76	~1.6	93% at 3 years	[26]
Prostate carcinoma	96 T3-4	76	1.9	92% local control	[30]
Prostate carcinoma	196	79	1.8	80% bNED at 5 years	[43]

sarcomas at various body sites. Outcome results are presented in Table 6.1. There has been intense interest in the potential efficacy of proton beam radiation therapy for pediatric subjects. The first patient and the final patient treated at the HCL in our program were pediatric, 1973 and 2002, respectively. Treatment of such patients was quite difficult due to complexities of performing anesthesia on a daily basis at a site so distant from the MGH. As a consequence, quite small numbers of pediatric patients requiring general anesthesia were treated at the HCL. At our new proton center there has been a very large expansion of the pediatric practice. There is excellent co-operation with anesthesia and we have a nurse to care for the pediatric patients. Currently the number of pediatric patients treated per day is ~12 with ~5 requiring anesthesia.

6.10 Development of the Francis H. Burr Proton Therapy Center (FHBPTC)

By the early 1980s, the clear need of our program for a proton therapy center on the MGH campus was obvious to all participants. Suit had multiple interactions with Dr. J.R. Buchanan, the MGH General Director,[9] regarding the anticipated gains for MGH patients were there a proton facility on the MGH campus. These interactions included discussing the rationale of proton therapy, results achieved, developments in progress, potential gains in outcome for MGH patients, publications, status of the hospital, grants to be obtained, as well as potential of NCI support for a new center. Buchanan consistently asked intelligent questions, expressed significant interest, and did describe the difficulties for the MGH to proceed with the program due to the projected cost.

In 1985, Goitein and I submitted a proposal to Buchanan for a timeline that would yield a proton medical facility in approximately 6 years, rather optimistic as we now know. Buchanan gave permission for Goitein and Suit to meet with L. Lederman, Director of the Fermi Laboratory, re a synchrotron for the MGH. We were offered a Fermi machine with an I year option. Then on September 20, 1988, J.R. Buchanan traveled with us to Bethesda, MD, to meet NCI officials. The senior NCI official was Bruce Chabner (later the Clinical Director of the MGH Cancer Center). Also present were J. Antoine, S. Link, and F. Mahoney. Their position was that NCI was committed to an additional 3 years of support for the fast neutron program. However, we were entirely free to submit an application to the NCI for support of the new proton center.

The MGH endorsed our proposal to apply to the NCI for funds for a proton center in January 1987. This included a commitment by the trustees to provide space on which it could be built. To cover other options, arrangements were made for Suit to meet with the President and VP of Shawmut National Ventures, Corp. They appeared to be interested and suggested a synchrotron and one gantry and three treatment bays. However, as I recall, they had only $3 M as a starter with expectation of getting additional investors. This was not judged by the hospital to be of serious potential or interest and was dropped. M. Goitein was the PI of the MGH grant application to the NCI for partial support of the construction of center planned to investigate the efficacy of proton radiation therapy. The finalist applicants were UCSF and MGH. Each group traveled to Bethesda for the 1 day reverse "Site Visit." We each had one half day for presentation. To our great and good fortune, the MGH was awarded the grant. The total NCI contribution to the construction and equipment of the new proton therapy center was $26.1 M and the MGH provided ~$20 M plus the land in the MGH campus. Clearly, this was a critical contribution. NCI funding was obtained effective September 1993.

---

[9] The title for that position was changed later to president of the hospital.

Goitein organized a comprehensive set of oversight and critical review committees to advise on vendor selection separately for the machine and the building and then for monitoring the progress of these two activities. MGH staff intensively participating in the review committees were as follows:

Director	M. Goitein
Co-director	A. Smith
Equipment	J. Flanz
Building	S. Durlacher
Hospital planning	J. Messervey
Grant management	S. Woods, A. Levine

Physician participants in several of the committee meetings included J. Munzenrider, M. Austen-Seymour, and H. Suit. There were a total of 44 outside experts. Ten of these comprised the principal review committee. These numbers do not include the MGH or HCL physicists. In addition there were representatives from the NCI at most of these meetings. Bill Turchinetz of MIT chaired almost all of the review committee meetings. There were 18 formal meetings with groups of 2–10 over the time from July 1993 to July 2001. Four responses were received from our request for proposals for a proton accelerator system that would meet our specifications. The most demanding of input from outside expertise was the review of the specifications for the desired machine (including the gantries) and evaluation of the responses of the individual vendors. Two were dismissed due to extremely high cost. The remaining two were reviewed by the committees by scoring for each specification. Both were very close to our listed specifications. Ion Beam Applications (IBA) in Belgium was the choice, largely on the basis of a more favorable price. The contract for the building was awarded to Bechtel Corp.

Despite this quite intensive effort by high-level experts to define the specifications, monitor the entire process from preliminary and final design, testing in the factory, and commissioning at MGH (the gantries, beam lines, and patient support systems), substantial delays were encountered in getting the facility into operational form with acceptable down-times. This is evident by the time from signing of the contract to start of commissioning and then to the first treatment, viz., September 1993 to November 2001. Recognition must be given to the fact that ours was IBA's first high-energy cyclotron and the control and QA requirements were stringent.

After the selection of the vendor, an oversight committee was appointed by the hospital composed of H. Suit (Chair), Hooks Burr (representing the trustees), R. Wilson (HCL), E. Gragoudas (MEEI), and N. Zervas (neurosurgery).

Funding for the center began in September 1993 and in short order construction of the machine and building

commenced in April 1994 and October 1995, respectively. The first beam testing of the cyclotron in Belgium was in October 1996. The cyclotron was shipped in April 1997 and the first gantry in November 1997. At the MGH, beam was tested in gantry 1 in April 1998 and the first double-scattered beam in June 1998. The first beam through gantry 2 was in September 1999. Commissioning was not quick and simple for this quite complex system, as reflected by the fact that the first treatment was not until November 6, 2001. Complete transfer of patient treatment from the HCL to the MGH was 6 months later. Figure 6.8 is a photograph of the exterior of the MGH proton therapy center at its opening in 2001. Note the Bragg peak painted on the wall of the foyer as seen through the window on the left. The proton therapy center was named the Francis H. Burr Proton Therapy Center in honor of Hooks Burr a very long term friend of the MGH who had served on the Board of Directors for many years and was a major participant in the development of the MGH proton therapy program, including serving on the Visiting Committee of the department.

This facility is complex and provides space on the treatment level for the technical components of the system, i.e., three treatment bays, the cyclotron, beam lines, and a machine shop. Also on the treatment level is the reception and waiting areas, examination rooms, anesthesia rooms, and office areas for nursing, social workers, and dieticians. The first floor provides physician and physicist offices, treatment planning, and two conference rooms. The area in gross ft^2 for each of the two levels is 16,500 and 27,500 ft^2 for a total of 44,000 ft^2. Suit and Loeffler made the decision to reinforce the building for potential further expansion. The \$500 K investment allowed for the construction of the 10 story Yawkey building above the FBPTC.

The floor plan for the two levels of the proton center are presented in Fig. 6.9.

Views of the magnets being assembled at the factory, the installed cyclotron, the magnet systems for the beam emerging from the machine, and the long beam line from which the beam may be deflected into gantry room 1 or 2 or sent straight ahead into one of the two rooms for fixed horizontal beam work: (1) a setup for treatment of lesions of the eye and

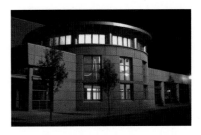

Fig. 6.8 The exterior of the MGH proton therapy center at its opening in April 2001

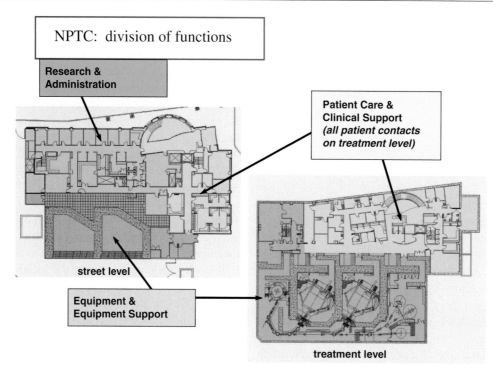

Fig. 6.9 Floor plans for the two levels of the FHBPTC

Fig. 6.10 (**a**) The magnets and
the cyclotron being positioned in
the MGH proton center. (**b**) The
long beam line that extends past
the two gantry rooms and into the
area of the fixed horizontal
beams. (**c**) The structural support
elements for one of the gantries.
Photograph by N. Osterweil.
Permission given for its use, 2008

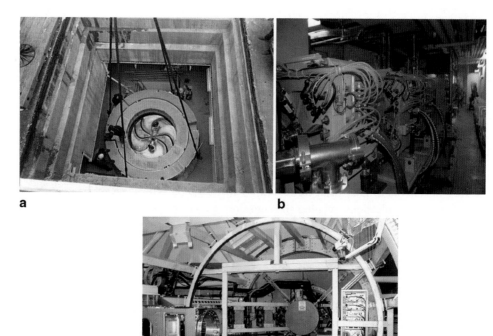

Fig. 6.11 (**a**) The 110 t gantry with the imaging system and patient support system. (**b**) A brass collimator for a proton beam used in the treatment of a patient. (**c**) A. Lucite compensator filter to achieve the desired penetration of each voxel for one of the fields used in treatment of an individual patient

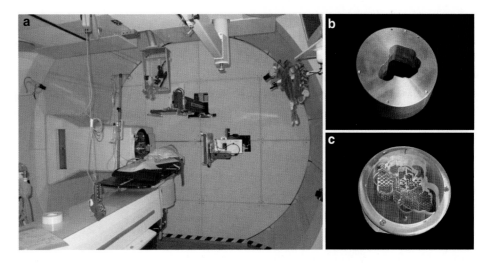

a separate unit for stereotactic radiosurgery and (2) for experimental studies (Fig. 6.10a–c). On the long beam line there are 39 magnet systems and 16 magnets in the secondary lines to the nozzle of each of the two gantries.

A gantry, the imaging system, and the patient support system are illustrated in Fig. 6.11a. Each gantry weighs 110 t. The patient support assembly can be moved in any of three axes in 0.1 mm increments and rotate about its long and short axis in 0.01° movements. Impressively, by the computer control of the gantry and patient support system, the gantry has a net error in rotation around a point in space of <0.5 mm. The patient support systems were designed by General Atomics in California and the cyclotron and gantries were manufactured by Ion Beam Application together with Cockerill Industries in Belgium.[10]

For each field, a beam collimator and a complex compensator example shown in Fig. 6.11b, c are prepared.

6.11 PET/CT Assessment of Dose Delivered to a Patient

T. Bortfeld has led an evaluation of the gain in treatment planning and in position verification by a commercial PET/CT scanner (positron emission tomography and computed tomography) [24]. Nine patients with tumors of the cranial base, spine, orbit, and eye were treated to 1.8–3 and 10 Gy (RBE) (for an ocular melanoma) per fraction. These doses were delivered in one or two fields. The scanning was started within 20 min following the start of treatment. "Measured PET/CT images were co-registered to the planning CT and compared with the corresponding PET expectation, obtained from CT-based Monte Carlo calculations

complemented by functional information." Excellent results were obtained for head/neck patients, viz., accurate range definition to within 1–2 mm. Substantial additional work is needed for application to additional sites.

6.12 Start of Operations of Proton Therapy at the Francis H. Burr Proton Therapy Center (FHBPTC) at the MGH

Birthing of the proton beams was not simple or straight forward as evident in the fact that although the first beams through gantry 1 and gantry 2 were in April 1998 and September 1999, respectively, the first patient treatment was not until 2001. Delays in commissioning and getting each of the components into good operational status included the following: (1) low extraction efficiency; (2) control of the nozzle components (especially software); (3) control systems for motion of the gantries; (4) lengthy process for validation and verification of safety features; and (5) a detailed QA program defined.

The first patient at the MGH facility was treated in 2001 for a meningioma by J. Loeffler.

There has been a gradual increase in the number of patients treated per day and reached 65 in February 2008 and has been stable since. There is sustained effort to increase the hours of operation to accommodate a larger number of patients. The major limitation in increasing the number of patients is the serious shortage of radiation therapists. The intent is to operate on a 14- to 16-h day as soon as feasible. There has been and is a significant shortage of radiation therapists.

The number of patients treated by the MGH team is 8935 as of February 2010. Of these 4564 were treated at HCL and 4371 at the FHBPTC (Delaney T and Kobayashi W, unpublished data). The total for the world is ~66,000.

[10] These specifications were provided by Jay Flanz and Steve Bradley.

6.13 Near-Term Goals for the FHBPTC

These include implementing IMPT and participating in an increasing number of clinical trials for protons therapy, viz., dose level, fraction number, inter-fraction interval, combinations with surgery, chemotherapy, and/or biological agents. Monte Carlo methods are expected to become standard for dose calculations, especially in patients with bone, air cavities, and/or hardware in the beam paths. An additional plan is to imbed biological models into the treatment planning system to predict response probability for TCP and NTCP. Special efforts are made to obtain follow-up examination or status reports on patients for ≥ 20 years post-treatment.

Recently, clinical studies have been started on low-grade glioma, hepatocellular carcinoma, early stage non-small cell carcinoma of the lung, retroperitoneal tumors, breast carcinoma, and additional sites in the head/neck region. Pediatric radiation oncology is expanding at a rapid rate with ~10 children treated/day and ~5 of these requiring anesthesia for each fraction. Follow-up studies of our patients continue and are planned to go to ≥ 20–30 years in assessing late normal tissue injury frequency and severity. Additionally, we expect to participate in trials of proton vs ^{12}C ion beam therapy. These trials should feature only one variable, viz., LET. That is, time between fractions and total number of fractions should be the same for the proton and ^{12}C treatments. The rationale for the trials is to determine if there is a benefit of the high-LET of ^{12}C beams and if found then quantitate that benefit.

The proton therapy center is a part of the 10 story Yawkey building. The entrance to the present facility after the addition of the Yawkey building is shown in Fig. 6.12.

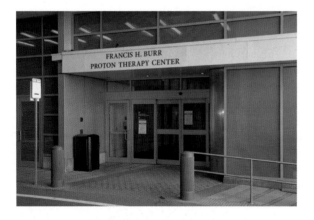

Fig. 6.12 The entrance into the Francis H. Burr Proton Center. The new 10 story Yawkey building was constructed over the FHBPTC. The Yawkey houses most of the MGH oncology program

6.14 MGH Results of Proton Therapy of Cancer Patients

Local control results in patients treated by protons ± x-rays for the chordoma and chondrosarcoma of the skull base, uveal melanoma, head/neck adenocystic carcinoma, and prostate carcinoma are given in Table 6.1.

These results are clearly impressive and constitute support for continued investigation of the efficacy of proton beam therapy. Clearly, there is need to examine future data for late morbidity frequency. A major emphasis in proton therapy has been and is the pediatric patients [15, 33, 42]. The pediatric patient numbers are at a high level as mentioned earlier. Proton beams have been employed in stereotactic radio-surgery for intracranial lesions [1, 18, 19]. These studies have been accompanied by a series of reports on radiation dose-related injury and these have been judged to be low [3, 12, 22, 29]. Further, with time, treatment planning has improved and dose to non-target tissues progressively decreased.

6.15 Management of the Proton Therapy Program

During the operation of the program at the HCL, A. Koehler managed the technical side of the treatment program. From 1997 to 2005 and from 2005 to the present, the clinical component has been managed by Jay Loeffler and by T. DeLaney, respectively. Clinical and the research physics segments of the programs have been directed by H. Kooy and T. Bortfeld from 2001 to the present. The technical aspects of the program at the MGH have been managed by J. Flanz from 1993 to the present. The PIs of the NCI grant supporting this program have been Suit, Loeffler, and DeLaney.

6.16 Proton Therapy Cooperative Oncology Group or PTCOG

By the mid-1980s, the MGH proton therapy program was a part of a small but growing group interested in proton therapy. Suit and Goitein decided that there was sufficient interest in proton therapy to warrant creation of a professional society to facilitate information exchange on the rapidly expanding knowledge base in this field, viz., clinical, physics, engineering, and biological. A meeting was called for all interested persons on September 18, 1985, at the MEEI (we could not get a meeting room on the MGH campus on short notice). The minutes list 17 participants plus some observers.

After discussion of the diverse problems, there was agreement that a society should be formed. The name was to be Proton Therapy Cooperative Oncology Group (PTCOG). Our plan was for this to be informal and that any interested person could become a member by simply asking to be a member. The first meeting with scientific and technical presentations was convened in St. Louis, MO, on October 24, 1985. The officers were H. Suit, Chair, and M. Goitein, secretary. The St Louis Meeting had some 40 attendees. There have been two or three meetings per year from 1985 through 2007, for a total of 45. The first 10 were held in North America and since 1989 they have been held alternately between North America and Europe, Asia and S Africa. Starting in 2007, there was to be only one meeting per year due to the substantial coverage of particle beam therapy in the annual scientific programs of ASTRO, ESTRO, JASTRO, and other organizations. As evidence of the growth of the scope of PTCOG program and interest of its members and the number of ^{12}C ion therapy facilities, the current President of PTCOG is Dr. Tsujii, Director of the ^{12}C ion program at Chiba, Japan. That is, the society has evolved into a Particle Therapy Co-Operative Oncology Group.

From February 1988 to July 2005, Janet Sisterson (MGH physicist) published 36 issues of PARTICLES, a PTCOG newsletter. In these she provided information on scientific presentations at PTCOG meetings, updates on existing and planned new facilities, general news items, etc. Martin Jermann is the present the editor of Particles.

6.17 Other Proton Radiation Therapy Facilities

6.17.1 First Hospital-Based Proton Therapy Facility

In 1986, Loma Linda Medical Center signed for a 250 MeV synchrotron from Fermi laboratory. Theirs was the first hospital-based proton therapy facility. Goitein and Suit talked with Jim Slater, the Director of the LLU program, at several PTCOG meetings. We made strong emphasis on the advantages of gantries in achievement of the best alignment of the beam on the target due to positioning of the patient in the most stable position, viz., supine and the use of all beam angles. This keenness for gantries was quite simple: the entire advantage of proton beams is that of a lesser dose to uninvolved normal tissues and, hence, every feasible effort should be made to place the beam accurately on the target. That is, the accuracy should be at least as good as the best in photon therapy and to plan for other than gantry-equipped facility was clearly not optimal. The final design of their center included three gantries and we judge that our discussions were non-negligible factors in the upgrade

of their plan to gantries. This had the effect of setting the standard for subsequent proton medical facilities.

6.17.2 Paul Scherrer Institute (PSI)

PSI was the first center to employ pencil beam scanning to achieve intensity-modulated proton therapy (IMPT) in 1999. This was accomplished under the physics direction of Tony Lomax and the clinical Chief, Gudrun Goitein. At present, ~30% of their patients are treated by IMPT techniques [20, 21]. The MGH has a large and intense team working to have IMPT available for our patients within the year. E. Hug, a graduate of our residency program, has had staff positions at MGH, Loma Linda, then chief at Dartmouth and currently is Chief at PSI.

There are some 30 active proton therapy centers worldwide and 8 in the USA with an impressive additional number in the planning stage. Further there are now some four active ^{12}C ion therapy centers and more planned (PTCOG web page, January 2010).

6.18 Biographical Sketches of Proton Therapy Staff

Brief biographical sketches of several of the team are alphabetically given.

6.18.1 Tom DeLaney

Tom is the Director of the MGH proton therapy program. He has a high-pressure life at the MGH, viz., in addition to responsibility for the proton therapy program (patient care, administration, and working to secure NCI funding); he heads the MGH Radiation Oncology component of the multi-disciplinary sarcoma center. The biographical sketch of DeLaney is in Chapter 10.

6.18.2 Judith Adams

Judy (Fig. 6.13) has served with great effect as the Head of the proton treatment planning team for 19 years. Her interest in radiology was a positive response to the excellent staff of the School of Radiological Sciences in Durban, South Africa, affiliated with Addington Hospital on the South Beach in Durban, a handsome location on the beach front. Admission to the school was highly competitive, viz., 30 of the 120 applicants selected. She specialized in radiation oncology.

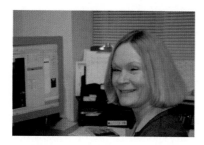

Fig. 6.13 Judith Adams, Head of the Proton Planning Group (1990–present)

After a few years she moved to Miami and then to Boulder, CO, as she was keen to have snow in the winter. There she co-chaired the annual meeting for the American Association of Dosimetrists in 1990. One task as co-chair was to invite Michael Goitein to discuss his paper on "Uncertainties in Radiation Therapy." He accepted. Judy impressed him as highly competent. Not long after the conference she accepted the invitation to join the proton program. Now, she is in her 19th year at the MGH.

Judy's assessment of her time here is quite positive. She states, "I took to the proton project quickly and also to Michael's treatment planning program. I discovered I had the ability to see things in 3D. Treatment planning is part art and part science and I found that I could look at a target's geometry and come up with unique ways to tackle the problem and get the dose where it was needed. This was very challenging. I was awed by what we could do with the proton beam and the great benefits we could afford our patients."

6.18.3 Thomas Bortfeld

Thomas (Fig. 6.14) grew up in Hannover, northern Germany. His father is a geophysicist and trained mathematician. This powerful role model in his immediate family was combined with the good fortune to have talented physics and math

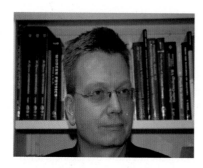

Fig. 6.14 Thomas Bortfeld, Director of Physics Research (2001–2008) and Head of the Biophysics Division (2009–present)

teachers in high school as important factors in his decision on a career in physics. As was standard requirement following high school, he spent 1 year in the German army, not in a science-related unit. He described the period as serving as a "useless truck driver" in a combat division. He entered university and studied at several universities, with a major in physics, with concentrations in geophysics and philosophy. He then moved to the University of Heidelberg and was awarded the equivalent of a Master of Science ("Diplom") degree in physics in 1988. At that point he decided to concentrate exclusively on medical physics. This resulted in his Ph.D. in Medical Radiation Physics at the German Cancer Research Center (DKFZ). His mentor was Wolfgang Schlegel. The time at the DKFZ affected his career positively in multiple ways. Very importantly, there he met his future wife. Thomas' Ph.D. thesis was on developments in intensity-modulated radiation therapy (IMRT), which was just a theoretical concept at that time (1988–1990). He showed that it is useful to formulate the inverse treatment planning problem in IMRT as an optimization problem, that it can be solved efficiently with "gradient" methods, and that in most cases less than 10 treatment beams suffice in IMRT. These developments and findings had critical impact on the clinical implementation of IMRT with commercial systems in later years and very wide adoption in clinical radiation oncology.

After developing IMRT treatment planning and optimization, he was eager to move on and to actually deliver IMRT. In 1992, Thomas accepted an invitation by Art Boyer[11] to work with him in radiation physics at the MD Anderson Cancer Center in Houston, Texas. There they implemented IMRT using a motor-driven multileaf collimator and treated phantoms with IMRT. In 1993, on his return to Heidelberg, he stopped in New York and presented this technology to the physicists at the Memorial Sloan Kettering Cancer Center. This visit led in short order to the first clinical IMRT treatment with a multileaf collimator in 1995 being delivered at Memorial Hospital.

Back in Heidelberg he completed the work on his habilitation thesis, then a requirement to become a professor in Germany. By this point Thomas had his own team and they succeeded in the implementation of IMRT clinically. This was followed by sustained and valuable refinement of IMRT treatment planning. These efforts had advanced the technique close to the physical limit for photon therapy. He judged in late 1990 that it was time to investigate an entirely different radiation beam, viz., protons. This reasoning coincided with a meeting with Michael Goitein, who had asked informally if he would be interested in a position at the MGH proton

---

[11] Art Boyer was our first Ph.D. physicist; he started in September 1971.

center. In 2000, George Chen formally invited Thomas to accept the position as director of physics research at the MGH. To our great good luck, he accepted.

During his 8 years with the physics program at MGH, Thomas has contributed importantly to several high interest projects. In the field of proton therapy, his overall goal is to make certain that the physical advantage of protons is fully translated into a clinical benefit for the patients. A particular aim is to determine with defined uncertainty the position of the end of range of the proton beam in the patient. To this end, he and the physics team are developing "4D" methods for proton treatment planning to address motion issues and to measure the dose delivered in vivo in the patient with PET/CT scanning immediately after the treatment. These efforts are components of the strategy for generation and delivery of "optimized" treatment plans. Specifically, he intends to develop and implement multi-objective optimization methods, as well as robust optimization strategies. These are to feature Pareto plots of how the risk of injury vs dose to a specific normal tissue varies with changes in the acceptable dose to other normal tissues of concern, i.e., a 3D display of the interplay of the change in risk to each of several tissues/structures of concern as dose to one is altered.

The research proposals by Thomas have been viewed quite favorably by the NCI in that both of these projects are funded through NIH by R01 grants. His clear plan is to continue the research along these lines and to create a teaching program in medical physics within the HST (Health Sciences and Technology) program at Harvard and MIT.

On January 1, 2009, Thomas was appointed Director of the Radiation Biophysics Section. One of his goals is to integrate the complex array of physicists working in the various divisions and pursue progressive each segment of the role of physics in our department of radiation oncology.

6.18.4 Steve Bradley

Steve (Fig. 6.15) manages the engineer group of the FHBPTC and is more than fully occupied in the daily operation of the cyclotron and related gear plus the continuous upgrading, especially the effort to implement IMPT.

6.18.5 George Chen

George Chen is the Head of the Division of Radiation Biophysics (1999–2008). A biographical sketch of George is given in Chapter 5. The direct operation of the physics component of the proton therapy program had been by Michael Goitein from 1972 to 2002. Since then Thomas Bortfeld and Hanne Kooy have had that responsibility under the general supervision of George Chen.

6.18.6 Jay Flanz

Jay (Fig. 6.16) is the Technical Director of the FHBPTC. He played an important role in the review process for selection of the cyclotron and gantries for the FHBPTC and then installing and bringing them into clinical service. He was actively involved in the application to the FDA. This involved several meetings with IBA and FDA. Following this, he spearheaded the validation and verification process at MGH.

Jay did his undergraduate studies at Rensellaer Polytechnic Institute including work at the RPI LINAC, as a National Science Foundation Fellow and his graduate work in nuclear physics at University of Massachusetts. He was very active in the design, fabrication, and commissioning of a system for measuring electrons scattered through 180° and performed the first experiment on that facility.

In 1979, as an MIT postdoc he worked at the Bates Accelerator Center in the design and construction of a Beam Recirculation Facility achieving almost double the 400 MeV energy from that electron linac. He was involved in preparing proposals for increases in the beam energy and duty factor at Bates. Later, Jay became project physicist responsible for the beam physics design and commissioning of the storage and high duty factor pulse stretcher ring.

Jay has serious interest in education, viz., supervised a number of high school students and worked with high school teachers. He conceived of and helped organize the first United States Particle Accelerator School (USPAS) course on beam measurement. This was the first course providing

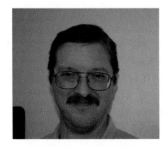

Fig. 6.15 Steve Bradley

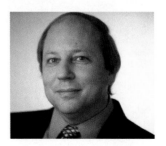

Fig. 6.16 Jay Flanz, Technical Director of the FHBPTC (1993–present)

"hands-on" experience in beam tuning and measurement of beam properties. He has given this course at several laboratories including FHBPTC. Recently he has taught the new USPAS course Medical Applications of Accelerators and Beams several times.

Jay joined the MGH during the proposal stages for the FHBPTC, viz., special contributions to the technical specifications required for vendor selection. He was responsible for the system integration of the accelerator and clinical systems. He contributed toward optimization of the proton equipment for clinical uses and played a leading role in the initial commissioning of the entire proton therapy system and in subsequent upgrades. He was central to the successful FDA 510(k) application. He has formed collaborations with MIT in areas of robotics and software to benefit the FHBPTC.

Presently he is continuing work at facility improvements, including the development of intensity-modulated proton beam delivery.

6.18.7 Michael Goitein

Michael Goitein (Fig. 6.17) has a record as a remarkably creative and productive physicist during his 30 years at MGH. He is considered by many to be the most innovative and creative medical physicist of our time.

Even as a boy, Michael was not intimidated by oversized tasks. This is evident in the above photograph of Michael at 4 years of age (Fig. 6.18). Michael started life in Broadway, a small village in the English Cotswolds, in 1939, close to Oxford. His education was physics and math all the way: 1 year in mathematics at the Sorbonne; B.A., Oxford; and Ph.D., Harvard. At Harvard, Richard Wilson was his mentor. After a 1-year post-doctoral fellowship, he moved to the University of California, Berkeley, where he was a staff physicist in the Moyer-Helmholtz group. Initially he worked

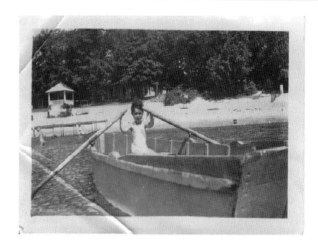

Fig. 6.18 Michael Goitein at 4 years of age

as an experimentalist in elementary particle physics, and then moved into applications of physics in medicine. Just as he was completing the design of a CT reconstruction algorithm with Cornelius Tobias, Hounsfield announced the first completed CT system. Michael judges that he and Tobias were something like the eighth group to "invent" CT. He then worked with Doug Boyd at Stanford in the development of a fan beam CT scanner.

Michael decided to move full time into medical physics. He discussed a position with Ted Webster of Radiology at MGH. There was no opening and Ted referred him to the new department of radiation medicine with positive comments. Richard Wilson, Professor of Physics at Harvard, enthusiastically endorsed his candidacy. Suit talked with Michael and was immediately and most favorably impressed. Michael accepted a position in December 1971. Initially he wanted to work in photon therapy, i.e., not to continue particle physics. He commenced work with Art Boyer and Merriam Gitterman. The accomplishments of this team are described in Chapter 4.

Michael's interest soon began to move toward protons. He organized a mini-symposium in the late spring of 1972 to consider the feasibility and rationale for fractionated dose proton therapy for cancer patients using the HCL 160 MeV proton beam. The participants included nuclear physicists from Harvard and MIT, the Princeton Particle Accelerator, and the MGH staff.

The recommendation was as anticipated, viz., proceed to use the HCL and to develop treatment planning skills, develop a large-field room, and get RBE assays started. Michael was active on each of these three goals in collaboration with A. Koehler and W. Preston of the HCL. This moved smartly, and treatment commenced in December 1973, viz., 2 years after Michael accepted the position at MGH. Major advances by Michael are described in Section 6.7.

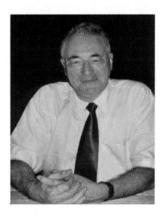

Fig. 6.17 Michael Goitein (1972–2002)

Michael served as Co-PI on the NCI grants for the support of the proton therapy program from 1976 to 2000 and PI on the NCI grants of $26.1 M as partial funding for the new MGH proton therapy facility. Further, he managed the contracts for the cyclotron and the building and the complex and lengthy processes of preparing the system for the start of patient treatments.

Additional research grants of Goitein included the following: (1) NCI Research Career Development Award; (2) NCI RO 1 grant, for 11 years, to investigate the "Assessment and Optimization of Radiation Therapy"; (3) NCI RO 1 grant for 3 years "3D Treatment Planning;" and (4) grants from two multiple institutional contracts one from the NCI and one grant from Siemens.

Of very high importance, he recruited an impressive group of physicists into the program. Those that he recruited directly to the MGH and are currently working here are Judy Adams, J. Flanz, A. Niemierko, H. Paganetti, and Janet Sisterson (from the HCL when it closed in 2001). Those whom he recruited and have moved are L. Verhey,[12] Marcia Urie,[13] K. Gall,[14] A. Smith,[15] Skip Rosenthal,[16] W. Neuhauser,[17] and M. Wagner.[18]

Michael has 152 papers in peer-reviewed journals. He has received several important awards, namely the ASTRO Gold Medal, 2003; Fellow of American Association of Physicists in Medicine, 2000; Honorary member of the Belgium Society of Radiotherapy and Oncology; Fulbright travel grant; Frank Knox Memorial; and IBM fellowships.

6.18.8 Hanne Kooy

Hanne Kooy (Fig. 6.19) was born in Brazil and had his childhood in Tilburg, southern Netherlands. He was a top-ranked student with interest in science and engineering. His father was an engineer. Hanne went to Delft University as a major in applied physics. He married a young American student in special education.

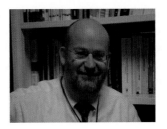

Fig. 6.19 Hanne Kooy, Director of Proton Clinical Operations (1997–present)

Hanne then went to Syracuse University. One of his projects was work on the upgrading of the Cornell University synchrotron to an electron positron beam machine. This proved to be a powerful learning experience. During that period he met both Richard Wilson and Robert Wilson. Hanne decided against a career in nuclear physics and worked for 1 year in the research division of Xerox in Rochester, NY. In 1982, Hanne joined the highly regarded medical physicist Larry Simpson who had recently moved to University of Rochester in Department of Radiation Oncology of Philip Rubin. Hanne used Monte Carlo methods to calculate the dose near density heterogeneities among several other activities. He then in 1987 moved to the JCRT in Boston with the B. Bjarngard Physics Group.

At the JCRT, he first participated in a major effort on electron beam dosimetry and treatment planning in 3D. Then he moved into treatment planning for the stereotactic radiosurgery (SRS) program. For Hanne and a few colleagues, this proved to be a major success, viz., transforming a quite complex planning procedure into one vastly more straightforward and much simplified. Another success was making brachytherapy under MRI guidance quite practical. This was accomplished with physicist Robert Cormack. The major use of the technique has been and is brachytherapy of prostate tumors. In addition, he became responsible for all of the treatment planning plus post-doctoral fellow training at the JCRT. The physician responsible for the SRS program was Jay Loeffler.

In 1996, Loeffler was recruited to the MGH and Hanne moved with him to develop the SRS program for photon and enhance the one based on protons. This he did in relatively short order. At that time Loeffler was the PI of the proton therapy program and Hanne devoted full time to develop the proton therapy center at the MGH. He made valuable contributions to the photon program of the department, especially his work with J. Kung to implement IMXT at the MGH.

Hanne worked with M. Goitein and J. Flanz to "birth" the cyclotron to operational status at the FHBPTC. He and a team commissioned the two gantry systems. He prepared the specifications for the new CT simulator and was central to its introduction into clinical service. Current efforts are dedicated to managing the clinical physics operation and

---

[12] Head Radiation Physics, University of California, San Francisco.

[13] Head Radiation Physics, University of Massachusetts, Worcester.

[14] Head Radiation Physics, Southwestern University Medical School, Dallas, TX, and then recently formed Stillwater, Inc. to build small cyclotrons that are to be installed on individual gantries.

[15] Head Proton Physics, MD Anderson Proton Therapy Center, Houston, TX.

[16] Staff at Stillwater Corp., Cambridge, MA.

[17] Staff, Proton Physics, MD Anderson Proton Therapy Center, Houston, TX.

[18] Stillwater Inc.

implementation of IMPT. This latter is a major task and involves a large fraction of the physics and engineering staff. The dose distributions are virtually certain to be superior to that by passive energy modulation used at present, especially in the near elimination of neutron scatter from the machine head.

6.18.9 Norbert Liebsch

Norbert (Fig. 6.20) was born in Germany in 1945, at the end of WWII and had his education in the midst of post-war reconstruction. He earned a Ph.D. in physics in July 1976 and then the Doctor of Medicine in 1982 from the University of Munich. Both the Ph.D. and the M.D. degrees were Summa Cum Laude. He decided to come to the USA for education in radiology. He entered the residency in diagnostic radiology at Washington University, St. Louis, and passed the American Board of Radiology in Diagnostic Radiology in June 1985. Then he moved to the Mayo Clinic for a separate residency in radiation therapy. He passed the boards examination in radiation oncology in May 1988, i.e., he has separate boards in diagnostic and therapeutic radiology.

Norbert was appointed to the MGH and the HMS in 1988 in radiation oncology with an assignment to the proton therapy program. His clinical performance has been rated outstanding by all observers. In addition to his appointment in radiation oncology, since 1991, he has served as a consultant in the Department of Diagnostic Radiology, Massachusetts General Hospital. At MGH, Norbert has specialized in management by proton radiation therapy of patients with sarcomas of the skull base and cervical spine. This interest is combined with high level of expertise in the interpretation of diagnostic imaging of the skull and upper spine. These talents are efficiently organized and have resulted in his being recognized as the top international specialist on this group of malignant neoplasms. He enjoys a very large international referral practice. Currently, the total number of patients treated for chordoma and chondrosarcoma of the skull base is ~800 and 400, respectively (personal communication from Norbert Liebsch, 2008).

He worked with John Munzenrider in this program. Earlier, Mary Austin-Seymour was active with this program. In the recent years, Norbert has treated most of these patients. This total experience is by far the largest number in any radiation oncology department. The 15-year local control rate results are given by Norbert to be 45% and 95% for chordoma and chondrosarcoma of the skull base, respectively. Radiation morbidity is estimated at ~5%. Liebsch has extended his practice to include lower spine and sacrum in collaboration with Tom Delaney.

6.18.10 Hsiao-Ming Lu

Lu (Fig. 6.21) is a native of Lingxian, Shandong Province, a small town about 300 km south of Beijing. His education was quite eventful in that it overlapped in time with the Cultural Revolution starting from 1966. He had the great good fortune while in the seventh grade to have a brilliant physics teacher, in exile from the capital for "anti-revolutionary crimes." This teacher introduced him to physics equations. Lu was particularly excited by one, viz., $F = ma$. He dreamed to study physics, even during the later "re-education" years working in farms and factories. This remained a dream until 1978 when colleges were finally reopened.

After receiving a B.S. degree from Nanjing University in 1982, he came to the USA by the CUSPEA (China-United States Physics Examination Application) program, which selects, through written and oral examinations, most qualified physics students (~100 per year) to enter U.S. graduate schools. Lu did mostly theoretical work on Raman scattering for his Ph.D. thesis at Arizona State University. This was followed by a post-doctoral fellowship and faculty position at the University of Nebraska investigating commensurate phase transitions. In 1993, he switched to radiotherapy physics and moved to the JCRT for training in medical physics and then appointment to faculty. In 2003 he joined the MGH proton group. Here he has worked on automatic planning optimization for radiosurgery, CT simulation, reducing cardiac toxicity for breast treatment, and

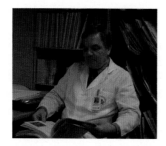

Fig. 6.20 Norbert Liebsch

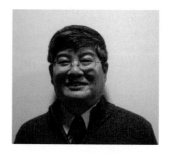

Fig. 6.21 Hsiao-Ming Lu

in recent years with protons, on dose distribution improvement, breast treatment, and respiratory gating for lung, liver, and other thoracic/abdominal lesions. His current areas of concentration are on range verifications for proton treatment and the clinical implementation of intensity-modulated proton therapy (IMPT). He has been promoted to be the Clinical Director of medical physics for our department

A biosketch of Munzenrider is given in Section 10.2.

6.18.11 Harald Paganetti

Harald (Fig. 6.22) spent his childhood in a small town near the Rhine River as an only child. After graduating from the public schools system in 1982, he served the obligatory 15 months in the German military. In high school he had decided on physics/math as he was the top student in those subjects. His next step was to attend the Rheinische Friedrich-Wilhelms University in Bonn. There he won his Ph.D. in 1992 with his thesis "The influence of meson-exchange currents in delayed fission and the direct nuclear excitation in muonic ^{209}Bi."

As a post-doctoral fellow, he worked in the Department of Medicine (Microdosimetry Group) at the Forschungszentrum Jülich, Germany, until early 1997 studying Monte Carlo simulations of the biological effects of proton beams. Next, he had a year as a research fellow in the Department of Ion-Beam Applications (Eye-Tumor-Therapy Group) at the Hahn-Meitner Institute, Berlin, Germany, investigating dose calculation for proton beam therapy. He was advised to join the clinical proton therapy program at the MGH. He was accepted and came as a research fellow in February 1998 to be with M. Goitein. His work has been highly regarded and he was promoted to Associate Professor in 2006.

Harald's main research areas have been and are Monte Carlo calculation of dose distribution in heterodense tissues. This is especially important for doses near tissue interfaces,

e.g., soft tissue to bone, air cavities, at points close to metallic support devices. An additional advantage is expected to be corrections for motion during the intra-fraction irradiation. Paganetti has worked extensively on biomathematical modeling of the effect of LET and fractionation. He and colleagues assessed the published in vivo proton RBE values and concluded that the mean RBE from the available data is 1.10 and that the use of this value as a generic RBE to be appropriate [32].

Harald is a member of the American Association of Physicists in Medicine (AAPM) and the American Physical Society (APS) and serves as consultant for the International Commission on Radiological Units and Measurements (ICRU) and the International Atomic Energy Agency (IAEA). Further, he is a member of the SBIR/STTR study section in ontological sciences of the US Department of Health and Human Services (NIH).

6.18.12 Alexi Trofimov

Alexi (Fig. 6.23) was born in Zaporozhye, Ukraine, an industrial city of 1 million located 700 miles south of Moscow. His father was an engineer and worked as a manager at a steel mill in charge of an entire division and his mother was a primary care physician. His interest in science was stimulated as a pre-schooler as his father got him engaged in scientific puzzles. Slightly later he had a subscription to the science journal *Quantum*. After his first 5 years in school, his parents transferred young Alexi to a special school that emphasized physics and math. Alexi commented that the general attitude in that city was the opposite of peer pressure to articulate a negative attitude toward science. In high school, he was taught differential and integral equations and performed physics laboratory experiments. For university he applied to Moscow State University, the number 1 in the Soviet Union. This was a real challenge in that were one to fail in the admission procedures and there was no admission to another university until one had served 2 years in the

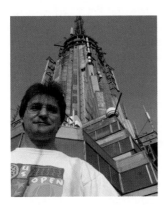

Fig. 6.22 Harald Paganetti

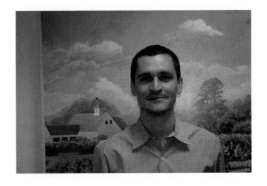

Fig. 6.23 Alexi Trofimov

army. Even in that situation, only one in three applicants were accepted to Moscow State.

He studied there for 5.5 years. For the final 2 years he specialized in high-energy physics in Protvino, south of Moscow, doing Monte Carlo simulations, prepared software to reconstruct particle decay kinematics and the signatures in the complex detector systems. His studies were predominately physics and math, almost no chemistry or biology. The system employed an extremely tightly focused curriculum.

On graduation in 1995 nearly all of his associates applied for and obtained admission to top US universities, several went to Yale, Princeton, Harvard, and Berkeley. He was admitted to Boston University with a scholarship. At no point was he asked by Russia to make any payment for his education. Namely, the USA got a very talented and educated young physicist absolutely with no cost.

At BU he became a participant in research on measurements of the magnetic moment of the moon. This work was performed at Brookhaven. The BU team had – five to seven persons on different aspects of this problem. His Ph.D. thesis was based on his work at Brookhaven.

Only at nearing the completion of his Ph.D. work did he learn of the field of medical physics. This appeared to be highly interesting. He applied to Thomas Bortfeld and came to the MGH. Here he has worked in the proton therapy research group of Bortfeld and also on projects with Hanne Kooy, Steve Jiang, and several physicians. A special research interest of Alexi is the physics of implementation of IMPT.

6.19 Proton Faculty Who Have Moved to Other Programs

6.19.1 Mary Austin Seymour

Mary Austin Seymour (1984–1988) was a very active and productive participant in the proton therapy program. Several significant papers on proton therapy were produced by her. She moved to the University of Washington Seattle, Washington.

6.19.2 Ken Gall

Ken Gall (1988–1996) developed "Repo Man" for patient positioning. Next he went to Southwestern University (Dallas) as head of radiation physics. Recently, he started Stillwater Corporation to manufacture gantry-mounted cyclotrons.

6.19.3 Wayne Neuhauser

Wayne Neuhauser (1997–2005) joined the MGH in 1997 to work on special proton therapy programs and participate in getting the FHBPTC operational. In 2002, he moved to the M.D. Anderson proton therapy program.

6.19.4 Skip Rosenthal

Skip Rosenthal (1991–1995) made major advances in systems for patient immobilization at HCL and at FBPTC. He left the MGH to join Stillwater Corp. and work with Ken Gall.

6.19.5 Al Smith

Al Smith (1992–2002) received his Ph.D. in physics in 1970 from Texas Tech University and accepted a post-doctoral fellowship at the University of Texas M.D. Anderson Cancer Center (MDACC) in Houston. He joined the MDACC faculty in 1971 and participated in the initial MDACC neutron therapy program.

In 1975 he moved to the University of New Mexico Cancer Center as Director of Negative Pi Meson (Pion) Clinical Physics at the Los Alamos National Laboratory. Then in 1982–1985 he was a Cancer Expert at the National Cancer Institute and from 1985 to 1992 he was Professor and Director of Clinical Physics, Department of Radiation Oncology at the University of Pennsylvania Medial School. He worked with Varian Medical Systems to develop their first multileaf collimator.

In 1992 he moved to MGH as Professor at the Harvard Medical School and Associate Director of the Northeast Proton Therapy Center. He directed the clinical proton physics activities at HCL, initiated an effort to obtain procedure codes and reimbursement rates for proton therapy, and was active in organizing the transfer of the proton clinical program from HCL to the MGH. There he participated in the development of the proton therapy center on the MGH campus. In 2002 he moved to Houston, Texas, as Professor at the University of Texas M.D. Anderson Cancer Center and Director, Proton Therapy Development.

6.19.6 Allan Thornton

Allan Thornton (1991–2002) concentrated on the radical treatment by proton beams of patients with paranasal sinus tumors. He was invited to lead the proton therapy program at the University of Indiana at Bloomington. This facility now is using gantries and treating ~50 patients per day. He was joined by Marcus Fitzek, a graduate of our residency program. Thornton has been named Medical Director of the Hampton University Proton Therapy Institute.

6.19.7 Marcia Urie

Marcia Urie (1980–1994) worked to great effect to plan and implement treatments at the HCL. Additionally she was a quite significant contributor to all phases of the program. She moved to Worcester MA to be the Head of radiation physics at University of Massachusetts.

6.19.8 Lynn Verhey

Lynn Verhey (1957–1991) performed basic and detailed proton dosimetry measurements and was very active in patient treatment. Further, he supervised Ph.D. student Paula Petti in her measurements of W values for a number of atoms. Lynn Verhey is currently the chief of radiation physics at the University of California, San Francisco.

References

1. Chen CC, Chapman P, Petit J, Loefler J. Proton radiosurgery in neurosurgery. Neurosurg Focus 2007;23(6):E5.
2. Chen GT, Kung JH, Rietzel E. Four-dimensional imaging and treatment planning of moving targets. Front Radiat Ther Oncol. 2007;40:59–71.
3. Debus J, Hug EB, Liebsch NJ, et al. Brainstem tolerance to conformal radiotherapy of skull base tumors. Int J Radiat Oncol Biol Phys. 1997;39:967–75.
4. Delaney T, Kooy HM. Proton and charged particle radiotherapy. Philadelphia, PA: Lippencott Inc; 2008.
5. Falkmer S, Fors B, Larsson B, et al. Pilot study on proton irradiation of human carcinoma. Acta Radiol. 1962;58:33–51.
6. Goitein M. Compensation for inhomogeneities in charged particle radiotherapy using computed tomography. Int J Radiat Oncol Biol Phys. 1978;4:499–508.
7. Goitein M. Calculation of the uncertainty in the dose delivered during radiation therapy. Med Phys. 1985;12:608–12.
8. Goitein M, Miller T. Planning proton therapy of the eye. Med Phys. 1983;10:275–83.
9. Goitein M, Abrams M, Rowell D, et al. Multi-dimensional treatment planning: II. Beam's eye-view, back projection, and projection through CT sections. Int J Radiat Oncol Biol Phys. 1983;9:789–97.
10. Gragoudas E, Li W, Goitein M, et al. Evidence-based estimates of outcome in patients irradiated for intraocular melanoma. Arch Ophthalmol. 2002;120:1665–71.
11. International Commission of Radiological Units and Measurements. Report 78: Prescribing, Recording, and Reporting Proton Beam Therapy. Oxford: Oxford University Press; 2008.
12. Kim J, Munzenrider J, Maas A, et al. Optic neuropathy following combined proton and photon radiotherapy for base of skull tumors. Int J Radiat Oncol Biol Phys. 1997;39(2 Suppl):272.
13. Kjellberg RN, Sweet WH, Preston WM, et al. The Bragg peak of a proton beam in intracranial therapy of tumors. Trans Am Neurol Assoc. 1962;87:216–8.
14. Koehler AM, Preston WM. Protons in radiation therapy. Comparative dose distributions for protons, photons, and electrons. Radiology. 1972;104:191–5.
15. Kozak KR, Adams J, Krejcarek SJ, Tarbell NJ, Yock TI. A dosimetric comparison of proton and intensity-modulated photon radiotherapy for pediatric parameningeal rhabdomyosarcomas. Int J Radiat Oncol Biol Phys. 2009;74(1):179–86.
16. Lawrence JH. Proton irradiation of the pituitary. Cancer. 1957;10:795–8.
17. Lawrence JH, Tobias CA, Born JL, et al. Pituitary irradiation with high-energy proton beams: a preliminary report. Cancer Res. 1958;18:121–34.
18. Loeffler JS. Can combined whole brain radiation therapy and radiosurgery improve the treatment of single brain metastases? Nat Clin Pract Oncol. 2004;1:12–3.
19. Loeffler JS, Niemierko A, Chapman PH. Second tumors after radiosurgery: tip of the iceberg or a bump in the road? Neurosurgery. 2003;52:1436–40.
20. Lomax AJ, Boehringer T, Coray A, et al. Intensity modulated proton therapy: a clinical example. Med Phys. 2001;28:317–24.
21. Lomax AJ, Pedroni E, Rutz H, et al. The clinical potential of intensity modulated proton therapy. Z Med Phys. 2004;14:147–52.
22. Marucci L, Niemierko A, Liebsch NJ, et al. Spinal cord tolerance to high-dose fractionated 3D conformal proton-photon irradiation as evaluated by equivalent uniform dose and dose volume histogram analysis. Int J Radiat Oncol Biol Phys. 2004;59:551–5.
23. Paganetti H, Niemierko A, Ancukiewicz M, et al. Relative biological effectiveness (RBE) values for proton beam therapy. Int J Radiat Oncol Biol Phys. 2002;53:407–21.
24. Parodi K, Paganetti H, Cascio E, et al. PET/CT imaging for treatment verification after proton therapy: a study with plastic phantoms and metallic implants. Med Phys. 1953;34:419–35.
25. Paterson R. The treatment of malignant disease by radium and X-rays. 4th ed. London, UK: Edward Arnold & Co; 1953.
26. Pommier P, Liebsch NJ, Deschler DG, et al. Proton beam radiation therapy for skull base adenoid cystic carcinoma. Arch Otolaryngol Head Neck Surg. 2006;132:1242–9.
27. Robertson JB, Williams JR, Schmidt RA, et al. Radiobiological studies of a high-energy modulated proton beam utilizing cultured mammalian cells. Cancer. 1975;35:1664–77.
28. Rosenberg A, Nielsen G, Keel S, et al. Chondrosarcoma of the base of the skull: a clinicopathological study of 200 cases with emphasis on it's distinction from chordoma. Am J Surg Pathol. 1999;23:1370–8.
29. Santoni R, Liebsch N, Finkelstein DM, et al. Temporal lobe (TL) damage following surgery and high-dose photon and proton irradiation in 96 patients affected by chordomas and chondrosarcomas of the base of the skull. Int J Radiat Oncol Biol Phys. 1998;41:59–68.
30. Shipley WU, Verhey LJ, Munzenrider JE, et al. Advanced prostate cancer: the results of a randomized comparative trial of high dose irradiation boosting with conformal protons compared with conventional dose irradiation using photons alone. Int J Radiat Oncol Biol Phys. 1995;32:3–12.
31. Suit H, Goldberg S, Niemierko A, et al. Proton beams to replace photon beams in radical dose treatments. Acta Oncol. 2003;42:800–8.

32. Suit H, Kooy H, Trofimov A, et al. Should positive phase III clinical trial data be required before proton beam therapy is more widely adopted? No. Radiother Oncol. 2008;86:48–53.
33. Tarbell NJ, Smith AR, Adams J, et al. The challenge of conformal radiotherapy in the curative treatment of medulloblastoma. Int J Radiat Oncol Biol Phys. 2000;46:265–6.
34. Tepper J, Verhey L, Goitein M, et al. In vivo determinations of RBE in a high energy modulated proton beam using normal tissue reactions and fractionated dose schedules. Int J Radiat Oncol Biol Phys. 1977;2:115–22.
35. Terahara A, Niemierko A, Goitein M, et al. Analysis of the relationship between tumor dose inhomogeneity and local control in patients with skull base chordoma. Int J Radiat Oncol Biol Phys. 1999;45:351–8.
36. Tobias CA, Anger HO, Lawrence JH. Radiological use of high energy deuterons and alpha particles. Am J Roentgenol Radium Ther Nucl Med. 1952;67:1–27.
37. Tobias CA, Van Dyke DC, Simpson ME, et al. Irradiation of the pituitary of the rat with high energy deuterons. Am J Roentgenol Radium Ther Nucl Med. 1954;72:1–21.

38. Urano M, Goitein M, Verhey L, et al. Relative biological effectiveness of a high energy modulated proton beam using a spontaneous murine tumor in vivo. Int J Radiat Oncol Biol Phys. 1980;6: 1187–93.
39. Urano M, Verhey LJ, Goitein M, et al. Relative biological effectiveness of modulated proton beams in various murine tissues. Int J Radiat Oncol Biol Phys. 1984;10:509–14.
40. Wilson R. A brief history of the Harvard University cyclotrons. Cambridge, MA: Harvard University Department of Physics; 2004.
41. Wilson RR. The radiological use of fast protons. Radiology. 1946;47:489–91.
42. Yock TI, Tarbell NJ. Technology insight: proton beam radiotherapy for treatment in pediatric brain tumors. Nat Clin Pract Oncol. 2004;1:97–103.
43. Zietman AL, DeSilvio ML, Slater JD, et al. Comparison of conventional-dose vs high-dose conformal radiation therapy in clinically localized adenocarcinoma of the prostate: a randomized controlled trial. JAMA. 2005;294:1233–9.

Chapter 7

Intraoperative Electron Radiation Therapy

7.1 Initial Use of Intraoperative X-Ray Therapy (IORT)

The earliest known use of the IORT was in Barcelona, Spain, in 1905 for a patient with an advanced carcinoma of the uterine cervix. The patient was treated by hysterectomy, partial cystectomy, and node dissection on February 18 and the wound left open until March 11. Five fractions were administered over a several week period. The patient also received external beam therapy. She was reported to have been a disease-free survivor at 10 years [2]. A small number of patients were treated by IORT in European centers prior to WWII. Six patients were treated at Stanford and reported in 1937. Frank Ellis employed 250 kVp x-rays for IORT at the London Hospital in ~1941. After the war, Ellis moved to Oxford and in ~1960 received funding for a linear accelerator. The unit was installed in an OR at the Churchill Hospital. To his serious regret the machine was never functional. In Japan, Abe of University of Kyoto began a study of IOERT in the 1960s, particularly for gastric and bladder carcinoma patients. Then, U. Henschke at Howard University commenced a major IOERT program in 1976.

7.2 Initiation of IOERT at MGH

Suit was keen to implement IOERT at the MGH because of the simple rationale, viz., dose distribution advantage due to ease of displacing normal tissues/organs from the beam path combined with depth dose characteristics of electron beams. He had heard this articulated forcefully by F. Ellis. For IOERT, the applicator can be placed directly on the target tissues. Further, for the PTV is literally a minimum, a clear advantage relative to that feasible by EBRT. This assumes no sensitive structures deep to the CTV in part or in toto within the electron's depth of penetration. A technique that avoids or reduces dose to normal tissue provides a gain.

HDS was very keen that we commence IOERT in the very near future using a linear accelerator in the Cox Ground Level. This would complement our efforts at improving dose distribution by proton beam therapy. Basis for this opinion were threefold. First, IOERT would increase the efficacy of treatment of several categories of cancer patients. Second, although IOERT would require transportation of the patient status post-resection or exposure of the tumor from an OR in the fourth floor to the department in the Cox Ground, we could readily provide time on a linear accelerator and have the room properly prepared. That is, the IOERT could be performed very shortly after the arrival of the patient at the linear accelerator. Importantly, we could perform IOERT at the MGH with virtually no increase in capitol costs. Third and critical, unless we have some clinical results, there was negligible probability of getting a new linear accelerator and the shielding and modification of an OR.

At approximately this time, while attending a meeting in Tokyo, HDS made a side trip to Kyoto University to examine their facility and discuss their experience. Following surgical exposure (with or without resection) the patient was transported to the electron beam room. The untidy state of the treatment room and the fact that the frequency of infection attributed to the IOERT procedure was near zero were most welcome news. On return to Boston, he talked with several surgeons re the feasibility of transporting the patient after the surgical procedure to our department for a single-dose IOERT and the associated risk of infection. In an air of puzzlement, one of the surgeons asked "Have you not heard or read of the Vietnam War? Do you not know that we operated regularly on wounded soldiers in simple tents in the jungle and that infections were quite uncommon? You need not worry about infections. Our interest is: will there be an increase in cure rate? If so, 'let us do it.' " With that unambiguous and quite positive surgical opinion, discussions commenced immediately by physicians, physicists, therapists, and nurses. In parallel, detailed discussions were held with anesthesia and administration. Approval was obtained from all concerned groups for an early start.

H.D. Suit, J.S. Loeffler, *Evolution of Radiation Oncology at Massachusetts General Hospital*, DOI 10.1007/978-1-4419-6744-2_7, © Springer Science+Business Media, LLC 2011

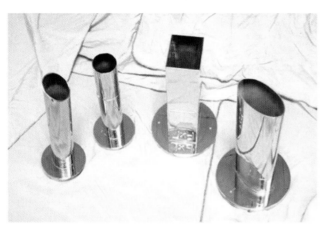

Fig. 7.1 Cones used for IOERT. These were designed by Biggs and made in our machine shop

Our basic concept was to employ IOERT as the boost dose (Fig. 7.1). The MGH was the first in the USA to employ IOERT exclusively as the boost dose. The plan was EBRT to ~50 Gy to the CTV at ~1.8–2 Gy per fraction followed by resection or tumor exposure for IOERT to the tumor BED or the GTV. IOERT has been single doses of ~15–20 Gy for gross tumor, ~10 Gy to the surgical bed with negative margins, and 12.5–15 Gy for suspected micro-positive margins. To no surprise, there have been positive results at the MGH and at other centers. Interestingly, this technique is analogous to the intra-oral cone treatment developed by C.C. Wang for intra-oral lesions.

7.3 IOERT at MGH

Our first patient had a non-resectable mass on the left pelvic side wall following prior radiation treatment at the MGH for a squamous cell carcinoma of the uterine cervix. In April 1978 she was given ~20 Gy by EBRT and then, after surgical exposure and careful protective draping, the anesthetized patient was transported through ~80 m of corridors, two elevators, and then to our Clinac 35 room. The procedure was uneventful. A significant action of the administration was to assign an MGH police officer at each of the two elevators to assure that an elevator was open for the patient and the medical team as we approached, i.e., zero delay at the two elevators. This extremely smooth transfer from the OR to Cox ground was 100% consistent and most impressive. The procedure went as planned and with no difficulty. For this first patient, local control was obtained but she did later develop significant sacral plexopathy and then fatal metastatic tumor.

Over the following 18 years, 1978–1996, there have been no infections attributed to the IOERT procedure in a total of

342 patients. One valuable development was the preparation of a QA program for IOERT by Joel Tepper [4]. Another contribution by Tepper et al. was the analysis of complications in patients treated by IOERT of their locally advanced rectal cancer [5]. No evidence was found for a higher morbidity rate in the pre-operative + IOERT than in the pre-operative radiation-alone patients.

From the start of our program, we wanted a linear accelerator in the OR. This was achieved after very lengthy negotiations and consideration of many different sites within the hospital, including a room in the sub-basement. A new linear accelerator in OR 43 in the new OR wing was realized in 1996. Our first patient there was treated on June 12, 1996. There have been 283 patients treated in that facility. Of the total of 625 patients, 437 (70%) were treated for lesions in the abdominal–pelvic regions.

This program has been broadly based with physicists, surgeons, medical oncologists, anesthesiologists, nurses, radiation therapists, hospital administration and security personnel, and radiation oncologists as participants. For an early paper on the MGH program, see [3].

7.4 Results at the MGH

Five very highly talented and effective clinicians have led this program: Leonard Gunderson, Joel Tepper, Chris Willett, Tom Delaney, and currently Ted Hong. They have worked with many surgeons and with medical oncologists for the management of the drug or biological agent administration. Importantly they have contributed to clinical and technical advances with this modality. The senior physicist leading this program over the entire period has been Peter Biggs. The results from this experience are viewed as positive. For selected series, see Table 7.1.

Willet et al. [6] reported the experience on patients with locally advanced rectal cancer who were treated at the MGH by pre-operative radiation (45 Gy/5 weeks) ± 5 FU and then resectional surgery and IOERT. The 5-year local control results were 89, 68, and 65% for margin negative, margin positive, and partial resections. The 5-year disease-free survival results were 63, 40, and 32%, respectively. This strategy (EBRT ± chemotherapy then surgery and IOERT, with postoperative EBRT for margin positive surgical specimens) is being employed in many centers and the results are indicating a gain in local control.

For retroperitoneal sarcomas, Gieschen et al. reported in 2001 that the 5-year local control result in a series of 16 patients was 83% following treatment by EBRT, resection, and then IOERT. In 13 patients treated by resection only, the local control result was 62% [1]. These data are not from a phase III trial. The MGH experience with IOERT for the

Table 7.1 Results in patients treated by IOERT at MGH

Site	Stage	# patients	Local control at 5 years	Survival at 5 years	References
Rectum locally advanced	Margins–	45	89%	63%	Willett et al. [6]
	Margins+	21	68%	40%	
	Gross residue	28	65%	32%	
Retroperitoneal sarcoma	No gross residual tumor	16	83%	74%	Gieschen et al. [1]
Pancreas	5–6 cm cone	26		17% at 3 years 0%	Willett et al. [7]
	~9 cm cone	11			

sarcomas at other sites remains too limited for comment. Results of IOERT for patients with pancreatic cancer were weakly positive for the smaller lesions. To achieve cure of patients with pancreatic carcinoma remains a most worthy challenge [7].

The efficacy of IOERT is being investigated for several additional sites, e.g., thoracic, H/N, extremity, and torso sarcomas of the soft tissues and bones, Gyn, GU, and pediatric [2]. There are as of this date quite limited patient outcome data for IOERT for tumors other than GI pelvic and connective tissue tumors.

For Biographical sketches of Gunderson, Tepper and Willett see Chapter 10 Section on GI tumors.

References

1. Gieschen H, Spiro IJ, Suit H, Ott M, Rattner D, Ancukiewicz M, Willett C. Long-term results of intraoperative electron beam radiotherapy for primary and recurrent retroperitoneal soft tissue sarcoma. Int J Radiat Oncol Biol Phys. 2001;50(1):127–31.
2. Gunderson l, Willett C, Harrison L, Calvo P. Intraoperative irradiation. Totowa, NJ: Humana; 1999.
3. Gunderson LL, Cohen AC, Dosoretz DE, Shipley WU, Hedberg SE, Wood WC, Rodkey GV, Suit HD. Residual, unresectable, or recurrent colorectal cancer: external beam irradiation and intraoperative electron beam boost + resection. Int J Radiat Oncol Biol Phys. 1983;9:1597–606.
4. Tepper JE, Gunderson LL, Goldson AL, Kinsella TJ, Shipley WU, Sindelar WF, Wood WC, Martin JK. Quality control parameters of intraoperative radiation therapy. Int J Radiat Oncol Biol Phys. 1986;12(9):1687–95.
5. Tepper JE, Gunderson LL, Orlow E, Cohen AM, Hedberg SE, Shipley WU, Blitzer PH, Rich T. Complications of intraoperative radiation therapy. Int J Radiat Oncol Biol Phys. 1984;10(10): 1831–9.
6. Willett C, Czito B, Tyler D. Intraoperative radiation therapy. J Clin Oncol. 2007;25(8):971–7.
7. Willett C, Fernandez Del Castillo C, Shih Helen, Goldberg S, Biggs P, Clark J, Lauwers G, Ryan D, Zhu A, Warshaw A. Long-term results of intraoperative electron beam irradiation (IOERT) for patients with unresectable pancreaticcancer. Ann Surg. 2005;241(2):295–9.

Chapter 8

Radiation Biology of Tumor and Normal Tissues

8.1 Goal for the Radiation Oncology Biology Research Laboratory

For the new department, the trustees wanted a program in laboratory research on the effects of radiation on animal cells and tissues, normal and malignant, and the whole organism.

8.2 The Defined Flora Pathogen-Free (DFPF) Mouse Colony

The mouse colony that Sedlacek and Suit had developed at the MDAH was virtually unique in academic centers in providing an experimentally useful supply of highly inbred mice that were defined flora and pathogen free (DFPF). The benefit to the researcher was virtually no loss of an experimental mouse due to infectious diseases. Having this colony at the MGH was essential to the research program of the new department. The result of having this quality of a mouse colony has served as a powerful attractant for an impressive number of investigators with special talents and as the basis for much of the substantial research conducted with other departments and institutions. An important fact is that the colony was a critical factor in Rakesh Jain's acceptance of the invitation to move his research program to the MGH in 1991.

The colony at MDAH had to be transferred to the MGH. This was recognized as no trivial task and was achieved due to the ingenuity, industry, and plain determination of Robert Sedlacek. He accomplished this assignment on time and within budget. The intent was to establish the colony in Temporary Building II (Temp II) and move it to the new Cox Cancer Center building as soon as space became available.

Suit met Sedlacek when visiting the Texas Inbred Mouse Company in Houston to consider the purchase of C_3H mice. He had become extremely disappointed by the low quality of mice available from one of the most highly regarded suppliers in the USA. During the negotiations, Bob discussed

his vision of a vastly improved experimental mouse colony, viz., a colony of mice with a defined bacterial flora that was pathogen free or DFPF. Bob's concept was judged feasible and extremely attractive. The effort to recruit Bob commenced immediately. Hospital funding was promptly obtained. The new colony was soon producing DFPF mice in useful quantities and full production in 2 years.

For the colony transfer to the MGH, Bob contracted for a Twin Engine Beech aircraft. The mice were C_3H and C_3H_f in cages fitted with filter tops. Additionally, there were four isolators for which he arranged for microbe-free air to be circulated through HEPA filters. This attention to detail assured that the 600 mice would arrive in Boston with negligible risk of infection. Bob flew with the mice. Figure 8.1a is a photograph of a mouse isolator cage similar to the ones used for the transfer of mice to the MGH. Figure 8.1b is a photograph of the plane at take-off on January 22, 1972, for the 12-h, one-stop flight to Boston. In conjunction with the transfer of the colony to Boston, Bob who had been a truck driver to earn money to go to university in Wyoming engaged a 14-wheeler truck, Fig. 8.1c, to bring a considerable collection of laboratory equipment including a special ^{137}Cs irradiator (3 cm diameter field, using parallel-opposed sources, collimated by uranium). This specialized piece of equipment had been made for our research. All of the equipment brought to the MGH had been purchased by Suit's NCI R01 and the transfer approved by MDAH administration. The truck also carried furniture, etc., for most of the staff moving to Boston.

Bob had carefully prepared the Temp II space to receive the mice. A group of us met the plane quite late one evening and took our marvelous cargo of mice to Temp II. Claire Hunt pitched in to assist with this effort that was not completed until 2:00 AM. One section of that temporary metal building had been modified so that all air entering the colony passed through HEPA filters (i.e., bacteria-free air). The air exhausted through vents at the floor level of each wall. Our requirements posed serious challenges due to the diverse occupants and condition of Temp II, namely, a holding area for sheep with the associated flies, a mycoplasma laboratory, and a laboratory with conventional mice, rats, and guinea

H.D. Suit, J.S. Loeffler, *Evolution of Radiation Oncology at Massachusetts General Hospital*, DOI 10.1007/978-1-4419-6744-2_8, © Springer Science+Business Media, LLC 2011

Fig. 8.1 (**a**) One of the isolator "cages" for the mouse transfer from MDAH to MGH. (**b**) The "take off" of the plane with Bob riding in the cockpit and 600 of our DFPF mice in the fuselage. (**c**) The truck Bob rented to transfer lab equipment and furniture of several of the staff to Boston

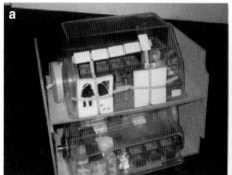
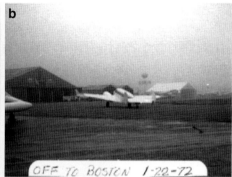
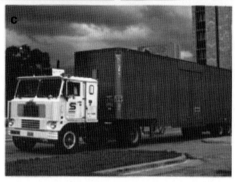

pigs. In that distinctly less than optimal environment, the colony functioned as planned. In addition to research space in the colony, there was an open research laboratory adjacent to the colony. Our laboratory and colony did not move to Cox 7 for 5 years and 4 months, viz., in 1977.

The required sanitation procedures have been and are that the mice are in filter cap cages ($\leq$5/cage), provided sterile food, water, and bedding. Importantly, each person entering the colony must wear a cap, a mask (exposing only a small part of the face, i.e., no visible hair), gowns, gloves, lab shoes and walk through a strong disinfectant footbath, disinfect the gloves after opening each mouse cage, and work with mice in a flow of HEPA-filtered air in a laminar flow bench. These requirements are exactly the same for researchers and animal caretakers. These conditions for reducing risk of infection to an extremely low level clearly are more stringent than those employed in the OR. One indicator of the impact of this pathogen-free status is the marked increase in tolerance of whole body irradiation (WBI). Specifically, the $LD_{50}s$[1] single dose irradiation for the acute GI syndrome of conventional and DFPF mice were ~3–4 vs 7–8 Gy.

The colony featured flow of HEPA filtered air from the ceiling toward the floor over the entire colony with exhaust via floor level vents in the walls of each room. Mice were in micro-isolator cages with $\leq$5 mice/cage. Bob gives a detailed description of the facility in his part of the Web Page.

Sedlacek was Director of the colony and also worked intensively side by side with the animal caretakers, always with an eye for improving the level of care and efficiency of the operation. This included special attention to general maintenance, equipment for sterilizing cages, bottles, etc., cage washing devices, the large sterilizer, and the performance of each animal caretaker. Importantly, he was active in teaching policies and rationale of animal care to new fellows and laboratory investigators. In addition, he participated in a goodly number of research projects that resulted in publications. Bob and Kathy Mason described the operation of the colony in Lab and Animal Science in 1977 [79]. Regrettably, Bob Sedlacek resigned his position at the MGH in 1988 because of back problems.

The present Director of the colony is Peigen Huang, a pathologist from Guangdong, China. He had been at the laboratory as a research fellow in 1992–1995 and produced six first-authored publications in referred journals. Peigen returned to the Steele Laboratory in 2000 to his present position. His prior experience in the laboratory gave him a very good understanding of the needs of the animal caretakers, research faculty, and fellows.

Peigen has managed a marked increase in complexity of the operation. The number of mouse strains and sub-lines (with specific "knock-out" or "knock-in" genes) has grown to 16. Weekly microbial testing of fecal samples (~150/week) for aerobic bacteria have shown growth in 174 of the 27,894 samples or 0.62% of samples for the period 2004–2007. In those rare instances of contamination, that cage and the mice are discarded immediately. Every 4 weeks there is a comprehensive testing of the mouse colony by an outside laboratory firm for aerobic and anaerobic bacteria and 18 adventitious viruses. These tests have also been negative,

---

[1] LD_{50} is the dose that is lethal to 50% of the irradiated mice.

i.e., only rare aerobic and virtually never anaerobic bacteria; additionally, all tests for the 18 viruses have been negative and no parasites detected. Thus, nearly all mice entered into an experiment survive free of infectious disease, viz., almost no risk of loss of an experimental animal due to infections. This includes mice with brain or subcutaneous "windows" for special visual monitoring of vascular physiology. The Steele Laboratory mice die predominately of cancer, viz., 99% of female and 80% of male C_3H mice in our colony die of spontaneous cancer. This cancer incidence varies between mouse strains.

Additionally, DNA analyses on mouse tissue of each fourth generation have consistently shown that the strains are inbred as planned. To date, there has been no instance of genetic contamination.

An impressive statistic for the C_3H mice is that the productivity index is 1.3 pups per breeding female per week, substantially higher than the 0.7 for conventional mice in colonies of commercial mouse supplier (personal communication, Sedlacek 2007). Our gain is the result of extremely low mortality among pups to weaning; the pups are weaned at 18 days in comparison to 28 days in conventional colonies. A valuable gain for the researcher is that life span increased from ~550 to 804 and 890 days for female and male C_3H mice, respectively. This virtual elimination of infection in the experimental mice is a tribute to the care with which the colony was and is directed and the positive attitude and attention to detail and pride in the colony by the animal caretakers and investigators.

The experiments of R. Jain and group had special requirements, viz., high technology observations of growth of tumor vasculature, the passage of agents and drugs from capillaries into the interstitium, and the use of special "windows" in the brain or in subcutaneous tissues as transplantation sites. These special animals survive infection free and for periods far beyond that feasible in a more conventional colony. Importantly, these mice can be repeatedly examined with complex measurements at negligible risk of loss of the animal.

8.3   Selected Experimental Findings by Several Research Groups Listed by Faculty

8.3.1   H Suit

8.3.1.1   Stromal Cell vs Tumor Cell Radiation Sensitivity and Tumor Response to Radiation

W. Budach et al. [13] determined the TCD_{50} for local irradiation of murine tumor allografts in 6 Gy whole body irradiated (WBI) nude and in normal or WBI SCID mice, viz., normal vs highly radiation sensitive (genetically determined) host mice. The TCD_{50}s were not lower for tumor transplants in SCID than nude mice, i.e., the stroma and capillaries of the tumors had no discernible impact on the tumor control probability (TCP) by radiation, i.e., TCP was determined by the sensitivity of tumor cells not the stroma. There was a greater growth delay in the SCID mice, but the probability of tumor regrowth was unaffected. Budach, a Fellow from Germany, is the Chief of Radiation Oncology at Dusseldorf.

8.3.1.2   Heterogeneity in Response Between Paired Organs

An examination for heterogeneity of radiation response in paired structures in an individual animal has been performed by S. Kozin et al. [53]. Length of the right and left tibiae of 5-day-old mice was measured on high resolution 30 kVp x-radiographs and then administered a highly uniform ^{137}Cs gamma dose in a single fraction and imaging repeated at 84 days post-irradiation. There was no difference in growth between the right and left tibia up to 16–18 Gy, but a significant difference at 20–22 Gy. The γ_{50}^2 was 7, viz., very steep. Serge, a Fellow from Russia, is now a senior fellow in the Steele Laboratory.

8.3.1.3   Therapeutic Gain Factors (TGF[3]) for Irradiation by Fast Neutron or by X-Rays + O₂ 3ATA

In 1988, a team determined TGFs for fast neutron (air breathing) and x-ray + O_2 3ATA irradiation in 5 of 15 dose fractions to 6 mm diameter tumors. The tumors were early generation syngenic transplants of three spontaneous C_3H tumors: MCaIV, a mammary carcinoma; FSaII, a fibrosarcoma; and SCCVII, a squamous cell carcinoma. Radiations were ^{60}Co or ^{137}Cs photons at MGH or d[25]Be or p[43]Be neutrons at the Cleveland Clinic. For the three tumors, there were positive therapeutic gain factors for photons + O_2 3ATA but none for fast neutrons [86].

8.3.1.4   Radiation Sensitivity of Cells of Sarcoma of Soft Tissue and Breast Cancer

The in vitro radiation sensitivity of seven soft tissue sarcoma and eight breast carcinoma cell lines were determined by W. Ruka et al. [78]. The mean SF2 values were 0.39 and 0.38 while the MIDs (mean inactivation dose) were 1.92 and 1.90 Gy, i.e., no difference between sarcoma and carcinoma

---

[2] γ_{50} is the percent point increase in response probability for a 1% increase in dose.

[3] TGF is the ratio of RBE tumor/RBE normal tissue.

cells. Ruka, a Fellow, from Warsaw and is now Head of the Sarcoma and Melanoma Surgical unit in the Marie Curie Cancer Center, Warsaw.

8.3.1.5 Metastasis

8.3.1.5.a J. Ramsay

J. Ramsay et al. [74] demonstrated that the incidence of metastatic tumor in mice with local control by radiation or amputation increased with tumor volume at primary treatment. The two spontaneous tumors studied were early generation transplants of a fibrosarcoma and a squamous cell carcinoma. Incidence of metastasis was substantially higher in mice that developed local regrowth and then achieved local control by salvage surgery. Jonathan, a Fellow from England, is now a staff radiation oncologist at the Cancer Center in Brisbane, Australia.

8.3.1.5.b P. Huang

P. Huang et al. in 1996 [42] determined the metastatic activity of locally recurrent xenografts from a human soft tissue sarcoma, a colon carcinoma and a glioblastoma. The tumors were growing in SCID mice. The tumors were unirradiated or had recurred after 90, 107, and 77 Gy, respectively, administered in 30 fractions. The recurrent tumors were transplanted into syngenic mice; the metastatic frequency was lower for two of the three recurrent tumor systems than the previously unirradiated tumors or their surgically treated counterparts. He and colleagues performed an assay of frequency of metastasis from xenografts of human tumors transplanted into SCID mice. The tumor types were five glioblastomas and nine other pathological types. The difference between the tumor types was small [41]. Peigen now is the Director of the animal colony of the Steele Laboratory.

8.3.1.5.c M. Baumann

M. Baumann et al. [5] assessed the metastatic frequency in mice with local control after 5 or 15 dose fractions of photon or fast neutron irradiation. The incidence of metastasis for FSaII was independent of fractionation but was increased for SCCVII following 15 but not 5 dose fractions. Although not significant, the frequency of metastases was higher for neutron than photon treatment at 15 fractions for both tumors. Further, in the study of the mouse mammary carcinoma, MCaIV, treatment was given in a single dose or in 9 photon fractions of 2 or 4 Gy at 24- or 48-h intervals and then a top-up dose to achieve local control. Metastasis frequency

was elevated for treatment at 48-h intervals, especially at 2 Gy/fraction relative to the frequency after single dose irradiation. Michael, a Fellow from Germany, is now the Chief at the Dresden Cancer Center.

8.3.1.5.d A. Allam

A. Allam et al. [1] reported in 1993 no correlation between the in vitro radiation sensitivity of tumor cell lines and metastatic activity. Allam, a Fellow from Egypt, is now practicing from Egypt and is now practicing radiation oncology in Saudi Arabia.

8.3.1.6 Post-irradiation Residual Tumor Cells and Risk of Regrowth

Most pathologists have accepted cytologically intact cells post-irradiation as proof of persistence of "viable tumor cells." An experiment by HDS and breast cancer pathologist Gallagher at the MDACC showed that tumor cells persisting after doses yielding very high and very low TCP were not distinguishable [85]. This was controversial in MGH weekly sarcoma conferences. Y. Chen et al. [14] examined this question using three tumor cell lines transplanted sc in nude mice. At 2 weeks post irradiation, the tumors were excised. The histological appearance did not correlate with dose or transplantability. Two MGH sarcoma pathologists performed the pathological examinations. Chen was a resident and is now at University of Rochester.

8.3.1.7 Tumor Regression and Local Control

N. Choi et al. [15] examined in 1979 the growth and radiation response of a radiation-induced osteosarcoma to local irradiation. Even at long times post irradiation at doses yielding high tumor control probability, there was almost no or only slight regression of the osteosarcoma mass. On pathology, the osteoid mass had no remaining tumor cells. Noah, a South Korean, is Professor of Radiation Oncology and Head of the MGH radiation oncology thoracic tumor group.

8.3.1.8 Metabolic Predictors of Response

P. Okunieff et al. [67] extensively examined the metabolic status of FSaII transplants at several volumes by ^{31}P NMR spectroscopy to estimate intra-cellular nucleotide triphosphates (NTP), inorganic phosphate (Pi), phosphocreatinine (PCr), and pH. The PCr/Pi was 1.03 for $\sim$38 mm^3 but decreased to 0.15 at 250 mm^3. The hypoxic fraction was 4 and 40% at these volumes. The change in NTP was much less than that of PCr. NMR examination was suggested as a non-invasive technique to estimate tumor metabolic status and pO_2. Paul was a resident and he is now Director of the Shands Cancer Center, University of Fla, and Chair of Department of Radiation Oncology.

8.3.1.9 Transplantation Site and TD$_{50}$

Zietman et al. determined the TD_{50}[4] values for two murine and three human tumors transplanted intracerebally (ic) and into subcutaneous tissues (sc). The TD_{50} was consistently lower for intra-cerebral transplantation [114]. This study was extended by determining TD_{50} values for transplantation of five human tumor and four murine tumor cell lines sc or IC of nude and SCID mice in 1993 by Taghian et al. [88]. The TD_{50}s ic were lower than the TD_{50} sc by factors of 1.7–1580. Anthony, a Fellow from London and later an MGH resident, is now an MGH senior staff in the GU group. Anthony is the newly elected president of ASTRO. Alphonse, a Fellow from Alexandria, Egypt, is Head of the MGH Breast Unit in radiation oncology.

8.3.1.10 Immune Status of NCr/Sed nu/nu Nude Mice

The immune status in the athymic nude mice, NCr/Sed nu/nu was examined by V. Silobrcic et al. [83]. Immune reactivity was significantly less in 4- than 12-week-old mice as determined by TD_{50} of a human squamous cell carcinoma. Similarly, immunity was suppressed by a single injection of cyclophosphamide. A greater suppression was achieved by a single dose of 6 Gy to the whole body (threefold reduction of TD_{50}). There was a marked and quite prolonged suppression of T cells. In contrast, B-cell suppression recovered in part within 2 weeks. Vlatko came from Zagreb Croatia, recently retired as Head of the Department for Clinical and Experimental Immunology and Chemistry of the Institute of Immunology, Zagreb.

8.3.1.11 Pre-operative Irradiation and TCD$_{50}$

In 1985, T. Todoroki et al. [90] assessed the efficacy of pre-operative radiation and conservative or radical surgery on syngenic transplants of the spontaneous fibrosarcoma, FSa II. Local excision achieved a $\sim$50% decrease in TCD_{50} for two tumor sizes. Extending surgery to radical resection reduced TCD_{50} by an additional $\sim$14%. Todoroki is a senior surgeon at the University of Tsukuba, Japan, who has developed an international reputation in the combination of surgery and IOERT for biliary and hepatic neoplasms.

8.3.1.12 Anti-coagulant and Radiation Therapy

In 1975, E. Röttinger et al. [77] considered the indications from several reports that microthrombus formation in tumors contributed to development of hypoxic regions. They determined the TCD_{50} (single or 10 dose irradiation) for 8 mm diameter early generation transplants of a spontaneous mammary carcinoma and a methylcholanthrene-nduced fibrosarcoma in control or warfarin-treated hosts. Warfarin caused a two- to threefold increase in prothrombin time but no discernible effect on radiation response. Erwin, a Fellow from Germany, became the Chief of radiation oncology at the University of Ulm.

8.3.1.13 Tolerance of Total Nodal Irradiation and Renal Allograft Acceptance by Cynomolgus Monkeys

Our only study based on non-human primates was conducted by resident E. Halperin et al. [37] on the effects of 20 Gy in daily fractions over a 4-week period to the cervical, axillary, mediastinal para-aortic, and pelvic lymph node chains of splenectomized cynomolgus monkeys. Renal allografts were transplanted into the monkeys following the irradiation. The four controls (transplanted but not irradiated) died at 8–11 days. The five monkeys transplanted immediately post-irradiation died at 11–56 days, four were judged due to infections, and one to rejection. Two monkeys were transplanted at 3.5 weeks. One died at day 42 of transplant rejection and one was alive at day 394. Ed was Chief of Radiation Oncology, then Associate Dean at Duke, and now Dean of the University of Louisville Medical School.

8.3.1.14 Hyperthermia

J. Overgaard et al. in 1979 [68] investigated the response to hyperthermia of the immunogenic fibrosarcoma (methyl-cholanthrene induced) isotransplants in the foot pad and reaction of the normal tissues (foot immersion in a temperature-controlled water bath). The therapeutic ratio (minutes to achieve a TCD_{50} divided by the time to produce a specified severity of reaction in the normal tissues) was independent of the water bath temperature over the range 42.5–45.5°C for a

---

[4] TD_{50} is the number of cells that transplant tumor into half of the recipients.

severe level of reaction. The duration of hyperthermia to produce the defined end-point decreased steeply over that range. In contrast, for a low level of normal tissue injury the therapeutic ratio decreased very steeply with temperature, going to less than 1.0 at higher temperatures. Jens, a resident from Aarhus, Denmark, now directs the cancer research program at Aarhus University Medical Center. Willet et al. measured blood flow and hypoxic fraction in a spontaneous fibrosarcoma as a function of temperature over the range 18–46°C. Maximum blood flow and minimum hypoxic fractions were at 35°C [104].

8.3.1.15 Life Shortening by Doxorubicin

Zietman et al. [113] determined the life span of C_3H mice after single doses of doxorubicin that produced no acute mortality within 30 days. The mean life spans were 690, 580, and 350 days after 0, 5, and 10 mg/kg. This was one of the very few published studies at that time of late toxicity of a chemotherapeutic agent in an experimental animal system.

8.3.2 Edward Epp

Epp moved his laboratory from the Memorial Sloan-Kettering Cancer Center in New York City to new research space on the sixth floor of the Cox Building in 1975–1976. He has conducted a long line of basic biophysical and biochemical investigations in cellular radiation biology. Funding for this research was by an uninterrupted 30-year series of RO1 NCI grants, starting at Sloan-Kettering in 1964. His MGH team was comprised of C. Ling, K. Held, H. Michaels, A. Fuciarelli, and E. Clark. Additionally, he collaborated on several large experiments with L. Gerweck of the Steele Laboratory and J. Biaglow of the University of Pennsylvania. Kathy Held, who arrived at MGH in 1985, took over the leadership of the laboratory on Dr. Epp's retirement in 1997.

For Epp's research program, the pivotal experiment was the irradiation of E. coli B/r in thin layers by 600 keV electrons at 10^{10} Gy/s in 3×10^{-9} s pulses under different pO_2 levels in 1968. The finding was the series of bi-phasic cell survival curves as shown in Fig. 8.2. The break points in these curves occurred at progressively higher doses as pO_2 was raised, i.e., higher doses are required to use the available oxygen [23]. Their interpretation was that the "break point" indicated the dose at which the pO_2 had been decreased to hypoxic levels. The experimental plan was expanded to split dose assays to measure the rate of diffusion of oxygen into bacterial and mammalian cells. The first dose reduced pO_2 to severely hypoxic levels and the second dose was administered after very carefully timed intervals. As the time interval

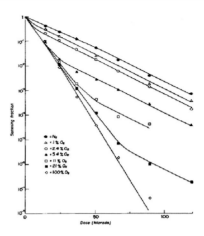

Fig. 8.2 Survival curves of E. coli B/r irradiated at extremely high rates under progressively lower pO_2 [23]

increased, oxygen diffused into the cells and radiation sensitivity increased sharply when the oxygen had diffused to the critical target(s). They found that sufficient oxygen diffused into the bacterial cell in $\sim 10^{-4}$ s to reach the critical target(s) and thereby modify radiation sensitivity. Similar experiments were performed on mammalian cells by Ling et al. in 1978 [57]. The diffusion time for CHO cells was $\sim 3 \times 10^{-3}$ s. For these exceptionally high-dose rate studies, a complex system for determining the absorbed dose was developed [58].

Michaels et al. (1981) demonstrated that the nitroimidazole compound misonidazole did sensitize CHO cells when exposed to the ultrahigh dose rate radiation but not at very low pO_2 levels [60]. Clark et al. found in 1983 that diamide sensitized CHO cells at low pO_2 levels by reducing shoulder [16]. At high diamide concentrations, the slope steepened in addition to shoulder reduction. Hydroxyl radicals secondary to radiolysis of water are an important component of the indirect effect of radiation, predominately by their reactions on DNA. Accordingly, a chemical strategy that reduces the extent of hydroxyl radical production or the life time of free hydroxyl radicals would reduce the effect of a defined radiation dose, viz., increase cell survival. The hydroxyl radical scavenger dimethyl sulfoxide at high concentrations was determined to be an effective radioprotective agent in severely hypoxic cells irradiated at ultrahigh dose rates as reported by Michaels et al. in 1983 [61]. Depletion of glutathione, the major non-protein sulfhydryl compound in mammalian cells, was predicted to increase the sensitivity of hypoxic tumor cells, viz., reduce the oxygen enhancement ratio (OER), provided aerobic cells were not affected by the compound. Radiation resistance of hypoxic cells constitutes a persistent constraint on success of radiation treatment for many tumors. There might well be a gain by strategies that deplete thiol levels of hypoxic cells selectively.

8.3.3 Leo Gerweck

Leo became a member of the laboratory research program in 1974 shortly after receiving his Ph.D. from Colorado State University with W. Dewey as his thesis advisor. For his Ph.D., he determined that sensitivity to hyperthermia increased inversely with pH. Further, at defined metabolic conditions, hyperthermic sensitivity was independent of pO_2. Additionally, S phase cells were of increased sensitivity to hyperthermia in contrast to their relative radiation resistance to radiation as shown by the paper with Dewey in 1977 [18]. Importantly, as solid tumors contain large fractions of hypoxic cells and those cells are at low pH levels, i.e., increased sensitivity to hyperthermia, there was a sound rationale to combine hyperthermia and radiation against human tumors judged or measured to have an important fraction of cells that are hypoxic. As we are aware, radiation is relatively quite effective against aerobic cells but much less so against hypoxic cells. See his papers of the early 1970s [31, 32]. This treatment strategy has not had serious clinical testing due to the great difficulty of achieving a known and reasonably uniform distribution of hyperthermia in human tumors.

Gerweck extended his studies on hyperthermia to determine the impact of pH on weakly acidic and weakly basic chemotherapy agents. The intra-cellular pH of tumor cells is similar to that for normal cells. In contrast, the extra-cellular fluid of tumors is more acid than that of normal tissues. He increased extracellular pH gradient in a tumor by 0.2 pH units. This caused the ratio of the chloroambucil to doxorubicin-induced delay in growth of tumor 54A in NCr/Sed/nu/nu mice to be increased by a factor of 2.1 as he reported in 2006 [33].

More recently, he has been quite active in the investigation of the role of radiation killing of tumor cells vs endothelial cells as determinants of tumor response. He and associates investigated a methylcholanthrene-induced sarcoma in SCID mice. The SCID mice are deficient in repair of DNA double-strand breaks and accordingly their normal tissues and tumors are more radiation sensitive than comparable tissues in normal mice by factors of 2–3. Gerweck et al. employed one cell line derived from a SCID sarcoma (sensitive) and two sub-lines that they had transfected with the repair gene DNA-PKcs. Thus, they had a sensitive cell line (DNA Pkse$^{-/-}$ negative) and two resistant cell lines (DNA Pkse$^{+/+}$), viz., FSC1−3 vs T53 and T43. The normal SCID cell line and the transfected cell lines differed in only one gene. The parent cell line, FSC1−3, was more sensitive than T53 and T43 cell lines in vitro by factors of 1.5 and 2.5. The tumor growth delay (TGD) for FSC1−3 tumors in NCr nu/nu mice was 1.5 that of T53. T43 was tested in SCID mice; the increase in TGD was by a factor of 2.1. They did not employ long-term local control as an end-point, but are currently examining this end-point. There was a similar ratio of tumor growth delay of transplants in NCr/Sed/nu/nu mice. These results were interpreted as indicating that tumor cell sensitivity and not the sensitivities of the stroma and capillary endothelial cells are the major determinants of tumor response in the reports of Gerweck et al. in 2006 [34] and with Ogawa et al. in 2007 [66].

8.3.4 Muneyasu Urano

Muneyasu joined the Steele Laboratory in 1977. For several years, his work concentrated on the biological effects of hyperthermia on mammalian cells in vitro and on murine normal and tumor tissues. Urano obtained an NIH RO1 grant within 18 months after joining the lab. He and colleagues published extensively on hyperthermia as a modifier of tumor and normal tissue responses to radiation, *C. parvum*, and several chemotherapeutic agents [96]. One of their findings was that a moderate increase in the temperature, e.g., to ~39°C significantly enhanced the effect of radiation and of alkylating agents. Muneyasu and team have investigated the impact of hyperthermia and chemotherapy on the radiation response of tumor and normal tissues in a series of papers, one being [95].

Urano et al. determined in 1980 and 1984 [94, 97] the RBE of the 160 MeV proton beam relative to ^{60}Co photons on these tissues of the C3Hf/Sed mouse: skin, small intestine, lens, lung, testes, tail vertebrae growth, and third-generation syngenic transplants of a mammary carcinoma and a fibrosarcoma. RBE values were 1.09–1.32.

He moved from MGH to a senior position at the University of Kentucky. After retirement, he began work as a part-time researcher with Dr. Clifton Ling and Gloria Li at Memorial Sloan-Kettering Cancer Center, NY.

8.3.5 Kathy Held

Prior to coming to MGH, Kathy had started work on the radiation chemical reactions between DNA and radioprotective thiols, work that she continued at MGH. At the MGH, she also began work emphasizing thiol-depleting agents and most especially thiol depletion of hypoxic cells. This work was performed in collaboration with Edward Epp of MGH and John Biaglow at the University of Pennsylvania. She and associates reported in 1988 that exposure of CHO cells to 5 mM dimethylfumarate (DMF) rapidly depletes intracellular glutathione by 90% in only 5 min resulting in a virtually complete reversal of sensitivity of hypoxic cells to that of aerobic cells [39]. Further the DMF was effective even when added very shortly after the irradiation [38].

In more recent times, Kathy has worked in a very imaginative collaboration with Barry Michael and Kevin Price from the Gray Cancer Institute in the UK in the study of the phenomena of bystander effects, viz., an effect by an irradiated cell on an unirradiated cell that is not necessarily in contact. This has resulted in several publications [73, 81].

Currently, Kathy has a large experiment in progress at the Brookhaven National Laboratory to assess the effects of space radiation on cells. This project is in collaboration with scientists of the MGH, principally H. Yang, and other institutions. She and her team have demonstrated the bystander effect (BSE) at doses lower than 10 cGy using 1 GeV protons, silicon, titanium, and iron ions. This BSE was found to be mediated by culture media, viz., the irradiated cells were not in contact with the unirradiated cells, and the effect was observed within 1 h of irradiation [110, 111]. Also in the studies with H. Yang and with A. Chakraborty of MGH, they have shown novel and important roles of reactive oxygen species in the BSE in several cell types. The work on BSE has been stimulated in part by the work at Columbia of Hall and Hei who demonstrated BSE by micro-beam irradiation of the cytoplasm. They found that the BSE included gene mutations.

With Bobby Redmond of MGH, Howard Liber of Colorado State, and Kevin Prise, Kathy's team has a large program to assess mechanisms for oxidative stress-induced damage in cells. They are using a unique live cell time lapse microscopy system to study timing of cell death, including apoptosis, in x-irradiated or photosensitizer-treated cells. Among several important findings, they have found that apoptosis may result from microbeam irradiation of an extremely small region of the cytoplasm, i.e., no part of the nucleus in the particle path, in both irradiated and bystander cells. This has provoked studies of the genetic pathways for apoptosis, viz., is direct damage to the DNA molecule required?

In a new effort, she and her team, especially H. Yang, have initiated studies of microbeam irradiation of model skin generated in vitro.

8.3.6 Peter Vaupel

Peter was recruited from the University of Mainz. He was the A. Werk Cook Professor of tumor biology. A clinical Fellow that came with him was Fred Kallinowski. They worked quite productively with P. Okunieff and getting results into the literature. After 2 years he returned to Mainz as the Professor and Chair of the Department of Pathophysiology of the Johannes Gutenberg University of Mainz.

8.3.7 Simon Powell

Simon was recruited in 1991 during a meeting at Lugano, Switzerland, when Suit heard him make a very fine presentation. Simon was very actively involved in the investigation of genetic factors that determine the repair of damaged DNA. He worked at the MGH for 11 years with research concentration on the role of P53, ATM, and BRCA1 in the kinetics, extent, and correctness of repair damage of DNA and the role of recombination. During his time here, he had three RO1 grants from the NCI and a total of eight M.D.–Ph.D. Fellows. Simon was also very active in clinical radiation oncology of breast carcinoma patients. He served as Director of the MGH Breast Cancer Center for a number of years.

Simon became Chief of Radiation Oncology at Washington University in St. Louis in 2004 and then moved to Memorial Sloan Kettering Cancer Center as Chief of Radiation Oncology in 2008.

8.3.8 Henning Willers

Henning joined the laboratory of Simon Powell as a postdoctoral fellow in November 1996. Over the ensuing $2\frac{1}{2}$ years, Henning's' work focused on the role of the tumor suppressor genes p53 and BRCA1 in the regulation of recombinational DNA repair, which is important for the maintenance of genomic stability and cell survival. These studies yielded several findings. The p53 gene, which has been mainly known to regulate cell cycle responses and apoptosis in response to genotoxic stress, limits the activity of homologous recombination, a major pathway for the repair of DNA double-strand breaks. This regulation is independent of p53's established function as a transcription factor, thus defining a novel regulatory role of p53. Similarly, p53 has a major role in regulating the fidelity of non-homologous end-joining. Together, these results have advanced the understanding of p53 as a protein with pleiotropic functions in the cellular response to DNA damage [17, 76, 89, 102]. Similarly, Zhang et al. discovered that the breast cancer susceptibility gene BRCA1 is involved in the regulation of homologous recombination and non-homologous end-joining [112, 117]. This was done in collaboration with Fen Xia [106]. In contrast to p53, BRCA1 promotes homologous recombination, suggesting that pro- and anti-recombinogenic factors exist to control the activity of DNA repair pathways. Thus, human cancers may harbor specific alterations in DNA repair depending on the particular gene mutations present. This has important implications for the effectiveness of much cancer therapeutics, including ionizing radiation, that kill tumor cells by damaging their DNA.

Following Powell's departure, Henning was appointed to the MGH Radiation Oncology faculty at the MGH in July 2005 to continue several of the DNA repair studies as a principal investigator. In collaboration with his home university in Hamburg, Germany (Jochen Dahm-Daphi), Henning has focused on the mechanisms of non-homologous end-joining, which is the major pathway for the repair of radiation-induced DNA breaks [80, 100]. These studies have utilized special plasmid substrates to model break repair in living cells. More recent translational research efforts are geared toward therapeutically exploiting altered DNA repair and pro-survival pathways in several tumor types, including lung and breast cancer, in collaboration with Lisa Kachnic [101] and Jeffrey Settleman (Center for Molecular Therapeutics at MGH).

8.3.9 Lisa Kachnic

Lisa has been active in the lab studies, effectively using her 1 day per week. This has been of high interest to her, but the expanding responsibilities at BMC requires that next year she devote all of her professional time to clinical issues.

8.3.10 David Kirsch

David developed model mouse soft tissue sarcoma systems that arise at the site of delivery of Cre recombinase. Approximately 20% of these sarcomas metastasize to lungs, not dissimilar to the figure for human soft tissue sarcomas. David et al. in 2007 [51] utilized these experimental tumors in evaluation of surgical, intraoperative molecular imaging and responses to radiation. These have been important to his genetic analyses of the molecular pathogenesis of sarcoma development. Ventura et al. in 2007 found that restoring normal p53 caused tumor regression in primary lymphomas and sarcomas in mice that lack p53 [98]. He also determined that the intrinsic pathway of apoptosis is not required for radiation killing of GI epithelial cells or endothelial cells in the GI syndrome.

Micro-CT to image primary lung cancers in mice has been employed by David in monitoring the response of pulmonary lesions to radiation therapy.

8.4 Rakesh Jain and the Steele Laboratory

8.4.1.a Rakesh Jain

Rakesh joined the department in 1991 and developed the Steele Laboratory. He brought with him three young scientists: Yves Boucher, Larry Baxter, and Bob Melder and Sylvia Roberge, a research technician. They promptly commenced an exceptionally productive and innovative research program. To employ experimental models that were defined genetically for special characteristics, Jain took two 2-week intensive courses in genetics, with heavy concentration on laboratory procedures. This facilitated the development of excellent working relations with Brian Seed and other geneticists at the MGH and outside laboratories. Jain and team now have a quite substantial array of mouse sub-lines with planned gene "knock out" and "knock in" for special studies.

During his 19 years here, Jain has vastly expanded his research team as is evident by Fig. 8.3. In addition to Rakesh, the Jain group now has three associate and four assistant professors and two instructors. Of major importance has been the energetic and creativity of the 10–20 post-doctoral fellows and 6–8 graduate students continuously. Significantly, he has had high yield collaborative research with clinicians within the department and with other departments. See Chapter 10 for clinical achievements.

His group has had extraordinary productivity as evidenced by a series of major advances in the understanding of the biology and physiology of normal and malignant tissues and their responses to radiation, drugs, and biologicals (immunological and genetic). The major focus has been on the basic tumor physiology, angiogenesis, and tumor vascular "normalization" after radiation, chemical and biological treatment. The concept of normalization of the vascular system originated with Jain. These researches have integrated remarkably elegant methods for quantitation of diverse physiological phenomena in genetically defined systems. Of

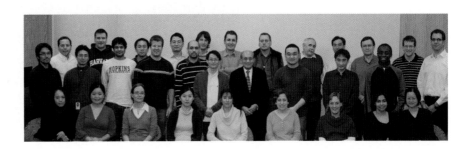

Fig. 8.3 Rakesh Jain and his laboratory research group at the MGH in 2006

special merit has been the extension of their findings to the design of clinical studies that have yielded quite positive patient outcomes, the *first* being for locally advanced rectal carcinoma.

The Steele Laboratory group's diverse investigations based on experimental animals and biomathematical model systems have resulted in a very large number of publications in the world's premier science journals. Consider that the laboratory has had 365 papers (peer reviewed, books, book chapters). Of special note are the 67 articles in very high impact journals, viz., *Nature* 7, *Nature Medicine* 19, other *Nature* journals 17, *Science* 5, *PNAS* 10, *Scientific American* 3, and other journals 6, an impressive record. One special note of this recognition is that of the soon to be published special issue of *Scientific American on Cancer*. Jain is the author of one of the 10 papers. Further, he has received grants from the NCI supporting this program (an Outstanding Investigator Grant, a PO1) and three of his staff have RO1 grants from the NCI. Thus, he and his team are recognized as one of the very top-ranked cancer biology research groups internationally.

A few of these research accomplishments by Jain and his team in the Steele Laboratories are mentioned here.

8.4.1.b Tumor Vessel "Normalization"

A major advance in tumor biology has been Jain's analysis and interpretation of extensive data on the anatomic and physiological changes in the vascular system in epithelial and mesenchymal tumors with growth and following certain treatments. There is a consistent pattern in untreated solid tumors in laboratory mice of progressive change from near normal vessel patterns in very small tumors to the quite abnormal capillary systems in larger tumors. Namely, the observed differences between capillary systems of tumors and normal tissues included decreased capillary number/unit of volume (increased inter-capillary distance), increased capillary length from arteriole to venule, large diameter, decreased flow rate (some instances of intermittent and even reverse flow); some portions of the blood flow track were without endothelial cells and the tumors had increased

interstitial pressure. The consequence of these abnormalities was accepted as clear evidence of decreasing nutrient availability and accordingly a related poor access of therapeutic agents to many regions of the tumor. One consequence of direct relevance to the radiation response is the development of regions of hypoxia. In many tumors these regions increase with tumor volume.

Jain observed that following treatment of some tumors with anti-angiogenic agents, the capillary system changes dramatically to one of more normal structure and function. He has designated this process "normalization" [44]. Contrary to standard wisdom, in many tumor systems anti-angiogenic agents reduce the number of capillaries but the remaining capillary system reverts to a quasi-normal functional status with a net gain in effective perfusion. For some tumors there is a gain in efficacy of radiation and chemotherapy. Jain and team have published a series of papers on the evidence for this concept. The *Scientific American* of January 2008 features a current summary article by Jain [45]. "Normalized" tumor vessels are shown in Fig. 8.4a, b. The tumor was an early generation transplant into a dorsal chamber of a syngenic C_3H mouse. The mouse was treated by daily injections × 3 of 40 mg/kg of DC101 (an anti-VEGFR-2). The image was taken at 5 days following the fifth dose.

Tong et al. [91] demonstrated that VEGF blockade effects a "normalization" of tumor vasculature yielding an improved nutrient perfusion and reduction in interstitial fluid pressure. This is a significant finding re the mechanism of the greater efficacy of certain therapeutic agents by use of multiple doses.

In a parallel study, Winkler et al. [105] observed that blocking VEGFR2 effects a "normalization" of the vascular system in a malignant brain tumor transplanted in mouse brain. During a relatively brief time "window" there is a substantially increased tissue pO_2. They reported that the hypoxic fraction fell from ~35 to 4%, but within 6 days had been partially reversed to ~15%. The clear implication is that the timing of administration of an additional treatment whose effectiveness is a function of pO_2 might well benefit by physiological monitoring during the course of treatment.

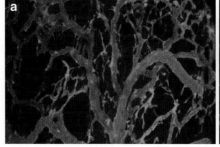 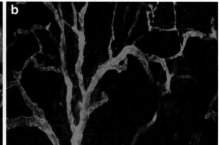

Fig. 8.4 (**a, b**) The grossly abnormal vessels of the tumor are exhibited on the *left* and the near-normalized vessels post-treatment on the *right panel*

Formation of stable blood vessels in vitro from umbilical endothelial progenitor cells (EPCs) and from peripheral blood and from human bone marrow mesenchymal stem cells (hMSCs) has been examined by Au et al. [2, 3]. Their finding was that the umbilical-derived EPCs could form stable (at least up to 4 months) vessels but not by peripheral blood EPCs. Further those derived from hMSCs were stable for the 4-month period also. Jain and Duda [47] found evidence of only a modest role of bone marrow-derived cells in the formation of endothelial cells of recurring tumors.

Perhaps the most impressive result from bench to bed research program by this department is that from the study of the efficacy of anti-angiogenic agents combined with radiation and chemotherapy in the treatment of locally advanced (T3-4) rectal cancer. The first and most dramatic clinical testing of this concept was the phase I clinical trial by clinician Chris Willett with Rakesh Jain and team of pre-operative treatment of locally advanced (T3-4) rectal carcinoma by bevacizumab, radiation (50.4 Gy in 5.5 weeks), and 5-FU followed by resection. In the initial report [103] responses of six patients were described. Five of the six had grossly complete response. All have had local control. Willett and Jain et al. treated 22 patients in this trial. Five patients had a complete pathological response. In 15 there were only scattered residual tumor cells in the surgical specimen and in two there were larger collections of residual tumor cells. Among these 22 patients, the 3-year actuarial results are 100, 100, and 91% for local control, overall survival, and disease-free survival, respectively (C. Willett, personal communication 2008). The wider potential of combining anti-angiogenic agents with radiation and/or chemotherapeutic agents has been assessed by Duda et al. [20].

Jain et al. reviewed the potential of anti-angiogenic agents in the management of patients with malignant tumors of the CNS [46]. Batchelor, di Tomaso, Duda, and others [4] have examined the response of the vascular system in recurrent glioblastoma multiforme (GBM) in 16 patients by the anti-angioenic agent AZD 2171. This is a tyrosine kinase inhibitor of VEGF receptors. The findings yielded evidence for a prompt but variable duration of normalization of the tumor vascular system. This was manifest by a rather sharp decrease in permeability index by the end of 4 weeks. In the absence of further treatment, the status soon reversed to the pre-treatment level. These findings have led to a phase III trial with AZD2171 as well as a number of studies with the AZD2171 combined with other agents.

Short summaries of selected additional accomplishments by faculty of the Steele Laboratory are given in the order that the faculty person joined the Steele Laboratory. These studies were conducted by faculty members and their post-doctoral fellows and graduate students.

8.4.2 Yves Boucher

Yves has had as his major area of concentration the increased interstitial fluid pressure (IFP) in solid tumors of experimental animals and human patients. His initial observations were made while at Carnegie Mellon University [8, 75]. In work with graduate students and post-doctoral fellows of the Steele Laboratory he has continued to unravel the complex mechanisms of this phenomenon and the impact on the efficacy of treatment by radiation, drugs, or biologicals. An unexpected finding was the absence of a clear correlation between IFP and pO_2 [9]. He has shown that tumor interstitial hypertension is associated with the development of angiogenesis [10] and the killing of tumor cells by radiation or taxanes reduces the intratumoral pressure [35, 115]. In other studies they demonstrated that the expression of vascular endothelial growth factor (VEGF) is a major cause of tumor interstitial hypertension [56]. Inhibition of VEGF signaling with blocking antibodies was found to increase the hydrostatic pressure difference across tumor vessels and the intratumoral penetration of large molecules [91].

Boucher has also done work on the effects of the tumor interstitial matrix on the transport of large molecules. With his colleagues they determined the rate of diffusion of macromolecules and liposomes in tumors as transplants in cranial window and dorsal chamber experimental systems [72]. The diffusion was significantly slower in the dorsal chamber model system. The slow diffusion was correlated with the increased level of collagen type I with organization into fibrils. In a subsequent study they showed that irradiation of a tumor was followed by a decreased hydraulic conductivity and an increase in collagen type I [116]. To overcome the transport hindrance imposed by the collagen in tumors, Boucher et al. tested the effects of the small hormone relaxin and bacterial and mammalian collagenases. The small hormone relaxin induced the modeling of collagen fibers by fibroblasts and improved the interstitial diffusion of large molecules in tumors [11, 72]. The remodeling of the interstitial/collagen matrix by bacterial and mammalian collagenases (matrix metalloproteinase-1, -8) improved the intratumoral penetration and anti-tumor efficacy of an oncolytic virus [59, 62].

Nagano et al. also reported that viral dispersion throughout a mouse mammary carcinoma was enhanced by tumor cell apoptosis induced by genetic manipulation or cytotoxic agents [64]. The induction of tumor cell apoptosis and void spaces lead to the formation of interstitial pathways, which facilitated the dispersion of large particles and virus. Kozin et al. [54] observed that growth rate of tumors regrowing after radiation treatment was slower than for the primary tumor. There was an associated reduced vascular density, more vessels with no perivascular cells, and an increased fibrillar collagen. Injection of the VEGF receptor blocking antibody, DC 101, resulted in a decrease in IFP and a 2.2 times longer growth delay than in primary tumors.

8.4.3 Lance Munn

Lance's research focuses on understanding the cellular mechanisms that control blood vessel formation and function in normal and pathological conditions. Current attention is directed toward development of original approaches for analyzing the diverse signals involved using novel imaging approaches, mathematical modeling, and microfabricated devices. A premise is that an endothelial cell responds to a few critical signals distributed spatially and produced dynamically in its neighborhood. Specific combinations of these signals are responsible for the full range of vessel function and remodeling including sprouting, pruning, lumen splitting, and anastomosis. The goal is to decipher these signals to identify new strategies for manipulating blood vessels in cancer and other pathologies.

Munn and group are also investigating the mechanisms of movement of tumor cells from the primary tumor into the blood or lymphatic vessels [63]. Despite the demonstrated large number of tumor cells that enter the vascular system on a daily basis, a very high proportion are killed by shear stress in the blood vessels and some are killed by the immune system. Further, the success in crossing the capillary wall at a distant site is low. To investigate this process, Munn and co-workers employed mouse kidney SN12C and a variant SN12CL1 (high frequency of metastasis) in an analysis of 23 genes judged to be involved in the metastasis process. Their finding was that the tumor cells that had gotten into the vascular system exhibited down-regulation of CD 44, alpha 3 integrin, and caveolin. Their findings were interpreted as consistent with the concept that CD44 and alpha 3 integrins suppress metastasis. Another important observation in this study by Bockhorn et al. was that the majority of cancer cells shed into the blood vessels were dead or dying [7]. Based on this finding, they proposed that tumor cells can get into the vascular system by being "pushed" through passive mechanisms, i.e., if even dead cells can enter the blood vessels, then active migration is not a prerequisite, and alternative, passive mechanisms must operate in some manifestations of metastasis [6].

To understand fully the physiology of blood vessels, Munn proposed that we must also understand the dynamics of the fluid that they carry. To this end, he has carried out pioneering analytical studies of how blood cells interact in flow [63]. Using state-of-the-art mathematical modeling and microfluidic devices, his group has shed light on how leukocytes and cancer cells interact with blood cells and with the blood vessel [7]. An extension of this work analyzed how blood cells redistribute in vessel networks in response to focal plasma leaks such as those seen in tumors. Sun et al. concluded that effective strategies to enhance tumor perfusion and drug delivery would be to reduce non-uniform plasma leakage and to inhibit leukocyte interactions and erythrocyte aggregations in capillaries [87]. This work has also led to novel technologies by Shevkoplyas et al. for separating blood cells for clinical applications [82].

8.4.4 Dai Fukumura

The long-term goal of Dai Fukumura's research is to uncover the fundamental nature of vascular biology in both physiological and pathophysiological settings and to utilize this knowledge for detection and treatment of a spectrum of diseases. Role of NO in tumor angiogenesis, microcirculation, and radiation therapy is a subject of major interest.

Nitric oxide (NO) is a highly reactive mediator with a variety of physiological and pathological functions [25]. NO increases and/or maintains tumor blood flow, decreases leukocyte–endothelial interactions, increases vascular permeability, and thus may facilitate tumor growth [29, 25, 49, 50]. Furthermore, NO mediates angiogenesis and vessel maturation predominantly through endothelial NO synthase [24, 49]. The Fukamura team recently found that creation of perivascular gradient of NO normalizes in part the structure and function of tumor vessels in human glioma xenografts in mice. As a result, tissue oxygenation and response to radiation therapy are improved [50]. Hagendoorn et al. also found that NO mediates lymphangiogenesis and metastasis (submitted) as well as function of lymphatic vessels [36, 55]. Role of tumor–host interactions in angiogenesis, tumor growth, and metastasis on tumor growth is assessed using transgenic mice harboring the green fluorescent protein (GFP) gene driven by vascular endothelial growth factor (VEGF) promoter. They found that VEGF promoter of nontransformed stromal cells is strongly activated by the tumor micro-environment [27]. Using tumor cells carrying the same gene construct Dai et al. and Xu et al. were the first to demonstrate that hypoxia and low pH independently up-regulate VEGF in vivo [28, 107]. Using VEGF$^{-/-}$ and wild-type ES cell-derived tumors, Tsuzuki et al. found that the host cells contribute approximately half of total VEGF production in this model [92]. Novel multiphoton laser scanning microscopy (MPLSM) allowed Brown et al. to observe deep inside the tumor at high spatial resolution; they found VEGF-expressing stromal cells closely associated with angiogenic vessels in the tumor [12]. Stroh et al. observed that the association of VEGF-expressing stromal cells spatially correlated with the extravasation of nanoparticles [84]. Furthermore, various anti-tumor treatments result in increased expression of host stromal cell VEGF and thus, Izumi et al. concluded that they may contribute to treatment resistance [43]. Their recent data indicate that stromal cells in the primary tumor travel with tumor cells and facilitate survival and growth of metastatic tumors (submitted). Finally, the study by Winkler et al. [105] and Kamoun et al. [48] indicated that the blockade of VEGF signaling can transiently normalize tumor vasculature and potentiate radiation therapy.

The inability to produce functional and lymphatic vessels is a major limitation of tissue engineering. First, they established in vivo system to investigate blood vessel formation during adipogenesis. Using genetic inhibition of PPARg and pharmacological inhibition of VEGFR2 signaling we found provocative reciprocal regulation of adipogenesis and angiogenesis, suggesting a novel strategy to treat obesity [26]. Next, Koike et al. established a model to monitor tissue-engineered blood vessels in vivo using MPLSM. The finding was that mesenchymal precursor 10T1/2 cells accelerate remodeling of 3D endothelial cell structure to functional blood vessels, differentiate into perivascular cells, and stabilize engineered vessel network for up to a year [52]. Au et al. and Wang et al. then showed that human ES cell, cord blood, and peripheral blood-derived endothelial cells form functional blood vessels in vivo using the tissue-engineered blood vessel model [2, 99]. Establishment of functional and stable blood vessels was advanced by the success of transplantation of human bone marrow-derived mesenchymal stem cells (hMSCs) that served as perivascular precursor cells [3].

8.4.5 Emmanuelle di Tomaso

An initial responsibility assigned to Emmanuelle was to set up the histopathology core due to her experience and knowledge of immunohistochemistry. Protocols were soon in place for staining for angiogenic markers, adding an additional technique to those in use in the Steele Lab. An important assessment was that for the character and extent of angiogenesis in the tissue samples from the Willett and Jain trial of Avastin plus chemotherapy, radiation, and surgery in the treatment of patients with locally advanced rectal carcinoma. She found that this anti-angiogenic therapy effected changes in microvascular density, vessel maturation, and tumor cells proliferation/apoptosis. Ultimately these data were the first clinical evidence of the normalization hypothesis put forward by Dr. Jain in 2001, i.e., anti-angiogenic therapy leads to improvement of vessels function, decrease in IFP, and better nutrient perfusion. This experience has been very positive and lead to Emmanuelle being part of the group that has developed some six protocols for clinical trials of several anti-angiogenesis clinical trials.

These include the trial by Bachelor and Jain and their teams on the effect of AZD2171, a tyrosine kinase inhibitor of the VEGFR on patients with recurrent glioblastoma [4]. The changes noted after this agent were similar to those observed earlier. Furthermore this trial gave her the opportunity to study the effect of long term treatment with AZD2171 on the tumor and adjacent tissue using autopsy material. She has been the first to report evidence of increased vessel co-option in human specimen in response to sustained anti-angiogenesis therapy. Her attention is currently directed to understanding the differences in angiogenic pathways between the benign Schwannoma (with the Plotkin group) and the high-grade CNS neoplasms. In particular her experience with immunohistochemistry lead to the identification of VEGF as a major player in NF2-related vestibular schwannomas. This prompted to treating some patients with recurrent schwannoma at risk for complete deafness with Avastin, which, ultimately turns out to be the first medical treatment with some improvement in all patients. This represents the first treatment to achieve hearing improvement in patients with recurrent vestibular schwannoma.

Earlier studies in the Steele laboratory indicated that there were gaps in tumor capillary "walls" due to missing endothelial cells over ~15% of the nominal "wall surface", i.e., the blood and plasma are in direct contact with tumor cells. To increase the accuracy of quantitation, Di Tomaso and associates employed CD31 and CD105 immunoreactivity and confocal microscopy for identification of endothelial cells in human colon cancer as orthotopic or ectopic xenografts. The score was 8 and 24% missing identifiable endothelial cells carrying these markers in the capillary walls, respectively [19].

In response to the observations of the importance of collagen to dispersal of macromolecules throughout a tumor [11]. She performed dynamic imaging of collagen and its modulation in tumors in vivo using second-harmonic generation. She participated in the development of a technique for estimating collagen content of tumors by a visual technique. This was proposed as a feasible means for assessment of collagen in the tumor as a factor to consider in treatment planning.

Emmanuelle has collaborated with Tyrrell and other faculty at Rensselaer Institute to model in 3D the tumor vasculature biomathematically. The Steele Laboratory uses intravital imaging with a multiphoton laser scanning microscope to investigate changes in tumor vasculature. These experiments result in images of the vessels over 200–300 μm depth. An accurate quantification of these images in 3D is prerequisite to a complete understanding of the vessel physiology. They developed cylindroidal superellipsoid models to allow quantification of the network. This is now used in every investigation of the Steele Laboratory to assess vessel length, diameter, and volume changes [93].

8.4.6 Dan Duda

Dan's central interest has been the origin and function of the endothelial cells that comprise capillaries of primary, recurring, and metastatic tumors. The endothelial cells of growing or recurring tumors may be derived, in part, from cells of the circulating blood or from bone marrow [47]. Quantitative studies by Duda demonstrated that the fraction of tumor capillary endothelial cells derived from peripheral blood or bone marrow to be variable and in most circumstances marginal. The magnitude varied with tumor type, tumor site, stage (primary or metastatic), and mouse strain and was most significant in brain tumors. These measurements were based on green fluorescent protein cell labeling, transparent window models, and intravital multiphoton laser scanning microscopy [21].

In local regrowth of irradiated tumors, the principal source of the blood-derived endothelial cells were myelo-monocytes (unpublished findings, 2008). Duda et al. [22] employed genetically labeled endothelial and other stromal cells in tumor fragments implanted into recipient mice. Endothelial cells became part of functional vessels and persisted for >4 weeks after transplantation, while the fibroblasts were gradually replaced by host cells.

Au et al. [2] achieved formation of stable and fully functional blood vessels in the mouse brain by endothelial progenitor cells derived from umbilical cord blood cells (more "primitive" cells) but not from adult blood cells (which had limited vasculogenic capacity due to rapid senescence). Another recent finding of Duda is that quantification of blood cells with endothelial cell markers appears to provide the basis for prediction of response to anti-angiogenic agents of advanced rectal carcinomas, recurrent glioblastomas, and hepatocellular carcinomas [4, and unpublished data, 2008]. This lead is being pursued in multiple NCI-supported trials [20].

8.4.7 Tim Padera

Tim pioneered the use of intravital multiphoton laser scanning microscopy [70] to image lymphatic vessels and study their function. They determined that lymphatic vessels found in solid tumors are non-functional [69]. The next finding was that a primary reason for non-functional intratumor lymphatic vessels is the compressive force generated by proliferating cancer cells, causing the collapse of intratumor lymphatic vessels [71]. The finding that intratumor lymphatic vessels are non-functional created a paradox, as it is known that tumors spread to lymph nodes through lymphatic vessels during the normal growth phase of tumor. Tim showed that altering the morphology and function of lymphatic vessels

surrounding the tumor could change the rate of lymphatic metastasis, implicating these vessels in the spread of cancer to lymph nodes. VEGF-C increased the arrival of cells in the peripheral lymph vessels. Further, blocking the VEGF-C receptor abrogated this effect [40]. By understanding that the lymphatics in the tumor margin are sufficient for lymphatic spread, these vessels have become targets for cancer therapies under development.

Nelson and Padera [65] completed transcriptional analyses of cultured endothelial cells of blood vessels and lymphatic vessels to examine for a genetic basis for the differences in appearance and function of the two categories of cells. They identified several new molecules associated with the blood vessel-derived cell lines, e.g., claudin-9, neurexin-1, neurexin-2, and neuronal growth factor regulator-1. In the lymph vessel-derived cell lines, they identified claudin-7, CD58, hyluronan, HALPLN1. These basic new findings do provide increased understanding of the cell and perhaps a basis for an advance in therapy or diagnosis. One subject of interest of Tim has been the near absence of intratumoral lymphatics vessels within the tumor mass, but exist in abundance at tumor periphery. VEGF-C does stimulate lymphangiogenesis at the periphery but not within the tumor mass.

8.4.8 Lei Xu

Lei Xu determined that reduced extracellular pH increased vascular endothelial growth factor in glioblastoma cells by way of the ERK1/2 MAPK pathway [107]. Xu has investigated the role of and the levels of PLGF (placenta growth factor) in angiogenesis and tumor growth. Xu and group showed that over-expression of PLGF suppresses growth of tumor and metastasis. She and Jain determined the level of PLGF in lung and colorectal tissues plus 45 cell lines (22 human lung cancers, 11 colorectal cancers, and 12 cell lines of diverse origin). PLGF was low in the lung and colorectal cancer tissue and cell lines. They found that the PLGF gene promoter is methylated and this is an important factor in the low rate of PLGF expression in these tumors and probably to the aggressiveness of these tumors. Namely, demethylation by treatment with 5-Aza-dc returned the PLGF expression toward normal [108]. Blocking platelet-derived growth factor-D/platelet-derived growth factor receptor beta signaling inhibits human renal cell carcinoma progression in an orthotopic mouse model [109].

8.4.9 Igor Garkavtsev

To investigate the exceptional angiogenesis observed in glioblastomas, Igor and team studied the tumor suppressor gene ING4 in glioblastoma. A major finding was that ING4 is reduced in glioblastoma tissue relative to tissue of normal brain. Of additional interest, ING4 levels declines with progression in malignancy, viz., glioma grade [30]. Recently, Igor has changed research focus to high-throughput screening for effective anticancer biological agents. Part of this effort has involved an ongoing collaboration with the Partners core facility in Cambridge, which has a library of some 120,000 chemical compounds. He now judges that he has a few compounds that show anticancer effect.

His search was for compounds that block focal adhesive kinase activity. The question is "does the blockage of focal adhesive kinase activity suppress metastatic activity"? He now has identified some compounds that destroy blood vessels in the zebra fish model and is investigating the mechanisms.

8.5 Biographical Sketches, Arranged Alphabetically[5]

8.5.1 Yves Boucher

Yves Boucher, French Canadian, was born in New Brunswick, Canada, on the border with the province of Quebec (Fig. 8.5). He comes from a literary family where his father was a teacher of French language and literature, and history. His mother, also a teacher, taught English and French. Based on his readings, he became fascinated with the concepts of Freud and elected to major in psychology when he entered Moncton University in New Brunswick. However, after several courses in psychology he did take courses in biology and decided that he much preferred the harder science of biology.

This led to a change in career plans toward medical school or a research degree in a science field. He was very powerfully stimulated by a course in histology/cytology that dealt

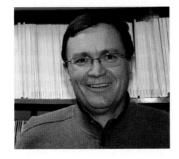

Fig. 8.5   Yves Boucher

with new aspects of cellular structure. He decided to enter a research program for a master's degree in experimental pathology and had to decide between a research or a medical future. He elected the Ph.D. research program. Yves became interested in the function of the lymphatic system and the mechanisms regulating the transport of water and proteins in the interstitial space and across the wall of lymphatic vessels.

In 1985, at a meeting in Oxford to present his research findings he met Rakesh Jain. After listening to Rakesh Jain's presentation on tumor pathophysiology, he approached Dr. Jain about a postdoctoral fellowship in his lab; the response was positive and with a fellowship from the Canadian Government he commenced work in the Department of Chemical Engineering at Carnegie Mellon University in Pittsburgh. At that time, he was quite involved in the measurements of tumor interstitial fluid pressure in patients and the study of the mechanisms of interstitial hypertension in solid tumors. In Pittsburgh, Yves worked with Larry Baxter, a graduate student doing biomathematics who had developed a mathematical model that yielded evidence for a flat or uniform interstitial pressure throughout the tumor mass but a sharp decline across the tumor edge. This was contrary to prior thinking and also to some limited published data. Yves and Larry confirmed with glass micropipette measurements that that there was a relatively flat pressure level across the tumor volume in accord with the model. Yves was also involved in making the first interstitial pressure measurements in human tumors. They found that the pressure within carcinomas of the uterine cervix and malignant melanomas was elevated in most cases with most being in the range of 15–60 mmHg vs near zero in most normal human tissues.

In 1991, he came to the MGH to work with Larry Baxter and Robert Melder to start the Rakesh Jain group in the Steele Laboratory. His wife, Sylvie Roberge, was and continues as a member working as a senior technician.

While in Pittsburgh he had completed studies which demonstrated that the pressure inside blood vessels of a tumor was similar to the interstitial fluid pressure in the center of a tumor. This project was completed and published in *Cancer Research* after his move to Boston. During his time at the Steele Laboratory, Yves served as an advisor to several graduate students and post-doctoral fellows, which he greatly enjoys. Another happy development of his work has been the involvement in anti-angiogenesis clinical trials based on ideas and concepts generated from laboratory studies by the Jain group.

Yves has been successful in obtaining independent financial support. In 2003 he received his first NCI RO1 and this was to evaluate the hypothesis that the induction of tumor cell apoptosis would improve the delivery of large therapeutic agents in tumors.

---

[5] The biosketch of Epp is in Chapter 5 and that of Suit is in Chapter 4.

8.5.2 Emmanuelle di Tomaso

Emmanuelle di Tomaso (Fig. 8.6) became a member of the Steele Laboratory group in 1998 after a complicated path. She commenced life in the famous Cote d'Azur region of France. An outstanding teacher in high school provided the first serious stimulus for her interest in the sciences. There she concentrated on biology, math, physics, and chemistry. She entered The University Claude Bernard in Lyon with a major in biology and biochemistry. As an aside, Lyon is recognized as the culinary capitol of France. The university degree program is usually of 3 years.

Due to the clear need of high level of skills in reading and speaking English for a career in science she had to have special education. To aid in this, she attended Kingston University in England resulting in a French and an English bachelors degree. She elected to stay in London for a Ph.D. research degree. Her supervisor was Prof. Magnus Hjelm at the Great Ormond Street Hospital, the famous pediatric hospital of the UK. She was in the very large department of metabolic diseases. This was her first appreciation of the existence of serious science in clinical biology. This added a special pleasure to the research effort by the knowledge of the clinical context. The title of her thesis was "Analysis of isoenzymes and isoforms of human alkaline phosphatase, hexosaminidase and transferrin, by microcolumn chromatography."

The goal was to develop technology to achieve protein separation from very small plasma samples, viz., ~50–100 ml from the new born patients. She was studying primarily CDGS or carbohydrate-deficient glycosylation syndrome. Her work resulted in a paper in *Lancet*. This was followed by joining a laboratory in San Diego concentrating on the pharmacology of endogenous cannabinoids, anandamide. This was at the Neuroscience Institute, headed by Nobel Prize winner Dr. Gerald Edelman. The whole focus of the NSI is to understand the biological foundation of consciousness. Emmanuelle wished to do fundamental research. One paper in *Nature* was on the addictive effect of chocolate. However, within 1.5 years she realized that her central interests were in more clinical research.

For this she moved to Hong Kong to work with her Ph.D. advisor who had become the head of Chemical Pathology Department at the Prince of Wales Hospital, teaching hospital of The Chinese University of Hong Kong (CUHK). There she focused on brain biochemistry. She decided that angiogenesis was the area of her most serious interest. Then at the annual AACR conference in New Orleans she met R. Jain. He invited her for an interview in Boston. She was offered a position by Jain by phone and quickly accepted.

This was her third post-doctoral position and the opportunity to learn about and investigate angiogenesis and drug delivery was powerfully appealing. She very much enjoyed the work with Willett and Jain on patients with advanced rectal cancer. This extended later to the studies on recurrent glioblastomas with Batchelor and Jain. This has now extended further to six additional clinical trials.

Emmanuelle really loves the laboratory research but not the Boston winters. On a clearly positive note is that she has married Lance Munn and they are greatly enjoying this laboratory, the medical/academic centers, and the city

8.5.3 Dan Duda

Dan Duda: Dan's parents were his main source of inspiration for pursuing a career in medicine. Both were outstanding physicians and teachers. Dan (Fig. 8.7) is a native of Lasi, Romania. His undergraduate work was at the Lasi University of Medicine. For his Ph.D. program, he ventured far from home; viz., in 1997 he applied for and received a Monbusho Graduate Research Fellowship from the Japanese Government to study tumor biology. He won his Ph.D. degree in Medical Science from Tohoku University Graduate School of Medicine in Sendai, Japan, in 2001, 1 year ahead of schedule. Tohoku is ranked among the top five medical schools in Japan.

Dan joined Dr. Jain's team after graduation in May 2001. He has worked closely with Jain and numerous collaborators within and outside the laboratory. The work in the Steele Laboratory is focused on the role of bone marrow-derived cells in tumor growth and relapse and has resulted so far in 16 original reports in high-impact journals.

His work is supported by individual grants from the Cancer Research Institute and the AACR and by grants from the NCI to Drs. Jain, Willett, Batchelor, and Rocco, on which he is co-investigator.

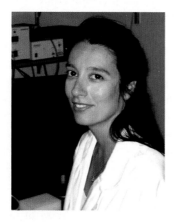

Fig. 8.6 Emmanuelle di Tomaso

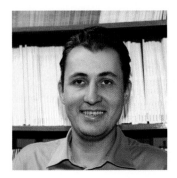

Fig. 8.7   Dan Duda

Dan's plan is to pursue a career as a researcher within the unique academic environment of Massachusetts General Hospital and Harvard Medical School. His ambitions are non-trivial, viz., to assemble a world-class research laboratory to train post-doctoral fellows and graduate students with the major goal being to elucidate the molecular and pathophysiological underpinnings of human tumor angiogenesis and metastasis and translate them to new therapies.

8.5.4 Dai Fukamura

Dai Fukamura (Fig. 8.8) had his childhood within a medical environment, as his father owned and operated a small private hospital in Yokohama with the family living in a residential quarter of the hospital building. Additionally, his father had served earlier as an assistant professor of internal medicine at Yokohama City University, School of Medicine. That Dai as a very bright boy became interested and involved in medicine was not unexpected. He enjoys the fact that although he is at present working full time in laboratory research it is in a hospital department within the main hospital building. As soon as he reached the age for university, he took and passed the entrance exam for medical school and entered Keio University School of Medicine, the oldest private university

in Japan, located in Tokyo. Keio University recently celebrated its 150th anniversary in 2008. Incidentally, the image on the 10,000 Yen bill (the highest denomination in Japan) is Yukichi Fukuzawa, founder of Keio. Mr. Fukuzawa opened Keio University during literally civil war, Meiji Restoration, and was known to continue his class under the artillery fire. Keio's school symbol represents its school philosophy – the pen is stronger than the sword.

Dai graduated in 1989 and took an Internal Medicine residency program, viz., the path of his father. Despite the family tradition in clinical medicine, after 1 year of the residency, Dai decided to pursue a Ph.D. program with Professor Masaharu Tsuchiaya, Chair of Gastroenterology. One of the professor's special research interests was microcirculation. This was intriguing to Dai and especially the potential of intravital microscopy. During 4 years of his Ph.D. study, Dai had studied the microcirculation in the stomach, liver, intestine, and mesentery following injury due to ischemia–reperfusion or endotoxin, as well as the roles of nitric oxide and endothelins. Additionally, he investigated the role of nitric oxide on host defense mechanism against metastasizing tumor cells in the liver sinusoid. Dai presented this latter work to the first Asia Congress on Microcirculation. There he met Rakesh K. Jain. This went very well and shortly Dai was invited to join the Steele Laboratory. He gladly accepted the invitation due to his interest in tumor microcirculation study and the well-known expertise of Jain and his laboratory in this field.

Dai joined Steele Laboratory in May 1994 and soon he obtained a Whitaker Foundation fellowship. Subsequently, he won an NCI R01 research grant. In addition he is a Project/core leader in Jain's P01 grant, and a leader of sections of other grants such as two BRP grants, viz., his work is very well recognized. Dai's long-term goal "is to uncover the fundamental nature of vascular biology in both physiological and pathophysiological settings and to utilize this knowledge for detection and treatment of diseases."

Teaching and mentoring post-doctoral fellows and graduate students has also been successful. This is evident by their publications in *Nature*, *Nature Medicine*, and *Journal of Clinical Investigation* as well as awards from NIH, DOD, Howard Hughes Medical Institute, American Association for Cancer Research, Institute for Cancer Research, Susan Komen Foundation, Deutsche Forschungsgemeinschaft, La Ligue Nationale Contre le Cancer, and Japanese Ministry of Health and Welfare.

Dai met with his wife Takako, a talented pianist and cembalo player, when Dai participated in a chorus performing Verdi's requiem. She was the pianist of that chorus. They married later and have one son (Taichi) and two daughters (Yoko and Yuriko). All of their children are young musicians and playing violin, piano, and cello, respectively. Taichi and Yuriko had a concert with Yoyo Ma recently.

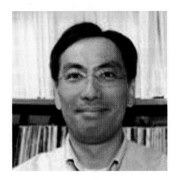

Fig. 8.8   Dai Fukamura

8.5.5 Igor Garkatsev

Igor Garkatsev (Fig. 8.9) comes from a small republic of the former USSR, close to Afghanistan. As a youth he moved to Moscow. His mother had the dominant influence on his career decisions. She is a Professor at the Cancer Research Center in Moscow and has a clinical genetics lab. They had frequent discussions about biology, medicine, and science. Interestingly, his memory of high school is not about science lectures or labs but a teacher of art who arranged for many visits to the first-class museums in Moscow and exceptional collections of impressionist paintings.

Igor was admitted to Moscow Medical University and graduated in 1983. Igor worked as a post-doctoral fellow at the Medical Institute and the Institute of Medical Genetics on *Drosophila*. This progressed to population genetics. Igor was a member of a team that went on an expedition to a small community near the Caspian Sea to investigate a very high incidence of Ehlers-Danlos syndrome, a collagen-related disease, and found a chromosomal linkage for this syndrome. He received his Ph.D. at the Cancer Research Center in Moscow in 1986. Igor's advisor was Andrei Gudkov who is now Vice President of Roswell Park Cancer Research Institute. His Ph.D. thesis was titled "Structural analysis of human ribosomal genes."

Igor met James Watson and described some of his experiments and was invited to come to the laboratories at Cold Spring Harbor. Igor worked there for 3 years, two determining the physical map of a yeast genome. Later he worked 1 year in Bethesda on computer analysis of whole genomes and protein structures. During that time he communicated with R. Jain and subsequently was invited to join the Steele Laboratory team and contribute in molecular biology and genetics. An initial task was to participate in the development of a fundamental understanding of angiogenesis. Together with Dr. Jain they discovered a new tumor suppressor gene involved in regulation of angiogenesis during development of glioblastomas, published in *Nature*.

In 2006, he began screening chemical compounds for effective anticancer biological agents. Working with the Partners core facility in Cambridge, he has screened a library with 120,000 chemical compounds to identify ones that block metastasis. He is now characterizing a few of these compounds that have some anticancer effect.

The favorite extra-curricular activity of Igor and his wife is hiking, especially in the White Mountains.

8.5.6 Leo Gerweck

Leo Gerweck (Fig. 8.10) hails from the very small town of Cheyenne Wells on the high plains of eastern Colorado, about 160 miles east of the Rockies. As a youngster he spent most summers as a farm laborer with typical working hours of 7:00 AM to dark. He also leased land, built a barn, and raised chickens and pigs during his high school years. These experiences clarified for Leo that he most certainly did not want to work as a hired-hand, but rather have a career that provided independence and the opportunity for problem solving. He succeeded in gaining admission into Regis College, a Jesuit institution in Denver, Colorado as a major in Biology with two minors, philosophy and chemistry. After graduation he spent 2 years as a graduate student in anatomy at the University of Colorado Medical School. At that point he decided to become a scientist and was admitted into graduate school at Colorado State University. There he was awarded a master's degree in Radiation Health Physics, and then a Ph.D. in radiation biology, with Bill Dewey as his advisor. There he met and interacted with Ed Gillette, a veterinarian radiation oncologist, and Mort Elkind, the first to quantitate on cells in vitro the kinetics of repair of sub-lethal radiation damage. Leo recalls that he was stimulated to come to the MGH following a lecture by H. Suit given at CSU.

During his initial years of research he showed by in vitro studies that low pH but not hypoxia enhanced the sensitivity of cells to hyperthermia. Gerweck became a member of the laboratory research program in 1974. He then studied pH levels in tumors and observed that pH declines as volume increases, viz., the more acidic lesions. As hypoxia increases with tumor volume and thus reduces the effectiveness of radiation but does not alter tumor cell's response to

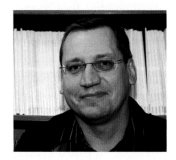

Fig. 8.9 Igor Garkatsev

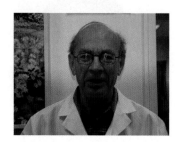

Fig. 8.10 Leo Gerweck

hyperthermia, he was interested in the combination of radiation and hyperthermia. This is potentially of serious clinical interest. However, at present the technology is not available to produce known and desired distribution of hyperthermia in human tissues. This has resulted in minimal clinical interest in hyperthermia. He is pursing other lines of study. Currently he is expanding his studies on the relative importance of tumor cell and capillary/stroma cell sensitivity on tumor control probability. He was recently a research fellow at the Cancer Center in Dresden, GE. Leo has had a number of post-doctoral fellow, residents and medical students working on projects. Additionally, he has been a regular lecturer in the course on radiation biology for the residents.

8.5.7 Kathy Held

Kathy Held (Fig. 8.11) became highly competitive as one of five children. Her home was in western Pennsylvania. Her mother was a school teacher and her father was employed by a steel company. The only member of her extended family that had any formal education in medicine or science was a physician whom Kathy held in very high regard. She became very interested in medicine and was contemplating medicine as a career when she entered college and majored in chemistry as a part of her pre-med program.

Kathy attended Theil College, a Lutheran school, with about 1200 students. Although small, the professors were very dedicated teachers. A chemistry professor, Richard Bennett, gave strong encouragement for her to follow chemistry. During her senior year Bennett urged that she go to the Argonne National Laboratory in Chicago. This she did and had a very stimulating year in the laboratory of radiation biologist Mort Elkind of split dose recovery fame. Tong Han, her advisor, convinced her that she had substantial future in basic science. She so enjoyed her time at Argonne that she decided to continue research as a Ph.D. student and not pursue medicine.

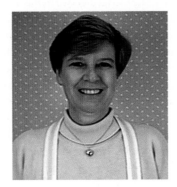

Fig. 8.11 Kathy Held

Kathy learned of the program of Larry Powers at the University of Texas at Austin and elected to go there for her graduate studies. She started in 1975 and her project was to examine "The Transforming DNA in Bacteria." Her program was to assay the effects of radiation-induced chemical changes in DNA by putting the irradiated DNA into bacterial cells and then determining alterations in their genetic characteristics. During her graduate studies she met and interacted with Barry Michaels and Jack Fowler from the Gray Laboratory at Mt Vernon, near London, one of the main centers in radiation biology in the world.

Kathy received a post-doctoral fellowship for 2 years of study at the Gray Laboratory. There was a quite impressive group of talented scientists, viz., Julie Denekemp, Adrian Begg, Anna Marie Rojas, Peter Wardman, Fiona Stewart, David Dewey. In addition, Kathy got to know and interact with Tikvah Alper and Jed Adams. Tikvah was a very impressive character as well as a significant scientist and did serve as a role model for young Kathy. Tikvah proved to be quite helpful, encouraging, and positive.

At the Gray Lab, Kathy worked with Barry Michael while continuing her studies of transforming DNA molecules particularly looking at radiation-induced chemical interactions between DNA, thiols, and oxygen. Several of the special techniques that she became familiar with were "Gas Explosion Technique" and "Rapid Mixing Technique" utilized in studies of the reaction of oxygen on DNA in very short time frames.

She moved from the Gray Lab to her first appointment as an independent researcher at the Mayo Clinic. There she continued her study of the mechanisms of action of thiols as modifiers of radiation response and began to work with mammalian cells. She obtained an NCI RO1 grant funding. Her research was combined with teaching of residents and technology students. After only a short while at Mayo she was invited by Ed Epp to join the group at the Massachusetts General Hospital. Kathy came to the MGH in 1985 and continued studies of thiol-depleting agents and oxygen in the Epp group. She also interacted productively with the research of the J. Biaglow team of the University of Pennsylvania and continued collaborative research with the Gray Laboratory group.

At present she is studying the by-stander effect and investigating the radiation biology of very heavy ions at the Brookhaven Laboratory.

8.5.8 Peigen Huang

Peigen Huang (Fig. 8.12) is a native of Guangdong, China, and is a member of an extended and well-educated family. There were no family members in science or medicine.

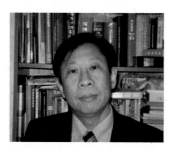

Fig. 8.12 Peigen Huang

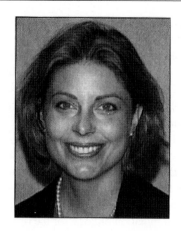

Fig. 8.13 Lisa Kachnic

His parents wanted "this gap filled" and encouraged young Peigen to pursue medicine or science. He rather easily became interested in the plight of those with illness and began study for admission to medical school. He was successful and graduated easily. For his specialization, he selected pathology hoping to contribute to understanding of human diseases. He was appointed to the faculty of the medical school and worked there for 10 years in research, teaching in addition to clinical pathology. Then he applied to the MGH and was accepted to a post-doctoral fellowship. He moved here in 1992 as a member of Suit's group and worked for 3 years. During his time his research resulted in six papers in referred journals. He then had a 1-year post-doctoral fellowship in Vancouver with Ralph Durand. Peigen returned to China to fulfill the service requirement to his country and then came back to Canada and worked for a biotech company for 2 years. He wished to return to the MGH. Jain engaged him as the Director of the DFPF mouse colony. He arrived back here in 2000 and has functioned extremely well in that capacity. He was aided by his knowledge of pathology and his research experience at MGH, Vancouver, and his medical school in China.

This large colony is operated with an excellent esprit and efficiency that results in abundant numbers of these most special mice. He not only operates the colony but participates in experiments.

8.5.9 Lisa Kachnic

Lisa Kachnic (Fig. 8.13) spent her childhood in Yonkers, NY, where she was educated through high school. She has a fascinating family history in that she has one brother who is 8 years her junior, but is a rock musical star. Lisa was among the first in her extended family to achieve a college education. She received a full scholarship to a Catholic high school outside of Yonkers and there became fascinated by science and creative writing. In fact, one of her career goals at the time was to become a science reporter. She decided to combine her interest in writing and science in a medical career. She

received a full scholarship to Boston College and Tufts medical school and graduated from medical school with no debt.

At Boston College she began a study of the gangliocide profile of glioblastoma in vivo and in vitro employing molecular and biochemistry techniques. This continued over 6 years, i.e., well into her medical school years. At Boston College she was very well recognized with a series of academic awards and was elected to be the Scholar of the College Program in her fourth year. She did spend a small amount of time in creative writing and had "a few detective stories (always with a science or laboratory spin) published in magazines." One of her fellow medical school students had family member in radiation oncology and was able to inform Lisa of the attractive features of radiation oncology as a career. Because of this interaction she was introduced to Hywel Madoc-Jones and Dave Wazer. Wazer actually became one of her medical school mentors. During that time and because of her interest in prostate cancer she was introduced to Bill Shipley. She elected to have her residency at the MGH. The opportunity of working with Shipley and Zietman with whom she did bladder cancer research and achieved two publications is a special point of pride. Gastrointestinal neoplasms fascinated her and she worked with Chris Willett on this. Additionally, she did an elective in the Steele Laboratory on a study of the immunological status of nude mice. She was especially pleased to have had the opportunity of working with Simon Powell on laboratory investigations.

At the completion of her residency, she selected the Medical College of Virginia where she was able to concentrate particularly on GI oncology and initiate her laboratory program. Lisa was invited to return to Boston as Chief at Boston University Medical Center when Delaney moved for full-time position at MGH. She has enjoyed this program very much and especially the one full day a week of time to work in the Steel Laboratory on repair of damaged DNA with S. Powell and H. Willers.

Lisa has been Chief at BUMC for 8 years and has recently seen the completion of a major new expansion with very impressive facilities with all the equipment being new, including two state-of-the-art image-guided therapy linear accelerators with cone beam and both cranial and extra-cranial radiosurgery capabilities. Additionally, there is a new high-dose brachytherapy suite and a Cyberknife machine.

Kachnic has worked with the national cooperative groups RDOG and SWOG. This is in addition to in-house studies on pancreas, esophagus, rectal, and anal cancers. Currently, she is serving as a national PI on a large phase II RTOG examining IMXT for anal cancer with the goal of decreasing dermatological toxicity that follows current by radiation and chemotherapy methods. Further, she has achieved two Centers of Excellence Grants with a total of approximately $11 M from the DOD for new image-guided and radiosurgery technologies. She is very much involved in the International Society of Gastrointestinal Oncology and was invited to be a candidate for presidency of the organization. Both she and Henning Willers have obtained independent funding and were able to continue their work on the repair of DNA even though Simon Powell had left.

8.5.10 David Kirsch

David Kirsch (Fig. 8.14) was born in Pietermaritzburg, South Africa. His family immigrated to the USA. David received his B.Sc., *summa cum laude*, from Duke University. Then he was awarded a Ph.D. and an M.D. from Johns Hopkins in 2000. During his residency at MGH (2001–2005) he commenced laboratory research and continued this intensively

through his time as staff radiation oncologist through August 2007. David was very productive of innovative laboratory research. Tyler Jacks at MIT was very supportive and provided David with lab space and some technical support. His time was on the basis of half time in the research laboratory at MIT and half time in the clinical sarcoma program with T. DeLaney.

8.5.11 Rakesh Jain

Rakesh Jain (Fig. 8.15) immigrated to this country after graduating with a B.S. in chemical engineering from one of the five founding Indian Institutes of Technology (IIT). These are intensely competitive institutions. Rakesh states that there were ~100,000 high school seniors taking the high school examinations in his state and that he ranked fourth among the ~100,000 students. IIT colleges are regarded internationally as first-class universities. They do educate extremely well a very small fraction of Indian students. Rakesh judges that this system of some absolutely first-class institutions of higher learning is one of the most significant of contributions to India by Nehru, India's first Prime Minister.

Rakesh started life in favorable circumstances, viz., first born and a son in an educated and prosperous family with parents who were absolutely devoted to their 10 children. For grades 1–5, he attended a local Catholic school, grades 6–8 a local middle school, and then transferred to a high school some 300 miles distant. He decided at a relatively young age that his career was to be an engineer reflecting his real joy in science, especially chemistry, math, and physics. He fortunately was admitted into an IIT Kanpur School of Engineering. After 5 years of study, he graduated with a degree in chemical engineering in 1972. For graduate study, the recommendation was that he go to the USA. He was admitted to the University of Delaware Department

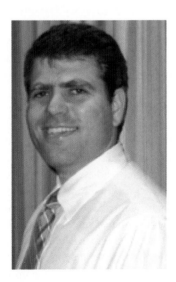

Fig. 8.14 David Kirsch

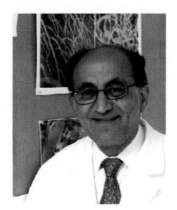

Fig. 8.15 Rakesh Jain

of Chemical Engineering on a fellowship. The faculty and facilities in chemical engineering were rated as among the top internationally. Not incidentally, this university was located very close to the Du Pont Chemical Company headquarters and they supported the chemical engineering program generously.

For his first study problem as a graduate student, he generated a mathematical model of the estuary of the Delaware River for control of the level of pollution. When considering the project, he talked with a Professor Wei (later Chair of Chemical Engineering at MIT and then Dean of Princeton School of Engineering) who asked of Rakesh's interest in biology. Rakesh had not studied biology. Even so, Wei gave him a copy of Guyton's textbook of human physiology and suggested that he read it with care. Guyton, a graduate of Harvard Medical School was the professor of physiology at the University of Mississippi. His book was for many years the highest rated physiology text for US medical students. Rakesh immediately became interested in physiology and the potential of study with an analytical approach. Professor Wei took him to the NCI to meet Dr. Pietro Gullino, who was chief of the Laboratory of Pathophysiology, and to observe his novel approach for studying tumor physiology. He had developed a model in which a small tumor grew in the rat supplied by a single artery and vein. Importantly for Rakesh's purposes, this allowed quantitative measurement of the input to the tumor and the output from the tumor. This appeared to be a superb model system for a chemical engineering approach. Thus, Rakesh enthusiastically adopted this model for his Ph.D. thesis project, viz., measuring the uptake of a drug by the tumor and performing biomathematical analyses of the process. This was a relatively unexplored area of study for engineers and even cancer researchers.

He received his Ph.D. in 1976 and Columbia University accepted him on their Faculty of Chemical Engineering. Starting in 1976, he taught chemical engineering courses such as thermodynamics, but he had no serious encouragement to pursue cancer research. Even so, he obtained NSF (National Science Foundation) funding and commenced cancer research in heat transfer and hyperthermia. This was of interest to the Carnegie Mellon University and in the fall of 1978 he transferred there to conduct cancer research and teach chemical engineering course, including graduate mathematics. His work progressed smartly and was rewarded by an NCI Research Career Development Award in 1980 and a Guggenheim fellowship in 1983. During his 1983–1984 sabbatical, he spent 6 months at MIT in chemical engineering department, where Prof Wei was now Chair of Chemical Engineering. There he taught a course "Transport Phenomena in Tumors." For the course, he had as guest lecturers Judah Folkman and David Baltimore. During his time at MIT, Suit first met Jain.

During further research at Carnegie Mellon, he proposed that high intratumoral pressure was an important factor in reducing drug access to tumors. Increased intratumoral pressure was confirmed in animal and then human tumors. He and team demonstrated that the abnormal vascular anatomy in murine tumors was similar to that in human tumors.

In 1990 he and several other candidates were interviewed for the position as Professor of tumor biology at Harvard Medical School and Director of the Edwin L. Steele Laboratories of the Department of Radiation Oncology at the Massachusetts General Hospital by the HMS search committee. Jain was the committee's unequivocal first choice. Suit then presented the rationale for the committee's decision to the medical school's committee on appointments, with Dean Tosteson as the Chair. During the proceedings, one of the most distinguished scientists on the faculty asked in a booming voice "Mr. Dean, are we to understand that you would consider appointing a person to an endowed professorship at this medical school who has no special education in modern genetics?" The Dean asked Suit to respond. Suit's response was that the Committee fully appreciated that the appointment of a chemical engineer to such an endowed professorship in tumor biology was an uncommon act at the school. The Committee judged that a basic fact of biology is that regardless of the detail with which the genetic characteristics of a tumor and normal tissues are known, the delivery of metabolites, drugs, and biologicals to and throughout a tumor will depend on the physiology and biochemistry of those tissues. That is, genetics alone will not be sufficient. There is a manifest requirement for major advances in our knowledge of the physiology combined with the most advanced genetics. There were no further questions. The recommended appointment was approved.

Jain accepted his appointment as the A Werk Cook Professor of Tumor Biology at the Harvard Medical School and the Director of the Edwin Steele Laboratory of this department. Jain and colleagues moved here in 1991 and commenced an exceptionally productive and innovative research program. Jain took two 2-week intensive courses in genetics and protein chemistry, with heavy concentration on laboratory procedures. This has led to excellent working relations with Brian Seed and other geneticist at the MGH and other laboratories. Jain and team now have a quite substantial array of mouse sub-lines with gene "knock out' and "knock in" for special studies. Other research faculty currently in Rakesh's group include three associate and four assistant professors and two instructors. Significantly, he has had high yield collaborative research with clinicians within the department and other departments (see, for example, the section on GI and CNS achievements). A point of quite special pride is the quality and success of the impressive number of graduate students and post-doctoral fellows. For details of these scholars are in Chapter 11 on Education.

Rakesh Jain is very widely regarded as a pioneer in the fields of tumor biology, drug delivery, in vivo imaging, bio-engineering, and bench-to-bedside translation. He uncovered the vascular, interstitial, and cellular barriers to the delivery and efficacy of molecular and nano-medicine in tumors; developed and tested new principles to overcome these barriers for improving treatment of cancer and non-cancerous diseases; and then translated these principles from bench to bedside, and in the process discovered new biomarkers and new strategies to improve the outcome further. His work has fundamentally changed the thinking of scientists and clinicians about how molecularly targeted therapeutics, especially anti-angiogenic agents, actually work in animal models and cancer patients and how to combine them optimally with cytotoxic therapies to improve survival rates in cancer patients. A seamless integration of engineering with biology and medicine is a hallmark of Jain's research.

Rakesh has served as mentor to more than 150 doctoral and post-doctoral students and fellows from multiple disciplines and a collaborator with a similar number of clinicians and scientists worldwide. He has 488 publications, including three in *Scientific American*, multiple in *Nature* and *Science*. As mentioned in the introduction, he is a member of all three US National Academies – the Institute of Medicine (2003), the National Academy of Engineering (2004), and the National Academy of Sciences (2009) – and the American Academy of Arts and Sciences (2005). He is one of only nine Americans and the only member of the faculty of HMS to hold this distinction.

Rakesh is very happily married to an attractive and very bright woman, Jackie. She is a clinical psychologist on the faculty of the McLean. Rakesh has twin daughters of six to whom he is totally committed and thoroughly enjoys.

Rakesh's name is Jain, the name of an important religion in India. It was founded around the same time as Buddhism and shares many common elements. He was brought up by a devout Jain family. Rakesh has noted that the Jain religion is quite attractive in that it is rare among religions in not only opposing killing but actually does not or rarely kills, e.g., Jainists are totally opposed to wars, capital punishment. Rakesh is not a practicing Jain but does carry the name.

8.5.12 Lance Munn

Lance Munn: Young Lance (Fig. 8.16) grew up near Dayton, Ohio, home of many pioneering engineers including the Wright brothers. He had an innate curiosity to understand the mechanisms of operation of the instruments and electronic devices around the house. This was stimulated in part by

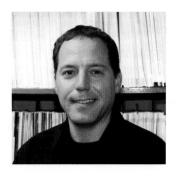

Fig. 8.16 Lance Munn

the influence of his tinkering grandfather who maintained an extensive workshop that Lance visited regularly. One of his earliest experiments involved the disassembly and reassembly of the vacuum cleaner to see how it worked – an exercise not completely approved of by his mother.

In high school, Lance's main interest was chemistry and physics, and he especially enjoyed "hands on" laboratory classes. Catalyzed by his fascination with chemistry laboratory experiments, he decided to major in chemical engineering at the University of Cincinnati. There, he excelled in the core engineering classes, but also took a few elective courses in the art department that cultivated what would later evolve into his interest in scientific illustration. During his final year at UC, he was asked to design a distillation column for a chemical plant – a common task for traditional chemical engineers. This experience led Lance to continue his training in another direction – bioengineering.

Lance went to Rice University to concentrate on basic biology. His project focused on the mechanics of leukocyte migration and required the development of novel imaging and analysis technologies. He obtained a post-doctoral fellowship with R. Jain and R. Melder in the Steele Lab. Lance was obviously an impressive candidate as he was offered a position after only a short phone interview. Lance began study of leukocyte trafficking in tumors, a project that quickly evolved into his main area of expertise: blood fluid dynamics. In addition, he is now trying to "disassemble and reassemble" tumors, tackling projects as diverse as blood vessel mechanics, angiogenesis and metastasis. On a side note, Lance is a prolific creator of scientific illustrations for publications and presentations; for a full and lucid discussion of this research and to appreciate some of his artwork, go to Lance on our Web page and to steele.mgh.harvard.edu.

8.5.13 Timothy P Padera

Timothy P Padera (Fig. 8.17) received his B.S. degree in chemical engineering and biomedical engineering from

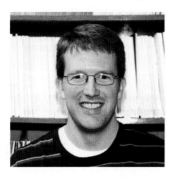

Fig. 8.17 Timothy P Padera

Northwestern University and then a Ph.D. in medical engineering from the Harvard-MIT Division of Health Sciences and Technology. He joined the Department of Radiation Oncology at Massachusetts General Hospital in February of 1998 working in the Edwin L. Steele Laboratory for Tumor Biology as a graduate student. In January 2006, Tim was appointed to the faculty at HMS and MGH Dr. Padera pioneered the use of intravital multiphoton laser scanning microscopy to image lymphatic vessels and study their function. Tim has married one of the special talents in the clinical faculty, Toruun Yock, who specializes in pediatric radiation oncology. They have two small children.

8.5.14 Robert Sedlacek

Robert Sedlacek *1971–1988* (Fig. 8.18) was born on February 1937 in Glendive, Montana, on the family ranch. Due to a prolonged drought, Bob's family moved to Riverton, Wyoming, and changed to raising sheep and farming irrigated land. His interests in school were science and agriculture. In a state competition, Bob won several Firsts Prizes. He won a scholarship at the University of Wyoming graduating with a B.S. in agronomy (1959) and an M.Sc. in soils (1961). Reflecting interest in chemistry, his thesis title was "*Effects of Titratable Alkalinity, Zink, Iron and Manganese on Chlorosis of Plants.*" To help pay for his education, he drove trucks

hauling feed and livestock during the school year and in summer he operated construction equipment and working in the shop welding and assisting the mechanics, i.e., one busy lad.

In September 1961, Bob and his wife Nelda moved to Houston. In February 1962 he started at the new Texas Inbred Mice Co., then in April 1967 to M.D. Anderson and December 1971 to MGH. A quite odd fact was that the salary at the MDAH was actually higher than that at the private company. Bob pursued the goal of perfecting his planned system of providing DFPF mice, based on the concept of the barrier at the cage level rather the room level leading to his micro-isolator, a system now used in many laboratories around the world.

At the MGH he continued to work on perfecting the Micro-Isolator, a patent granted in 1982. He quickly demonstrated the success of the Micro-Isolator to produce and maintain gnotobiotic mice consistently. Bob worked with researchers in the development of techniques and procedures, so they could maintain this gnotobiotic status throughout experiments of several years of duration. The number of strains was expanded to include immunodeficient mice (also defined flora). Bob proved that the DFPF reproduce extremely well and can be employed in long-term research.

Bob retired on September 1988 due to significant back problems. He and Nelda "hit the road." They have traveled over 400,000 miles in their Beaver Marquis motor coach and fished in New Zealand, Mexico, and Canada and are planning their ninth visit to Alaska. He built a double deck trailer which carries their boat and SUV behind the motor coach. They now have a house at Lake Ashton, FL, for winters.

8.5.15 Muneyasu Urano

Muneyasu Urano (Fig. 8.19) was born in Osaka, Japan (1936). He went to the Kyoto Prefectural University for his medical education (M.D. in 1961 and Ph.D. in 1968). He had a 3-year fellowship at the MD Anderson with Suit in the 1960s and returned to Japan. He joined the Steele

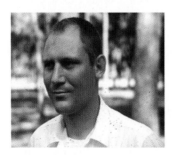

Fig. 8.18 Robert Sedlacek

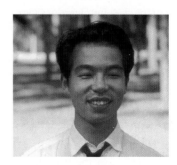

Fig. 8.19 Muneyasu Urano

Laboratory group in 1977 and performed experiments on the defined flora mice examining hyperthermia, radiation carcinogenesis, proton RBE, dose fractionation, repopulation, and more. His research was fully supported by his NCI RO1 grant. In 1989, he moved to the University of Louisville. After his retirement he has continued to work on a part-time basis with the Clift Ling group at Memorial Sloan Kettering Hospital on genetic factors, oxygen distribution in xenografts. His actual residence is in Oceanside, California.

8.5.16 Henning Willers

Henning Willers: The biographical sketch is in Chapter 10 section on thoracic radiation oncology.

Lei Xu: Beijing is the birthplace and education of Lei (Fig. 8.20). Her family was medical and science oriented. Specifically, her father was a professor of immunology at Beijing University and also worked at the Beijing Cancer Center. Lei planned on medicine and went to Capital University Medical School. While an intern at the Beijing Children's hospital, she was involved in the care of a number of children with leukemia and other childhood cancers. She became fascinated with the potential of her contributing significant improvements in the care of cancer patients. She decided to make oncology her career. She determined that to advance oncology she must study basic science. For this she entered the graduate program of Joshua Fidler at MD Anderson Cancer Center. The main interest of the Fidler group was and is the biology of metastasis. Her Ph.D. study was on ovarian cancer in nude mice. She then came to R. Jain's groups as a postdoctoral fellow to work on tumor–host interaction at the micro-environmental level.

She now is serving as co-director of the molecular core in the Steele Laboratory program. She has greatly enjoyed working closely with a number of post-doctoral fellows and the supervision of two Ph.D. students. Xu received the Claflin Distinguished Scholar Award in 2005. Her long-term goal is to become an independent researcher and return to the specific study of ovarian cancer.

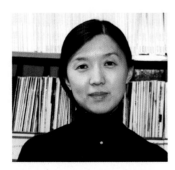

Fig. 8.20 Lei Xu

8.6 Faculty that Moved to Other Centers

8.6.1 Laurence Baxter

Laurence Baxter (*1991–1998*), a chemical engineer, headed the mathematical modeling efforts in the early days of the Steele Lab. He constructed a series of mathematical models for analyzing blood perfusion and interstitial pressure in tumors. He also used these models to predict how drugs are distributed in tumor tissue and to work on the design and treatment strategies. Larry has moved to Advanced Process Combinatronics as VP.

8.6.2 David Berk

David Berk (1992–1998) has a serious interest in drug delivery. He developed and implemented microscopic techniques for measuring the diffusion and convection of drugs within tumor tissue. University of Manchester, UK, attracted David to their faculty and he is now Senior Lecturer in the School of Pharmacy.

8.6.3 Ed Brown

Ed Brown (1999–2005), an expert microscopist, constructed a multiphoton microscope in the Steele Lab. Using this novel and powerful technology he was the first to image several aspects of tumor biology and physiology. Ed is currently Assistant Professor in the University of Rochester medical center.

8.6.4 Edward P. Clark

Edward P. Clark joined the Epp Laboratory Group in 1980. His Ph.D. from the State University of Colorado; W. Dewey was his thesis supervisor. He participated in studies the outcome of competitive reactions between oxidizing and reducing species for radiation-induced radicals in critical molecules such as DNA leading, respectively, to either damage fixation (e.g., by peroxy radicals) or damage repair (e.g., by hydrogen atom donation from a sulfhydryl group such as glutathione). Thus, instead of trying to sensitize the radioresistant hypoxic cells by addition of oxygen or chemical agent acting as an oxygen mimic, the concept is to try to interfere with the hydrogen-donating mechanism which act to protect the hypoxic cells. Ed left MGH in the late 1980s to accept a senior leadership position at the Armed Forces Radiobiology Research Institute in Bethesda, Maryland.

8.6.5 Cliff Ling

Cliff Ling had worked with Epp from 1971 and joined Epp at the MGH in 1975. His Ph.D. was from the University of Washington in nuclear physics. They employed extremely high instantaneous dose rates, viz., 10^{10} Gy/s in 3 ns pulses to investigate fast radiochemical processes occurring in cells immediately after irradiation. This was relevant to the mechanism of the oxygen effect. At MGH he contributed importantly to the research on chemical radiosensitizers. Clinically he contributed to development of use of I-125 seeds in brachytherapy and the intraoperative electron therapy program.

Clift became successively the chief of radiation physics at George Washington Medical Center, University of California at San Francisco, where he was Professor and Vice-Chair in the Department of Radiation Oncology and then in 1989 to Memorial Sloan-Kettering Cancer Center succeeding Dr. John S. Laughlin.

8.6.6 Robert Melder

Robert Melder (1989–1998) led the effort on leukocyte biology in the Steele Lab. He was interested in the ability of solid tumors to evade the immune response and performed intravital experiments to determine the physiological mechanisms that prevented leukocytes from localizing in tumors. He also developed novel approaches for using activated leukocytes to treat tumors. Bob has joined Medtronics and he enjoys the comfortable climate in Santa Rosa, CA.

8.6.7 Howard B. Michaels

Howard B. Michaels joined the Epp Laboratory Group in 1977. His Ph.D. project was under J. Hunt at the Ontario Cancer Institute. Howard studied the oxygen sensitization of mammalian cells irradiated at ultrahigh dose rates and oxygen diffusion rates in mammalian cells. He then engaged in a series of studies related to the combined effects of oxygen of various concentrations with different electron affinic agents on the radiosensitization of mammalian cells. During his 6 years he published nine papers in peer-reviewed journals. Michaels returned to Canada and is now at the Ontario Cancer Institute in Toronto.

Simon Powell 1991–2002: For the biographical sketch, see Section Section 10.5.

8.6.8 Vlatko Silobrcic

Vlatko Silobrcic came for two fellowships to work in the Steele Laboratory. He was the first immunologist post-doctoral fellow to work in the lab at the MDACC. He had been a fellow with immunologist J. Trentin at Baylor Medical School where Suit and Silobrcic met during an immunology conference at Baylor. Vlatko is a native of Zagreb, Croatia. The two fellowships at MGH were quite productive working very well with post-doctoral fellows and residents.

He has received numerous awards and prizes. These include the following: the Annual Prize of the Republic of Croatia for outstanding scientific achievements (1974); membership of the Medical Academy of Croatia (1974); Professor of immunology at the Medical Faculty, University of Zagreb; Head of the department for clinical and experimental immunology and chemistry, Institute of Immunology, Zagreb (1987); full member of the Croatian Academy of Sciences and Arts (1991); appointed General Director of the Institute of Immunology (1992); the Gold Medal of the Gilbert Fletcher Society (2003).

8.6.9 Fan Yuan

Fan Yuan (1991–1996) had been educated as a biomathematician who rapidly evolved into a first-class experimentalist. He used animal window models to make a number of seminal observations and measurements of tumor blood vessel function. Fan moved to Duke University and is an Associate Professor of biomedical engineering.

References

1. Allam A, Gioioso D, Taghian A, et al. Intrinsic radiation sensitivity: no correlation with the metastatic potential of human and murine tumor cell lines. J Natl Cancer Inst. 1993;85(23):1954–7.
2. Au P, Daheron LM, Duda DG, et al. Differential in vivo potential of endothelial progenitor cells from human umbilical cord blood and adult peripheral blood to form functional long-lasting vessels. Blood. 2008;111(3):1302–5.
3. Au P, Tam J, Fukumura D, et al. Bone marrow-derived mesenchymal stem cells facilitate engineering of long-lasting functional vasculature. Blood. 2008;111(9):4551–8.
4. Batchelor TT, Sorensen AG, di Tomaso E, et al. AZD2171, a pan-VEGF receptor tyrosine kinase inhibitor, normalizes tumor vasculature and alleviates edema in glioblastoma patients. Cancer Cell. 2007;11(1):83–95.
5. Baumann M, Suit HD, Sedlacek RS. Metastases after fractionated radiation therapy of three murine tumor models. Int J Radiat Oncol Biol Phys. 1990;19(2):367–70.
6. Bockhorn M, Jain RK, Munn LL. Active versus passive mechanisms in metastasis: do cancer cells crawl into vessels, or are they pushed? Lancet Oncol. 2007;8(5):444–8.

7. Bockhorn M, Roberge S, Sousa C, et al. Differential gene expression in metastasizing cells shed from kidney tumors. Cancer Res. 2004;64(7):2469–73.

8. Boucher Y, Kirkwood JM, Opacic D, et al. Interstitial hypertension in superficial metastatic melanomas in humans. Cancer Res. 1991;51(24):6691–4.

9. Boucher Y, Lee I, Jain RK. Lack of general correlation between interstitial fluid pressure and oxygen partial pressure in solid tumors. Microvasc Res. 1995;50(2):175–82.

10. Boucher Y, Leunig M, Jain RK. Tumor angiogenesis and interstitial hypertension. Cancer Res. 1996;56(18):4264–6.

11. Brown E, McKee T, diTomaso E, et al. Dynamic imaging of collagen and its modulation in tumors in vivo using second-harmonic generation. Nat Med. 2003;9(6):796–800.

12. Brown EB, Campbell RB, Tsuzuki Y, et al. In vivo measurement of gene expression, angiogenesis and physiological function in tumors using multiphoton laser scanning microscopy. Nat Med. 2001;7(7):864–8. Erratum in: Nat Med. 2001;7(9):1069.

13. Budach W, Taghian A, Freeman J, et al. Impact of stromal sensitivity on radiation response of tumors. J Natl Cancer Inst. 1993;85(12):988–93.

14. Chen Y, Taghian AG, Rosenberg AE, et al. Predictive value of histologic tumor necrosis after radiation. Int J Cancer. 2001;96(6):334–40.

15. Choi CH, Sedlacek RS, Suit HD. Radiation-induced osteogenic sarcoma of C3H mouse: effects of *Corynebacterium parvum* and WBI on its natural history and response to irradiation. Eur J Cancer. 1979;15(4):433–42.

16. Clark EP, Michaels HB, Peterson EC, et al. Irradiation of mammalian cells in the presence of diamide and low concentrations of oxygen at conventional and at ultrahigh dose rates. Radiat Res. 1983;93(3):479–91.

17. Dahm-Daphi J, Hubbe P, Horvath F, et al. Nonhomologous end-joining of site-specific but not of radiation-induced DNA double-strand breaks is reduced in the presence of wild-type p53. Oncogene. 2005;24(10):1663–72.

18. Dewey WC, Hopwood LE, Sapareto SA, et al. Cellular responses to combinations of hyperthermia and radiation. Radiology. 1977;123(2):463–74.

19. di Tomaso E, Capen D, Haskell A, et al. Mosaic tumor vessels: cellular basis and ultrastructure of focal regions lacking endothelial cell markers. Cancer Res. 2005;65(13):5740–9.

20. Duda DG, Batchelor TT, Willett CG, et al. VEGF-targeted cancer therapy strategies: current progress, hurdles and future prospects. Trends Mol Med. 2007;13(6):223–30.

21. Duda DG, Cohen KS, Kozin SV, et al. Evidence for incorporation of bone marrow-derived endothelial cells into perfused blood vessels in tumors. Blood. 2006;107(7):2774–6.

22. Duda DG, Fukumura D, Munn LL, et al. Differential transplantability of tumor-associated stromal cells. Cancer Res. 2004;64(17):5920–4.

23. Epp ER, Weiss H, Santomasso A. The oxygen effect in bacterial cells irradiated with high-intensity pulsed electrons. Radiat Res. 1968;34(2):320–5.

24. Fukumura D, Gohongi T, Kadambi A, et al. Predominant role of endothelial nitric oxide synthase in vascular endothelial growth factor-induced angiogenesis and vascular permeability. Proc Natl Acad Sci USA. 2001;98(5):2604–9.

25. Fukumura D, Kashiwagi S, Jain RK. The role of nitric oxide in tumour progression. Nat Rev Cancer. 2006;6(7):521–34. Review.

26. Fukumura D, Ushiyama A, Duda DG, et al. Paracrine regulation of angiogenesis and adipocyte differentiation during in vivo adipogenesis. Circ Res. 2003;93(9):e88–97. Erratum in: Circ Res. 2004;94(1):e16. Circ Res. 2005;96(9):e76.

27. Fukumura D, Xavier R, Sugiura T, et al. Tumor induction of VEGF promoter activity in stromal cells. Cell. 1998;94(6):715–25.

28. Fukumura D, Xu L, Chen Y, Gohongi T, Seed B, Jain RK. Hypoxia and acidosis independently up-regulate vascular endothelial growth factor transcription in brain tumors in vivo. Cancer Res. 2001;61(16):6020–4.

29. Fukumura D, Yuan F, Endo M, et al. Role of nitric oxide in tumor microcirculation. Blood flow, vascular permeability, and leukocyte-endothelial interactions. Am J Pathol. 1997;150(2):713–25.

30. Garkavtsev I, Kozin SV, Chernova O, et al. The candidate tumour suppressor protein ING4 regulates brain tumour growth and angiogenesis. Nature. 2004;428(6980):328–32.

31. Gerweck LE, Gillette EL, Dewey WC. Killing of Chinese hamster cells in vitro by heating under hypoxic or aerobic conditions. Eur J Cancer. 1974;10(10):691–3.

32. Gerweck LE, Gillette EL, Dewey WC. Effect of heat and radiation on synchronous Chinese hamster cells: killing and repair. Radiat Res. 1975;64(3):611–23.

33. Gerweck LE, Vijayappa S, Kozin S. Tumor pH controls the in vivo efficacy of weak acid and base chemotherapeutics. Mol Cancer Ther. 2006;5(5):1275–9.

34. Gerweck LE, Vijayappa S, Kurimasa A, et al. Tumor cell radiosensitivity is a major determinant of tumor response to radiation. Cancer Res. 2006;66(17):8352–5.

35. Griffon-Etienne G, Boucher Y, Brekken C, Jain RK, Suit HD. Taxane-induced apoptosis decompresses blood vessels and lowers interstitial fluid pressure in solid tumors: clinical implications. Cancer Res. 1999;59(15):3776–82.

36. Hagendoorn J, Padera TP, Kashiwagi S, et al. Endothelial nitric oxide synthase regulates microlymphatic flow via collecting lymphatics. Circ Res. 2004;95(2):204–9.

37. Halperin EC, Haas G, Dosoretz DE, et al. 1982 resident's essay award: the immunologic effects of lymphoid irradiation in human and non-human primates: cellular changes and the potential for renal transplantation. Int J Radiat Oncol Biol Phys. 1983;9(7):1083–9.

38. Held KD, Epp ER, Awad S, et al. Post irradiation sensitization of mammalian cells by the thiol-depleting agent dimethyl fumarate. Radiat Res. 1991;127(1):75–80.

39. Held KD, Epp ER, Clark EP, et al. Effect of dimethyl fumarate on the radiation sensitivity of mammalian cells in vitro. Radiat Res. 1988;115(3):495–502.

40. Hoshida T, Isaka N, Hagendoorn J, et al. Imaging steps of lymphatic metastasis reveals that vascular endothelial growth factor-C increases metastasis by increasing delivery of cancer cells to lymph nodes: therapeutic implications. Cancer Res. 2006;66(16):8065–75.

41. Huang P, Allam A, Taghian A, et al. Growth and metastatic behavior of five human glioblastomas compared with nine other histological types of human tumor xenografts in SCID mice. J Neurosurg. 1995;83(2):308–15.

42. Huang P, Taghian A, Hsu DW, et al. Spontaneous metastasis, proliferation characteristics and radiation sensitivity of fractionated irradiation recurrent and unirradiated human xenografts. Radiother Oncol. 1996;41:73–81.

43. Izumi Y, Xu L, di Tomaso E, Fukumura D, Jain RK. Tumour biology: herceptin acts as an anti-angiogenic cocktail. Nature. 2002;416(6878):279–80.

44. Jain RK. Normalizing tumor vasculature with anti-angiogenic therapy: a new paradigm for combination therapy. Nat Med. 2001;7(9):987–9.

45. Jain RK. Taming vessels to treat cancer. Sci Am. 2008;298(1):56–63.

46. Jain RK, di Tomaso E, Duda DG, et al. Angiogenesis in brain tumours. Nat Rev Neurosci. 2007;8(8):610–22.

47. Jain RK, Duda DG. Role of bone marrow-derived cells in tumor angiogenesis and treatment. Cancer Cell. 2003;3(6):515–6.

48. Kamoun WS, Dan Ley C, Farrar CT, et al. Edema control by cediranib, a VEGF targeted kinase inhibitor, prolongs survival despite persistent brain tumor growth in mice. J Clin Oncol. 2009;27:2542–52.

49. Kashiwagi S, Izumi Y, Gohongi T, et al. NO mediates mural cell recruitment and vessel morphogenesis in murine melanomas and tissue-engineered blood vessels. J Clin Invest. 2005;115:1816–27.

50. Kashiwagi S, Tsukada K, Xu L, et al. Perivascular nitric oxide gradients normalize tumor vasculature. Nat Med. 2008;14(3):255–7.

51. Kirsch DG, Dinulescu DM, Miller JB, et al. A spatially and temporally restricted mouse model of soft tissue sarcoma. Nat Med. 2007;13(8):992–7.

52. Koike N, Fukumura D, Gralla O, Au P, Schechner JS, Jain RK. Tissue engineering: creation of long-lasting blood vessels. Nature. 2004;428(6979):138–9.

53. Kozin SV, Niemierko A, Huang P, Silva J, Doppke KP, Suit HD. Inter- and intramouse heterogeneity of radiation response for a growing paired organ. Radiat Res. 2008;170(2):264–7.

54. Kozin SV, Winkler F, Garkavtsev I, et al. Human tumor xenografts recurring after radiotherapy are more sensitive to anti-vascular endothelial growth factor receptor-2 treatment than treatment-naive tumors. Cancer Res. 2007;67(11):5076–82.

55. Lahdenranta J, Hagendoorn J, Padera TP, et al. Endothelial nitric oxide synthase mediates lymphangiogenesis and lymphatic metastasis. Cancer Res. 2009;69:2801–8.

56. Lee CG, Heijn M, diTomaso E, et al. Anti-vascular endothelial growth factor treatment augments tumor radiation response under normoxic or hypoxic conditions. Cancer Res. 2000;60:5565–70.

57. Ling CC, Michaels HB, Epp ER, et al. Oxygen diffusion into mammalian cells following ultrahigh dose rate irradiation and lifetime estimates of oxygen-sensitive species. Radiat Res. 1978;76(3):522–32.

58. McDonald J, Pinkerton A, Weiss H, et al. Dosimetry for thin biological samples irradiated by nanosecond electron pulses of high intensity. Radiat Res. 1972;49(3):495–506.

59. McKee TD, Grandi P, Mok W, et al. Degradation of fibrillar collagen in a human melanoma xenograft improves the efficacy of an oncolytic herpes simplex virus vector. Cancer Res. 2006;66(5):2509–13.

60. Michaels HB, Ling CC, Epp ER, et al. Interaction of nitroimidazole sensitizers and oxygen in the radiosensitization of mammalian cells at ultrahigh dose rates. Radiat Res. 1981;85(3):567–82.

61. Michaels HB, Peterson EC, Epp ER. Effects of modifiers of the yield of hydroxyl radicals on the radiosensitivity of mammalian cells at ultrahigh dose rates. Radiat Res. 1983;95(3):620–36.

62. Mok W, Boucher Y, Jain RK. Matrix metalloproteinases-1 and -8 improve the distribution and efficacy of an oncolytic virus. Cancer Res. 2007;67(22):10664–8.

63. Munn LL, Dupin MM. Blood cell interactions and segregation in flow. Ann Biomed Eng. 2008;36(4):534–44.

64. Nagano S, Perentes JY, Jain RK, Boucher Y. Cancer cell death enhances the penetration and efficacy of oncolytic herpes simplex virus in tumors. Cancer Res. 2008;68(10):3795–802.

65. Nelson GM, Padera TP, Garkavtsev I, et al. Differential gene expression of primary cultured lymphatic and blood vascular endothelial cells. Neoplasia. 2007;9(12):1038–45.

66. Ogawa K, Boucher Y, Kashiwagi S, et al. Influence of tumor cell and stroma sensitivity on tumor response to radiation. Cancer Res. 2007;67(9):4016–21.

67. Okunieff PG, Koutcher JA, Gerweck L, et al. Tumor size dependent changes in a murine fibrosarcoma: use of in vivo 31P NMR for non-invasive evaluation of tumor metabolic status. Int J Radiat Oncol Biol Phys. 1986;12(5):793–9.

68. Overgaard J, Suit HD. Time-temperature relationship in hyperthermic treatment of malignant and normal tissue in vivo. Cancer Res. 1979;39(8):3248–53.

69. Padera TP, Kadambi A, diTomaso E, et al. Lymphatic metastasis in the absence of functional intratumor lymphatics. Science. 2002;296(5574):1883–6.

70. Padera TP, Stoll BR, So PT, Jain RK. Conventional and high-speed intravital multiphoton laser scanning microscopy of microvasculature, lymphatics, and leukocyte-endothelial interactions. Mol Imaging. 2002;1(1):9–15.

71. Padera TP, Stoll BR, Tooredman JB, et al. Pathology: cancer cells compress intratumour vessels. Nature. 2004;427(6976):695.

72. Pluen A, Boucher Y, Ramanujan S, et al. Role of tumor-host interactions in interstitial diffusion of macromolecules: cranial vs. subcutaneous tumors. Proc Natl Acad Sci USA. 2001;98(8):4628–33.

73. Prise KM, Schettino G, Folkard M, Held KD. New insights on cell death from radiation exposure. Lancet Oncol. 2005;6(7):520–8.

74. Ramsay J, Suit HD, Sedlacek R. Experimental studies on the incidence of metastases after failure of radiation treatment and the effect of salvage surgery. Int J Radiat Oncol Biol Phys. 1988;14(6):1165–8.

75. Roh HD, Boucher Y, Kalnicki S, et al. Interstitial hypertension in carcinoma of uterine cervix in patients: possible correlation with tumor oxygenation and radiation response. Cancer Res. 1991;51(24):6695–8.

76. Romanova LY, Willers H, Blagosklonny MV, Powell SN. The interaction of p53 with replication protein A mediates suppression of homologous recombination. Oncogene. 2004;23(56):9025–33.

77. Rottinger EM, Sedlacek R, Suit HD. Ineffectiveness of anticoagulation in experimental radiation therapy. Eur J Cancer. 1975;11(10):743–9.

78. Ruka W, Taghian A, Gioioso D, et al. Comparison between the in vitro intrinsic radiation sensitivity of human soft tissue sarcoma and breast cancer cell lines. J Surg Oncol. 1996;61(4):290–4.

79. Sedlacek R, Mason K. A simple and inexpensive method for maintaining a defined flora mouse colony. Lab Anim Sci. 1977;27(5 Pt 1):667–70.

80. Schulte-Uentrop L, El-Awady RA, Schliecker L, Willers H, Dahm-Daphi J. Distinct roles of XRCC4 and Ku80 in non-homologous end-joining of endonuclease- and ionizing radiation-induced DNA double-strand breaks. Nucleic Acids Res. 2008;36(8):2561–9.

81. Shao C, Folkard M, Held KD, Prise KM. Estrogen enhanced cell-cell signaling in breast cancer cells exposed to targeted irradiation. BMC Cancer. 2008;8:184.

82. Shevkoplyas SS, Yoshida T, Munn LL, Bitensky MW. Biomimetic autoseparation of leukocytes from whole blood in a microfluidic device. Anal Chem. 2005;77(3):933–7.

83. Silobrcic V, Zietman AL, Ramsay JR, et al. Residual immunity of athymic NCr/Sed nude mice and the xenotransplantation of human tumors. Int J Cancer. 1990;45(2):325–33.

84. Stroh M, Zimmer JP, Duda DG, et al. Quantum dots spectrally distinguish multiple species within the tumor milieu in vivo. Nat Med. 2005;11(6):678–82.

85. Suit HD, Gallager HS. Intact tumor cells in irradiated tissue. Arch Pathol. 1964;78:648–51.

86. Suit HD, Sedlacek R, Silver G, et al. Therapeutic gain factors for fractionated radiation treatment of spontaneous murine tumors using fast neutrons, photons plus O2(1) or 3 ATA, or photons plus misonidazole. Radiat Res. 1988;116(3):482–502.

87. Sun C, Jain RK, Munn LL. Non-uniform plasma leakage affects local hematocrit and blood flow: implications for inflammation and tumor perfusion. Ann Biomed Eng. 2007;35(12): 2121–9.

88. Taghian A, Budach W, Zietman A, et al. Quantitative comparison between the transplantability of human and murine tumors into the brain of NCr/Sed-nu/nu nude and severe combined immunodeficient mice. Cancer Res. 1993;53(20):5018–21.

89. Tang W, Willers H, Powell SN. p53 directly enhances rejoining of DNA double-strand breaks with cohesive ends in gamma-irradiated mouse fibroblasts. Cancer Res. 1999;59(11):2562–5.

90. Todoroki T, Suit HD. Therapeutic advantage in preoperative single-dose radiation combined with conservative and radical surgery in different-size murine fibrosarcomas. J Surg Oncol. 1985;29(4):207–15.

91. Tong RT, Boucher Y, Kozin SV, et al. Vascular normalization by vascular endothelial growth factor receptor 2 blockade induces a pressure gradient across the vasculature and improves drug penetration in tumors. Cancer Res. 2004;64(11):3731–6.

92. Tsuzuki Y, Fukumura D, Oosthuyse B, Koike C, Carmeliet P, Jain RK. Vascular endothelial growth factor (VEGF) modulation by targeting hypoxia-inducible factor-1alpha--> hypoxia response element--> VEGF cascade differentially regulates vascular response and growth rate in tumors. Cancer Res. 2000;60(22):6248–52.

93. Tyrrell JA, di Tomaso E, Fuja D, et al. Robust 3-D modeling of vasculature imagery using superellipsoids. IEEE Trans Med Imaging. 2007;26(2):223–37.

94. Urano M, Goitein M, Verhey L, et al. Relative biological effectiveness of a high energy modulated proton beam using a spontaneous murine tumor in vivo. Int J Radiat Oncol Biol Phys.

95. Urano M, Kahn J, Kenton LA. Thermochemotherapy (combined cyclophosphamide and hyperthermia) with or without hyperglycemia as an adjuvant to radiotherapy. Int J Radiat

96. Urano M, Overgaard M, Suit H, Dunn P, Sedlacek R. Enhancement by *Corynebacterium parvum* of the normal and tumor tissue response to hyperthermia. Cancer Res. 1978;38(3):862–4. 1980;6(9):1187–93.

97. Urano M, Verhey LJ, Goitein M, et al. Relative biological effectiveness of modulated proton beams in various murine tissues. Int J Radiat Oncol Biol Phys. 1984;10(4):509–14. Oncol Biol Phys. 1986;12(1):45–50.

98. Ventura A, Kirsch DG, McLaughlin ME, et al. Restoration of p53 function leads to tumour regression in vivo. Nature. 2007;445(7128):661–5.

99. Wang ZZ, Au P, Chen T, et al. Endothelial cells derived from human embryonic stem cells form durable blood vessels in vivo. Nat Biotechnol. 2007;25(3):317–8.

100. Willers H, Husson J, Lee LW, et al. Distinct mechanisms of non-homologous end joining in the repair of site-directed chromosomal breaks with non-complementary and complementary ends. Radiat Res. 2006;166(4):567–74.

101. Willers H, Kachnic LA, Luo CM, et al. Biomarkers and mechanisms of FANCD2 function. J Biomed Biotechnol. 2008;2008:821529.

102. Willers H, McCarthy EE, Wu B, et al. Dissociation of p53-mediated suppression of homologous recombination from G1/S cell cycle checkpoint control. Oncogene. 2000;19(5):632–9.

103. Willett CG, Boucher Y, di Tomaso E, et al. Direct evidence that the VEGF-specific antibody bevacizumab has antivascular effects in human rectal cancer. Nat Med. 2004;10(2):145–7.

104. Willett CG, Urano M, Suit HD, et al. Effect of temperature on blood flow and hypoxic fraction in a murine fibrosarcoma. Int J Radiat Oncol Biol Phys. 1987;13(9):1309–12.

105. Winkler F, Kozin SV, Tong RT, et al. Kinetics of vascular normalization by VEGFR2 blockade governs brain tumor response to radiation: role of oxygenation, angiopoietin-1, and matrix metalloproteinases. Cancer Cell. 2004;6(6):553–63.

106. Xia F, Taghian DG, DeFrank JS, et al. Deficiency of human BRCA2 leads to impaired homologous recombination but maintains normal nonhomologous end joining. Proc Natl Acad Sci USA. 2001;98(15):8644–9.

107. Xu L, Fukumura D, Jain RK. Acidic extracellular pH induces vascular endothelial growth factor (VEGF) in human glioblastoma cells via ERK1/2 MAPK signaling pathway: mechanism of low pH-induced VEGF. J Biol Chem. 2002;277(13):11368–74.

108. Xu L, Jain RK. Down-regulation of placenta growth factor by promoter hypermethylation in human lung and colon carcinoma. Mol Cancer Res. 2007;5(9):873–80.

109. Xu L, Tong R, Cochran DM, et al. Blocking platelet-derived growth factor-D/platelet-derived growth factor receptor beta signaling inhibits human renal cell carcinoma progression in an orthotopic mouse model. Cancer Res. 2005;65(13):5711–9.

110. Yang H, Anzenberg V, Held KD. The time dependence of bystander responses induced by iron-ion radiation in normal human skin fibroblasts. Radiat Res. 2007;168(3):292–8.

111. Yang H, Asaad N, Held KD. Medium-mediated intercellular communication is involved in bystander responses of X-ray irradiated normal human fibroblasts. Oncogene. 2005;24(12): 2096–103.

112. Zhang J, Willers H, Feng Z, et al. Chk2 phosphorylation of BRCA1 regulates DNA double-strand break repair. Mol Cell Biol. 2004;24(2):708–18.

113. Zietman AL, Suit HD, Okunieff PG, et al. The life shortening effects of treatment with doxorubicin and/or local irradiation on a cohort of young C3Hf/Sed mice. Eur J Cancer. 1991;27(6): 778–81.

114. Zietman AL, Suit HD, Ramsay JR, et al. Quantitative studies on the transplantability of murine and human tumors into the brain and subcutaneous tissues of NCr/Sed nude mice. Cancer Res. 1988;48(22):6510–6.

115. Znati CA, Rosenstein M, Boucher Y, et al. Effect of radiation on interstitial fluid pressure and oxygenation in a human tumor xenograft. Cancer Res. 1996;56(5):964–8.

116. Znati CA, Rosenstein M, Mckee TD, et al. Irradiation reduces interstitial fluid transport and increases the collagen content in tumors. Clin Cancer Res. 2003;9(15):5508–13.

117. Zuang J, Zhang J, Willers H, et al. Chk2-mediated phosphorylation of BRCA1 regulates the fidelity of non-homologous end-joining. Cancer Res. 2006;66:1401–8.

Chapter 9

Biomathematics and Biostatistics

9.1 Establishment of the Division

The division of biomathematics and biostatistics was established in 2004 with A. Niemierko as the Head. The intent was to provide an organized program in biomathematics in clinical radiation oncology. The principal function is to collaborate with clinicians in the design of clinical studies, analysis of the resultant data, and development of new model systems and concepts for clinically related biomathematics and statistics. Further, the faculty is to contribute biomath and biostatistics lectures in the educational courses for residents and pre- and post-doctoral fellows.

One of the clinically new concepts in understanding the impact of dose heterogeneity on tumor control probability (TCP) was by Niemierko who proposed the concept of the equivalent uniform dose (EUD) from which the TCP could be computed for a tumor irradiated by a heterogeneously distributed dose. Basically, the concept is to consider the tumor as consisting of (1) a large number of voxels of uniform volume; (2) uniform tumor clonogen number per unit of volume of each voxel; (3) uniform dose within each voxel; and (4) constant distribution of radiation sensitivity of the clonogens for all voxels. Namely, the variable is dose to voxels. From these parameters, the EUD and, hence, the TCP can be computed on the same basis as for a tumor of the same volume that is irradiated uniformly to the nominal EUD. His method provides a convenient means of estimation of the impact of a cold or a hot spot within the tumor on TCP. This has proven to be clinically useful in planning treatment of lesions in close proximity or abutting sensitive tissues/organs, viz., estimating the impact of dose "cold spots" and "hot spots" [9, 11].

Niemierko was an important participant in the assessment of the power of ^{18}F-FDG uptake in locally advanced NSCLC in prediction of the pathological response following pre-operative radiation treatment in their study of 29 patients [4].

An additional study is the assessment of the risk of secondary radiation cancer in patients following SRS [8]. This study was a review of the world's literature and concluded that a total of six tumors have been reported. The implication is that the high single radiation dose to the quite small volumes of normal tissue carries a quite small, but non-zero, risk of induced cancer. This point will almost certainly be re-evaluated in another decade or so with the increase in numbers of treated patients and greater length of follow-up times.

Marek Ancukiewicz came to the MGH from Poland as a Ph.D. in biostatistics from the U of Warsaw and 8 years at Duke working on the biostatics of cardiovascular studies. Here he has been very effective in a quiet manner working with several clinicians. In addition, he has contributed by analysis of modeling the relationship between continuous covariates and clinical events using isotonic regression [1]. Three of his papers on clinical studies are [2, 3, 7] in the reference list.

Analysis of error on interpretation of biostatistical analysis of clinical data is and has been of special interest to Saveli Goldberg [5]. He has used most of his time in the statistical analysis of clinical outcome and clinical trial data. He has been productive in this area. See [6, 10, 12].

9.2 Biographical Sketches (Arranged Alphabetically)

9.2.1 Marek Ancukiewicz

Marek (Fig. 9.1) originated in Sroda, a town of 20,000 near Poznan, Poland. There were good public libraries and he was a frequent visitor.

Marek's parents had a high respect for science; he loved to study on his own and considered school an obstacle to learning. Thus there was substantial time and freedom to learn things on the individual student's interest. Students were given a set of new books at the start of summer for the coming school year and the eager young Marek regularly finished reading the lot during the summer. His interests

H.D. Suit, J.S. Loeffler, *Evolution of Radiation Oncology at Massachusetts General Hospital*,
DOI 10.1007/978-1-4419-6744-2_9, © Springer Science+Business Media, LLC 2011

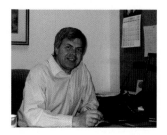

Fig. 9.1 Marek Ancukiewicz

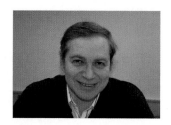

Fig. 9.2 Saveli Goldberg

ranged widely but with time centered on physics and math. He did obtain and read university-level books. He acquired scientific instruments, a chemistry lab, telescope, and others. In Poland, the standard was 7 years of physics classes starting at grade 6 (age 12 years); the students were doing linear equations and differential equations by the end of high school.

Also in high school, he read a book on mathematical modeling of biology that stimulated significant interest. He had high success in national physics, math, and astronomy examinations and was admitted to the university of his choice, with no examination. In 1979, he entered Biomedical Engineering at Technical University in Warsaw to study biomedical engineering and medical physics at U Warsaw. The later included a 1 year internship in a French company, Cardio France, doing medical devices. He received a Masters degree in 1985. Then he had 1 year in the Polish army, in anti-aircraft artillery.

This was followed by his Ph.D. program at the Polish Academy of Sciences. However, regular admission into the Ph.D. program was blocked by the Communist Party; they objected to his political activities while a master's student. He could not attend any classes but was given permission to study under the direction of a professor and then take the exams. He did this readily.

His studies included a year as an intern. While there, visiting cardiologists from Duke cardiologists invited Marek to Duke to do some of their biostatistics. This he did and learned much biostatistics. in 1988 he returned to Poland and won his thesis with a special distinction.

In 1991, he returned to Duke for 6 years. This was a good additional learning experience. He was then brought to the MGH to work with A. Niemierko and many clinicians especially, Chris Willett, Ira Spiro, and Simon Powell. This involved learning about tumor biology and radiation oncology.

9.2.2 Saveli Goldberg

Saveli (Fig. 9.2) had his childhood in Sverdlovsk, Russia, a large town with high-quality schools, universities, and

several scientific institutes. Probably an important factor in Saveli's passion for mathematics and physics was that his father was an engineer in charge of a major department in the manufacture of turbines. He enjoyed real success and had received special government prizes. There was a cultural balance in that his mother was a teacher of languages and literature.

As a high school student, Saveli concentrated on physics and math and mastered calculus. He won second place in the Mathematical Olympiad in his province. This provided him the opportunity to attend any university in Russia. He elected a university in Sverdlovsk. His studies were principally math and philosophy with a lesser emphasis on physics. He continued to excel in the very competitive university environment, being in the top 15% of the students.

Ambitions for a graduate degree were quite complex and he worked independently for a period. This was, however, very productive. He submitted a paper and it was accepted for presentation at a math meeting in Moscow. A senior scientist at that meeting judged that the work would constitute a very good project for a Ph.D. thesis. He was admitted forthwith into the Institute of Mathematics in Sverdlovsk and was awarded a Ph.D. degree in 1985. He began to work in a physiological laboratory as a member or a cardiac research team. He confronted the fact that there was such a plethora of parameters and a serious paucity of data and the available data on humans had wide but unquantified uncertainty bands. He changed from cardiac research to special studies of intensive care for pediatric patients. The resulting monitoring system was sold to many medical centers in the Soviet Union.

Saveli presented some of his material at a conference in Vancouver. This caught the attention of the president of Hewlett Packard (HP) who invited him to join the firm. By the time Saveli arrived at HP the president had moved. Not long afterward he came to the MGH in 1998 as a biostatician. His interest was analysis of error frequency, type of error, and its impact on outcomes of analysis. He is expanding his study of this problem in his examination of the various departmental databases. Saveli has provided support for many of clinical outcome studies in the department.

9.2.3 Andrjez Niemierko (1987–Present)

Andrjez (Fig. 9.3) was born near Warsaw and his family moved to Warsaw when he was in the third grade. Even at that age he was keen on math but in the fifth grade, classes in physics commenced and he immediately liked it. His family was especially well educated, viz., both parents have Ph.D.s. His father is in education and his mother in biology. His father was very interested in getting Andrjez involved in math and complex puzzles. He was fortunate in having a very good teacher (he had an M.Sc. in physics). In junior and high school his majors were math and physics. He competed and got to the regional final exams. Warsaw University accepted him into physics in 1974, his choice. His scholarly performance was excellent excepting philosophy, predominately Marxist. He elected medical physics for graduate study for 5 years. The course was 3 years in experimental physics and then 2 years in medical physics. Some of the final courses were at the Warsaw Cancer Center. He especially enjoyed the physics of radiation oncology. He obtained a position, while a student at the Warsaw Cancer Center.

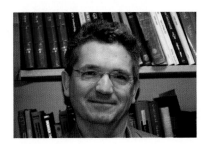

Fig. 9.3 Andrjez Niemierko

After receipt of the Ph.D. he applied for and was awarded an NIH grant for his physics project. At that time he applied for a post-doctoral fellowship with Michael Goitein. He came here with his 1-year grant and his salary from Poland. His research got to a very good start. Michael proposed that they prepare an application for an NCI RO 1. This was approved and meant that Andrjez could settle into a relatively long-term research plan. This work has enjoyed an impressive record of advances, i.e., his RO 1 is in its 21st year without interruption.

References

1. Ancukiewicz M, Finkelstein DM, Schoenfeld DA. Modeling the relationship between continuous covariates and clinical events using isotonic regression. Stat Med. 2003;57:701–8.
2. Batchelor TT, Sorensen AG, di Tomaso E, et al. AZD2171, a pan-VEGF receptor tyrosine kinase inhibitor, normalizes tumor vasculature and alleviates edema in glioblastoma patients. Cancer Cell. 2007;11:83–95.
3. Brower RG, Lanken PN, MacIntyre N, et al. Higher versus lower positive end-expiratory pressures in patients with the acute respiratory distress syndrome. N Engl J Med. 2004;351:327–36.
4. Choi NC, Fischman AJ, Niemierko A, et al. Dose-response relationship between probability of pathologic tumor control and glucose metabolic rate measured with FDG PET after preoperative chemoradiotherapy in locally advanced non-small-cell lung cancer. Int J Radiat Oncol Biol Phys. 2002;54(4):1024–35.
5. Goldberg S, Niemierko A, Turchin A. Analysis of data errors in clinical research databases. AMIA Annu Symp Proc. 2008;32:242–6.
6. Kepka L, Suit HD, Goldberg SI, et al. Results of radiation therapy performed after unplanned surgery(without re-excision) for soft tissue sarcomas. J Surg Oncol. 2005;92(1):39–45.
7. Lee CG, Heijn M, di Tomaso E, et al. Anti-vascular endothelial growth factor treatment augments tumor radiation response under normoxic or hypoxic conditions. Cancer Res. 2000;60:5565–70.
8. Loeffler JS, Niemierko A, Chapman PH. Second tumors after radiosurgery: tip of the iceberg or a bump in the road? Neurosurgery. 2003;52(6):1436–40.
9. Niemierko A. Reporting and analyzing dose distributions: a concept of Equivalent Uniform Dose (EUD). Med Phys. 1997;24(1):17–26.
10. Suit H, Goldberg S, Niemierko A, et al. Secondary carcinogenesis in patients treated with radiation: a review of data on radiation-induced cancers in human, non-human primate, canine and rodent subjects. Radiat Res. 2007;167(1):12–42.
11. Terahara A, Niemierko A, Goitein M, et al. Analysis of the relationship between tumor dose inhomogeneity and local control in patients with skull base chordoma. Int J Radiat Oncol Biol Phys. 1999;45(2):351–8.
12. Willett CG, Del Castillo CF, Shih HA, et al. Long-term results of intraoperative electron beam irradiation (IOERT) for patients with unresectable pancreatic cancer. Ann Surg. 2005;241(2):295–9.

Chapter 10

Clinical Advances by the MGH Department of Radiation Oncology

According to anatomic site and age,

CNS	Uveal melanoma
Head and neck	Breast
Lung	GI
GYN	GU
Pediatric	Mesenchymal tumors

The unambiguous goal of the MGH Department of Radiation Oncology is to work intensively to substantially increase the proportion of treated patients who are free of tumor and of treatment-related morbidity. There is acute awareness of the high incidence of cancer each year and the fact that we do not achieve our goal of cure in a significant proportion of patients. Thus, we are definitely sensitive to the fact that there are many questions to be posed and that the answering of those questions requires imaginative and thoughtful laboratory and clinical research. Importantly, there is no ambiguity that time is moving on without the slightest delay. The need for critical questions and the relentless progress of time are clearly illustrated by Fig. 1.

10.1 CNS

Clinician specialists:

Helen A. Shih (adult), **Head of the unit**
Jay S. Loeffler (adult and pediatrics)
Kevin Oh (adult)
Norbert Liebsch (base of skull and spine adult and pediatrics)
Nancy Tarbell (pediatrics)
Shannon MacDonald (pediatrics)
Torunn Yock (pediatrics)

The department has a long and rich history of efforts in the management of patients with full array of brain tumors combined with comprehensive program of clinical and laboratory research. This has been based on a productive and collaborative work with the Neurosurgical and Neurology Services. Ten years before the establishment of an independent department of radiation oncology, William Sweet of the Neurosurgical Service had initiated an active program in boron-neutron capture therapy (BNCT) for patients with malignant glioma (using the MIT reactor). In parallel, Sweet with R. Kjellberg (neurosurgery) developed the largest radiosurgery program in the USA using the Harvard Cyclotron proton beam. Both programs were on the cutting edge of radiation delivery during the 1960s for treating patients with a wide range of intracranial pathologies, by single dose. While the BNCT program enjoyed great notoriety, the clinical results were disappointing and the program was discontinued. The proton radiosurgery program has been highly successful and has continuously expanded. Initial treatment applications included benign indications of pituitary adenomas and arteriovenous malformations by Kjellberg et al. [48–50]. This utilization of the HCL kept the clinical program in operation and the HCL was thus available from the early 1970s to 2001 for our program in fractionated proton therapy of patients with both benign and malignant conditions as described by Fitzek et al. [28], Hug et al. [43], Wenkel et al. [100], and Chan et al. [9, 10]. Expertise within radiation therapy for brain tumors involved management by photon-based therapy as well, including roles for LINAC-based stereotactic radiotherapy such as for optic nerve sheath meningiomas by Arvold et al. [2], management of rare diseases such as the role for salvage therapy for primary CNS lymphoma by Nguyen et al. [63] or treatment for adult medulloblastoma patients by Chan et al. [9], and understanding of normal tissue toxicity of the pituitary axes by Pai et al. [66], brain by Barker et al. [3], and hair by Lawenda et al. [59].

Our department has played a fundamental role in the management of patients with cranial base chordomas and chondrosarcomas, uveal melanoma, and spinal and paraspinal tumors. The results of the treatment of thousands of such patients have proven to be superior to those published from photon therapies in terms of local control as well as toxicity. The opening of the Francis H. Burr Proton Therapy

H.D. Suit, J.S. Loeffler, *Evolution of Radiation Oncology at Massachusetts General Hospital*,
DOI 10.1007/978-1-4419-6744-2_10, © Springer Science+Business Media, LLC 2011

Center in November 2001 allowed the proton effort to expand rapidly into the field of pediatric neuro-oncology, with particular emphasis on the cranio-spinal treatment of children with medulloblastoma.

Intra-operative therapy using a dedicated linear accelerator within an operating room, interstitial therapy for brain and para-spinal tumors, radioactive dural plaques for spinal chordoma patients as well as a unique miniature kilovoltage stereotactic treatment device have allowed the department to constantly modify localized therapy for the individual patient. These intra-operative techniques have been due to collaboration with surgeons from a wide variety of disciplines.

Working with our colleagues within the Pappas Brain Tumor Center, the scientific discoveries with R. Jain and the Steele Laboratory have led to clinical and translational trials that exploit anti-angiogenic therapies given concurrently with radiation and chemotherapy. The results of a recent trial led to highly cited papers in *Cancer Cell* and the *Journal of Clinical Oncology* by Batchelor et al. [4, 5]. The clinical results have circulated back to the laboratory with results that are leading to modifying future trials. A major effort in the molecular genetics has been supported by the Brian Silber Fund.

The current neuro-oncology efforts within the department involve three full-time adult neuro-oncologists, three full-time pediatric neuro-oncologists, and a cranial-base oncologist. The volume of patients treated for benign and malignant intracranial tumors is unparalleled within the USA. The research portfolio in neuro-oncology involves basic science efforts, clinical trials, and medical physics. We also participate in the Radiation Therapy Oncology Group as well as the North American Brain Tumor Consortium clinical and translational trials.

10.1.1 Biographical Sketch

10.1.1.1 Jay Loeffler

Please see the autobiography of Jay Loeffler in the Introduction and comments on the future of radiation oncology at MGH in Chapter 18.

10.1.1.2 Helen Shih

New Jersey is Helen's place of birth and where she spent her young life (Fig. 10.1). Her parents emigrated from Taiwan. Helen's father earned a doctorate in education, specializing in industrial arts. He taught for over 30 years at Trenton State College in New Jersey, which has been renamed the College

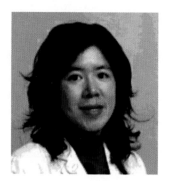

Fig. 10.1 Helen Shih

of New Jersey. His teaching evolved and later included electronics, electrical engineering, and robotics. Helen has two brothers and all three of the children are physicians. This emphasis on medicine is of interest in that these three are the first members of her extended family to be in modern medicine. She does have a paternal grandfather who was an herbalist.

She became interested in medicine while a high school student, based on a long-term interest in biology and medicine. This was recommended by her family and her high school counselor for her career. While in the 12th grade she saw a medical science TV program featuring Steve Rosenberg discussing advances in oncology and the efforts to employ immune rejection reactions against the tumor. This gave her a significant push toward oncology as a career. Her plan to be involved in translational research and to become a pioneer in the development and use of more effective patient management for the cancer patient became final.

Helen won a scholarship at Brown. She states that she "loved Brown" and her years there as a biology major. Her mentor was Marjorie Thompson, the Dean of Biological Science in the undergraduate school and who also taught embryology and histology at the medical school. Helen rated her advice and encouragement as invaluable. Her laboratory research was with Lundy Brown investigating human papillomaviruses (HPV) and cervical cancer. At the U Penn medical school she had an exceptionally fine interaction with Barbara Weber, a very prominent breast cancer geneticist and who was central to the development of the cancer center at U Penn. Helen so enjoyed her research that she spent an additional year and was awarded an M.Sc. in molecular and cell biology.

Helen decided on a career in oncology. To become familiar with the field she took an elective in radiation oncology and really enjoyed the ability to employ physics and technology in medicine. This resulted in her decision to become a radiation oncologist. For a research elective, she investigated photodynamic therapy with S. Hahn, her mentor. For this she received an RSNA award during her fourth year.

She decided to apply to the MGH for the residency as it was judged the best suited for her career aims. One rotation was with Choi during which she examined the problem of target motion. She also participated in a study of genetic markers in glioblastoma. A highly significant contribution was her study using iron oxide nanoparticles to define the position of the pelvic lymph nodes relative to the major vessels. The result was a map of the nodes and vessels demonstrating that absent quite enlarged nodes a margin of 2 cm around the vessel group would be adequate. She collaborated with Mukesh Harisinghani of radiology on this project.

On completion of the residency she was offered a staff position in the CNS program by J. Loeffler. She accepted and is now full time and has responsibilities for skull base tumors with N. Liebsch and uveal melanomas with two other staff. Helen is the lead radiation oncologist in the uveal melanoma program. In addition, she has general CNS patients plus a small number of patients with skin lesions. Helen is participating in an evaluation of very late morbidity in proton-treated patients with low-grade gliomas because of their long survival.

Helen is the Medical Student Clerkship Director in Radiation Oncology, viz., overseeing medical students and giving introductory lectures on radiation oncology for the residents in diagnostic radiology who take a rotation in the department.

Helen is the very happy mother of a lovely daughter.

10.2 Uveal Melanoma

Specialist clinicians:

Helen A. Shih, Head of the unit
John Munzenrider
Helen Shih,
Yen L. Chen
Shannon MacDonald
Evangelos Gragoudas, MEEI

The interest of the department in the use of proton beams for irradiation of uveal melanoma developed from the early interest of ophthalmologist Ian Constable of the MEEI. His proposal for pre-clinical investigation of the radiation response of monkey eye was judged feasible and was of clear interest. M. Goitein worked with Constable and developed the experimental plan to assess the tolerance of the monkey eye to large single doses of proton irradiation starting in 1972. They employed single doses up to 100 Gy and observed only modest changes, but for very short follow-up periods. Constable accepted a professorship in Perth, Australia, in 1974. Evangelos Gragoudas was appointed to be the ophthalmologist on this project and has continued in this role to the present. Michael Goitein commenced development of plans for proton treatment of uveal melanoma. J. Munzenrider became the radiation oncologist of this program shortly after his appointment to the staff in 1977 and he worked with Gragoudas through 2006. Currently, the radiation oncologists on this program are H. Shih, Y.L. Chen, and Shannon MacDonald. The treatment-planning physicist has for many years been Michael Collier.

As part of the planning for the start of the clinical program of patient treatment, Goitein designed the first 3D computer-based treatment-planning system for external beam therapy [31]. The clinical preparation of the patient for the treatment planning included these procedures: Gragoudas examines the eye; takes wide-angle photographs; measures the two dimensions of the tumor base and the height; and sutures four 2.5 mm tantalum rings onto the sclera over the margins of the *trans*-illuminated tumor. Then bi-planar (orthogonal, or AP and Lt Lat) radiographs are taken with the eye in a defined direction of gaze. The rings serve as fiducial markers permitting the proton treatment planner to reconstruct the position of the tumor in 3D relative to each of the rings. Similarly, the positions of the macula and disc are determined relative to the rings. The physicist measures distances from an edge of each ring to a defined point in the tumor or to the macula and disc. These measured distances are used in the 3D treatment planning, viz., determining the position of the tumor in 3D relative to the rings. From these are determined the exact angle of gaze at irradiation.

The treatment plan specifies the required position and gaze direction of the eye; the latter is achieved by having the patient look intently and directly at a very small light source so placed that the gaze direction would position the markers and thus the tumor in the planned beam path. To document that the eye is in correct position, bi-planar radiographs are taken of the eye. Any deviation from the plan of ≥ 0.5 mm results in the patient and eye being re-positioned until the correct position is achieved. During actual treatment, a camera is focused on the eye and the stability of the eye position is monitored by observing the position of the iris relative to marks on the monitor screen at the treatment console. Any change in eye position results in the beam being stopped and the eye and patient repositioned. Thus, as the position was monitored continuously during each fraction, the result was an early version of 4D IGRT with tracking.

The first patient was treated in 1976 by Gragoudas, Goitein, and Suit. The latter decided that treatment be started using 5 fractions of 10 Gy (RBE). The dose was rapidly increased from 50 to 70 Gy (RBE) in 5 fractions, viz., 14 Gy (RBE)/fraction. This 70 Gy RBE schedule has been employed in almost all of the patients and continues to be our standard treatment. A photograph of the first patient treated

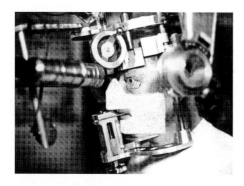

Fig. 10.2 The first patient treated by proton beams for uveal melanoma is shown in the immobilization system

period or ~ 150 per year. This program (the technique and planning system) has been adopted in several centers. The total number of uveal melanoma patients treated worldwide by proton techniques is >8000, with results comparable to those obtained here (J. Sisterson, personal communication, 2007).

10.2.1 Biographical Sketch

10.2.1.1 John Munzenrider

by protons for uveal melanoma in the RT position at the Harvard Cyclotron is presented in Fig.10.2.

Figure 10.3 presents a view of a uveal melanoma with isodose contours from three perspectives for a different patient. The patient was a 48-year-old man who had a uveal melanoma located close to the macula and optic disc. The tumor was measured to be 13.3 mm × 11.4 mm × 3.9 mm with a volume of 0.28 ml, calculated by EYEPLAN. The distances from the closest tumor margin to the macula and disc were 3.3 and 6.4 mm, respectively. The PTV was 3 mm wider than the drawn target and the SOBP was 23 mm.

A dose of 70 GyRBE in 5 fractions has been well tolerated and quite effective, viz., local control at 15 years is 95% [33]. One of our completed clinical trials randomized small- to intermediate-sized lesions to be treatment by 5 × 14 vs 5 × 10 Gy RBE. No difference in outcome has been observed for relatively short-term follow-up in either local control or the status of the eye [32].

As of 2008 the total number of uveal melanoma patients treated in this program is ~3000. From the start of eye treatment at the FHBPTC, 937 patients have been treated for uveal melanoma through May 2008, viz., over a 6.25 year

John (Fig. 10.4) first developed a serious interest in medicine as a high school student. He attended Belmont Abbey College in North Carolina and found chemistry to be his favorite subject. This tilted him from medical school to a graduate program in physical chemistry. There was an additional consideration in that he perceived medical school as too costly. He was accepted into a physical chemistry Ph.D. program at Duke. After getting into the graduate courses, he realized that he wanted something else for his professional life. He did well in the exams but did not really enjoy the subject material. There were quite positive aspects to his 2 years at Duke. There he met a wonderful young woman and they married. They have three children and four grandchildren.

John's less-than-intense interest in a career in physical chemistry prompted a serious re-assessment of the career plans. The conclusion was that he wanted to go to medical school. This plan met with success and he entered Washington University Medical School in St. Louis and was there for 5 years including some special electives. He had a clinical rotation in radiology. At that time, students were encouraged to spend additional time in radiation therapy. This came about as several faculties had just been recruited to UCSF. John spent several weeks in radiation therapy and met

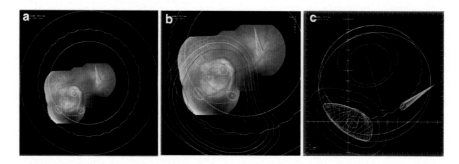

Fig. 10.3 (**a**) A wide-angle fundus view of a uveal melanoma with the four tantalum rings (*white*) and the target contour (*green*) shown. (**b**) The same view with the isodose contours on the retina displayed.

(**c**) Beam's eye view of the eye showing the tumor (*red*), the aperture (*green*) which also corresponds to the 50% isodose line, and the 90% isodose line (*magenta*). These were provided by Michael Collier, 2008

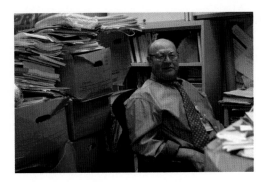

Fig. 10.4 John Munzenrider

Bill Powers.[1] On John's first visit to the department, Powers was virtually in the betatron removing the donut. Bill happily explained the mechanism of operation of betatron and many aspects of radiation therapy. John had a very informative time seeing patients being treated, new and follow-up patients, etc. He found Bill to be a very dynamic individual who manifestly loved what he was doing. The decision to enter radiation oncology was made. His strong background in chemistry, physics, and math were factors making radiation oncology an especially attractive medical specialty as it was a fascinating combination of clinical oncology and substantial component of relatively high technology.

Fernando Bloedorn was a very well known and admired clinician with special interests in head/neck cancer patients and a specialist in brachytherapy. John applied and was accepted by Fernando and moved to the University of Maryland. There was an upset in the plans, in that after 1 year he was drafted. Fernando told John about the opportunities in the US Public Health Service and that he should consider applying for an appointment and for an assignment at a government research institution. This he did and the application was approved. He then had two informative years at the National Cancer Institute. He worked in the same office as Nora Tapley, who later was a specialist in electron beam therapy at the MDACC. His work was largely administrative in the handling of grant applications and participating in the complex grant review process. This included site visits and meetings of the Radiation Study Section. During that period he met several luminaries in our field, viz., Simon Kramer, Henry Kaplan, Luther Brady, and many others.

During this period, Bloedorn moved to Tufts University in Boston. John rejoined Fernando after the NCI. Most saddening was Fernando's death quite soon after John's completing the residency. One very positive feature of the time at Tufts

was the frequent visits (at least six) and lectures of Gilbert Fletcher, whom he got to know. John was appointed to the staff and continued there for 2 years. At that point he was recruited to the MGH in 1977. John was soon working near full time on the proton therapy program at the Harvard Cyclotron Laboratory in Cambridge. Proton therapy was soon being applied to a number of tumor sites from 1976 when the major NCI grant was funded. This subspecialty was especially attractive to John with his solid background in physics and math. A very valuable and new program was Goitein's 3D computer-based treatment-planning system. A special area of interest was the management of uveal melanoma patients with Evangelos Gragoudas and Michael Goitein. The dose was 70 Gy RBE in 5 fractions in ≤ 8 days. Local control at 15 years on ~ 2000 patients is 95%. This was the first computer based treatment planning system used clinically. Initially, this was specifically designed for the eye program and was then quickly modified for all body sites. John was also quite involved in the treatment of skull base sarcoma patients. He was a participant in several publications on the experience with proton radiation therapy for a spectrum of tumors with reference to not only TCP but also risk of radiation injury to critical normal tissues.

An activity of which John is especially proud is his interaction with the residents and fellows. He served as Director of the Resident Program from 1980 to 1998. He was rated very highly by the residents for his personal interest and positive attitude and efforts on their behalf. We sent a questionnaire 1 year asking the residents to rank the staff as teachers. John won that by a large margin. Virtually all of his 65 papers in referred journals since joining the MGH have been with residents and fellows. John has more recently helped in the general radiation oncology programs at BMC, Jordan Hospital, and Emerson Hospital.

10.3 Head and Neck

Specialist clinicians:

Paul Busse, Head of the unit
Annie Chan
C.C. Wang (Head of this unit from 1970 to 2002)
Milford Schulz was active in head/neck therapy from 1942 to 1976

10.3.1 Milford Schulz

Milford Schulz was a general radiation oncologist but contributed importantly to this area. In his early career, CC

---

[1] Bill Powers was the first to use tomography in the assessment of glottic carcinoma.

practiced general radiation oncology with concentration on head/neck patients, but for the later three decades he limited his work primarily to head/neck.

10.3.1.1 Early Special Techniques

Early Special Techniques. Milford Schulz was innovative in his techniques for shielding normal tissues in EBRT and interstitial brachytherapy [40]. Figure 10.5a, b illustrates a special lead cut-out that provides an open area for direct orthovoltage irradiation of the exposed lip tumor and a tongue of lead folded to slip behind the lip to protect the gingiva and oral cavity.[2] He also used radium needle implantation of residual cervical nodes after EBRT, a substantial boost dose, Fig. 10.5c.

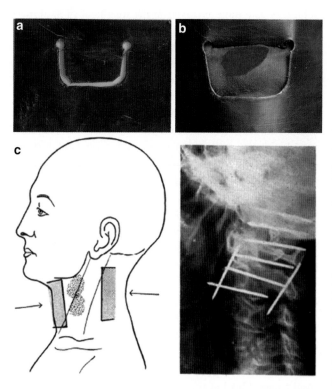

Fig. 10.5 (**a**) A lead cut-out designed so that a "tongue" of lead would fit behind the lip and shield the gingiva from the x-irradiation. (**b**) The shield in place. (**c**) A radium implant for a boost dose to residual nodes after 250 kVp EBRT [2]

---

[2] These images are based on a lead cut made in our machine shop and placed in an employee's mouth to simulate the technique of Schulz. This was necessary as the quality of the two images illustrating this technique in the Holmes and Schulz book was not adequate for publication. The colored area on the lip is to indicate the position of a model tumor.

10.3.2 C.C. Wang

The H/N group of tumors was especially interesting to C.C. Wang (Cure Cancer Wang) who led this area from 1970 until his retirement in 2002. He worked closely with MEEI surgeons and MGH medical oncologist Phil Amrein. CC wrote one of the important texts on head/neck cancer and their management by radiation, *Radiation Therapy for Head and Neck Neoplasms*. The third and final edition was published in 1997 [96].

10.3.2.1 IOC

IOC. CC developed the technique of intra-oral cone electron beam therapy [6, 96, 98], principally for lesions of the anterior two-thirds of the tongue and to a lesser extent for patients with tumors of the floor of mouth, soft palate, and buccal mucosa (especially in edentulous patients). He employed this as an upfront boost dose to the gross tumor before EBRT. The merits of the technique are that the cone is placed directly on the observed lesion, i.e., greatly reduced incidental irradiation of normal tissue. This technique is analogous to IOERT. The local control results were judged to be higher than for EBRT, e.g., 5-year local control rates were 90 and 81% for 44 T1 and 79 T2 carcinomas of the oral tongue patients, respectively. Soft tissue ulceration and osteoradionecrosis was less frequent than tongue implant. CC developed the sub-mental boost technique with EBRT for tumors of the floor of mouth and base of tongue to decrease dose to the mandible.

10.3.2.2 BID

BID. Another early strategy, in the late 1960s, of Wang was his use of BID dose fractionation, viz., two fractions on each treatment day with ≥4 h between fractions. The rationale was to decrease the potentially negative impact of tumor cell proliferation during the 24–72 h between once-per-day fractions [96]. His BID treatment administered 1.8 Gy BID to ~38 Gy and then a rest period for ~10–12 days to reduce the severity of the acute mucosal reactions. The treatment was completed using 1.6 Gy/fraction, BID. For early-stage squamous cell carcinomas of the oral cavity and oro-pharynx, there was an indication of a gain relative to QD treatment. The gain was judged to be important for most sites by BID radiation treatment of T3–4 carcinomas. Many centers are employing a variant of the accelerated treatment. At present, a common protocol is QD fractionation for the initial component (treatment of the CTV), and then BID for the boost dose for the final component of the treatment. By this approach, there is no rest period or break in treatment. This is accepted as providing a gain in local control.

10.3.2.3 Intracavitry

Intracavitary Therapy for Nasopharyngeal Tumors. CC was among the first to employ intracavitary therapy as a boost for nasopharyngeal carcinoma. In addition, he effectively adopted angiocatheters for interstitial brachytherapy. These were readily available, were inexpensive, and came in a range of lengths and diameters. These were utilized with great effect and almost entirely with ^{192}Ir.

Another active clinician in head/neck tumors was Alan Thornton in the proton program.

10.3.3 The Busse and Chan Era

The Busse Era After the retirement of CC in 2002, Paul Busse, a graduate of our residency program, was recruited by Jay Loeffler to direct the head/neck program in radiation oncology. Paul works collaboratively with Annie Chan, a full time head/neck radiation oncologist, in the MGH/MEEI Cancer Center. Several of the advances are noted here.

10.3.3.1 Locally Advanced Paranasal Sinus Cancer

These patients present very difficult treatment problems due to the immediate proximity of the target to sensitive and critical normal tissues and the need for high target dose levels. Happily, the data available from our proton treatment program indicate clearly improved local control rates relative to photon therapy. Treatment for most MGH patients has been high-dose proton ± photon treatment. The principal clinicians on this project have been Annie Chan, Alan Thornton, and James McIntyre. Alan was the lead staff in the management of these patients prior to his move to the University of Indiana, Bloomington, to be the director of their proton therapy center.

Between 1991 and 2002, 102 patients with advanced sinonasal cancers received proton radiation therapy at the MGH. There were 33 squamous cell carcinomas, 30 carcinomas with neuroendocrine differentiation, 20 adenoid cystic carcinomas, 13 soft tissue sarcomas, and 6 adenocarcinomas. The median dose was 71.6 Gy RBE and median follow-up was 44 months. The 5-year actuarial local control and disease-free survival rates were 86 and 54%, respectively [8, 70, 71]. For adenocystic adenocarcinoma in 23 patients treated for gross disease, local control at 5 years was 93% [70].

Distant metastasis was the predominant pattern of relapse for squamous cell, neuroendocrine, and adenoid cystic carcinomas. These results compare very favorably to that achieved by IMXT.

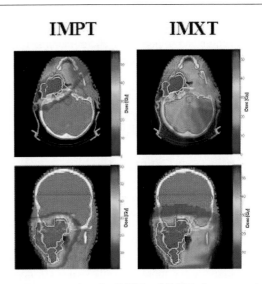

Fig. 10.6 Treatment plans for IMXT and IMPT of a paranasal sinus cancer were prepared by N. Liebsch, R. Houlihan, and J. Adams using Kon Rad

A comparison of dose distributions for IMXT and IMPT are presented in Fig. 10.6. There is a striking reduction in the volumes of normal tissues beyond the PTV receiving radiation by IMPT.

The long-term ocular and visual toxicities in 36 patients treated with accelerated hyperfractionated proton ± x-ray therapy for advanced stage sinonasal malignant tumors at the MGH were reported [99]. The median dose to the gross tumor target was 69.6 Gy RBE and mean follow-up was 52 months. The LENT/CTC grade ≥2 toxicity at 5 years was 15.8%. Late visual morbidity after these high-dose levels by proton techniques is judged acceptable.

10.3.3.2 Base of Tongue

Base of Tongue Karakoyun-Celik, Busse, and colleagues reported results in 2005 [45] of treatment of 40 patients with carcinoma of the base of tongue by 61.2 Gy EBRT plus 17.4 Gy BRT. Median follow-up was 56 months. Adjuvant chemotherapy was given to 24 patients. Local control and survival rates at 5 years were 78 and 62%, respectively.

10.3.3.3 Locally Advanced Nasopharyngeal Carcinoma (NPC)

At the MGH, proton radiation therapy has been used to treat advanced NPC. Between 1990 and 2002, 17 patients with newly diagnosed T4 N0-3 tumors received 73.6 Gy RBE by proton and photon beams [8, 68]. For 11 patients, treatment was on a BID schedule and 10 also had chemotherapy. At a median follow-up time of 43 months, the 3-year results are local control at 92% and disease-free survival at 79%.

The group led by Annie Chan has an on-going phase II study of proton combined with chemotherapy for locally advanced nasopharyngeal carcinoma. Quality of life will also be assessed.

These results for several sites are judged to be quite good, especially for advanced lesions located in sites with important normal structures in close proximity.

10.3.4 Biographical Sketches

10.3.4.1 Paul Busse

Paul (Fig. 10.7) has a very special history in that he is from a family of multigenerations of florists, viz., have operated florist businesses for more than 70 years. He appreciated quite clearly that he was expected to follow this career path. However, he was very strongly influenced by a high school biology teacher who provided Paul a quite special experience to work in microbiology and perform anatomic dissections on laboratory animals. Clearly, this was an exceptional exposure to science in high school. The impact on Paul was far more than the family anticipated. Because of his serious interest in science he majored in biology at Southern Illinois University on a scholarship. Paul was determined to be as independent as possible despite the fact that he came from a quite affluent family. He did win scholarships right along the way and was close to being independent. At Southern Illinois University he received yet another scholarship to do a Ph.D. degree in microbiology. This was transformed slightly in that his interest became rather involved in viruses associated with tumors involving some 2.5 years of study. At that point, his advisor lost RO1 funding. Fortunately, Paul was put in touch with Len Tolmach, the famous radiation biologist at Washington University in St. Louis. Paul completed his Ph.D. degree in Tolmach's group with emphasis on understanding radiation sensitivity and the cell replication cycle and the kinetics of the cell population growth. Tolmach was among the earliest in the study of potential lethal damage repair. While in St. Louis he became acquainted with William Powers, Chief of Radiation Oncology. Powers had worked closely with Tolmach on the quite significant series

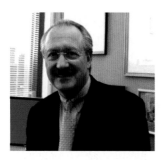

Fig. 10.7   Paul Busse

of experiments that quantitated the fraction of cells in a tumor that were hypoxic, i.e., their analysis of the break point in their famous cell survival curve. This was an intense, thoroughly stimulating, and productive period for Paul. Hywel Medoc Jones was a fellow student who later became Chief of Radiation Oncology at Tufts Medical School.

After graduation in 1978, Paul attended medical school at St. Louis University. He very much enjoyed medical school and was the president of his class for his junior and senior years. For an internship, he had 1 year in internal medicine at the Barnes Hospital, finishing in 1986. Upon graduation he came to the MGH for a 3-year residency in radiation oncology and performed extremely well there. He was rated very highly as a resident. He accepted an invitation from Normal Coleman for position at the Deaconess Hospital and the JCRT. There he initiated the program of intra-operative x-ray therapy (IORT) based on a 250 kVp Chief of Surgery at the Deaconess was keen to have IORT available for irradiation post grossly complete but very close resection margins. Accordingly, the penetration of the 250 kVp beam was reasonable. Paul also worked effectively with John Chaffey, head of the radiation oncology service. Chaffey shortly left the Deaconess to work at Framingham, in a unit of the JCRT. Paul became Head of the Deaconess unit at age 36. Another major interest of Paul was head and neck oncology and he worked closely with surgeon Dan Miller, who had recently moved there from the MEEI where he had practiced for many years in very close collaboration with C.C. Wang. Also, these two worked very actively with Tom Frei, Chief of Medical Oncology at the Dana Farber, to assess the efficacy of 5 FU and radiation protocols for head and neck cancer patients.

Another major activity of Busse was boron neutron capture therapy (BNCT) performed in collaboration with R. Zamenhof, a physicist who had transferred from Tufts to work on this project. Treatments were performed at the reactor facility at MIT. The program there had been inaugurated by Bill Sweet, MGH neurosurgeon. The basic concept was to administer a boron-containing compound with preferential uptake in the tumor tissue. There was some evidence that this might obtain for the highly malignant brain tumors. BNCT was being studied especially for CNS tumors by Paul and by other centers in Japan and Europe. During the challenging work with the BNCT, Paul became the PI of the BNCT program grant. Results were less than expected and the program was closed. There is a continuing effort in Japan and Europe in search for compounds that concentrate much better in tumors.

Paul was recruited by Jay Loeffler to be responsible for the MGH Head/Neck Unit after the retirement of C.C. Wang. Not long after Paul's start at the MGH, Chris Willett accepted the Chair at Duke and Simon Powell left to become Chair at Washington University in St. Louis, and Paul was appointed to head the MGH clinical program in the department.

Paul states that he is very impressed with the difficulty of trying to work in the "shadow of CC Wang." He has developed very effective and good working relationships with the head and neck surgeons at MEEI. The head and neck radiation oncology service now treats about 30 patients per day and this is shared with Annie Chan. Further, they have initiated studies on proton beam therapy for head and neck patients. With respect to photon therapy, substantially more than 50% of the patients are now treated by IMXT and for some of the anatomic sites there is expectation of some definite gains by 4D image-guided therapy. Paul is very impressed by the strength in physics and the effort being led by George Chen and Thomas Bortfeld.

Paul has found that a quite significant effort is required to head the clinical service with the large expansion of staff and the increasing interactions with other departments of the hospital, the various Harvard hospitals, and affiliated centers the in and beyond Boston.

10.3.4.2 Annie Chan

Hong Kong lost a young star when Annie Chan (Fig. 10.8) decided at age 18 to come to UCLA for her university-level education in chemistry and general pre-med. She had been at the top of her high school class in chemistry and biology. Her years at UCLA were a time of sustained excitement, especially in chemistry. In those classes and laboratories the interaction with many keen students and a Nobel Prize professor proved to be an exceptional time.

Annie won a scholarship to University of Chicago Pritzker School of Medicine and thereby did not need to obtain any funding from her parents. The 4 years in medical school were clearly interesting and also productive. She learned of the existence of radiation oncology as a medical specialty when hearing that the President of the University of Chicago hospital, Samuel Hellman, was a radiation oncologist. He had previously been Chief of the JCRT (Brigham, Beth Israel, and Deaconess Hospitals) and then Head of the Memorial Sloan Kettering hospital prior to moving to Chicago as Dean. Curiosity directed her to the radiation oncology department where she met excellent people and found the discipline to be of serious interest. Annie decided that she would become a radiation oncologist. She had become especially interested in head/neck oncology and wished to spend time with C.C. Wang. She came to the MGH for her residency. During that period she completed projects with C.C. Wang and Jay Loeffler. On completion of her residency she became a member of our faculty and works with the head/neck group. Her clinical interest is on improving therapeutic ratio with proton beam radiation therapy in head/neck and skull base malignancies. She is the principal investigator of two phase II studies at MGH, one on nasopharyngeal cancer and one on sinonasal malignancy.

Annie has a daughter, Alessandra, who is a source of enormous pleasure.

10.4 Breast

Specialist clinicians:

Alphonse Taghian, Head of the unit
Shannon Mac Donald, Angela Robertis
Simon Powell, former Head of the unit

Simon Powell was recruited in 1991 to initiate a strong program in the study of repair of double-strand breaks in DNA combined with the development of an innovative academic program in breast tumors. His clinical work was highly regarded and he was appointed to serve as Director of the MGH Breast Tumor Center. This he did effectively for several years. However, time pressure required a choice of time for laboratory research or an expanding administrative role. He chose the laboratory. Simon was joined by A. Taghian in 1998 who became Head of the breast program when Simon moved to Washington University in 2004. This chapter considers the history during the Powell and Taghian years. The basic DNA research initiated by S. Powell is described in Chapter 8.

The current Breast Team of Taghian, Katz, and McDonald work closely with physicists and the extensive team of medical oncologists, surgeons, radiologists, pathologists, biostatisticians, and scientists. This breast cancer program has had sustained growth. Currently ~350–400 breast cancer patients are seen per year for radiation treatment.

Powell and Taghian initiated an evaluation of partial breast irradiation in a prospective trial for patients with ≤2 cm

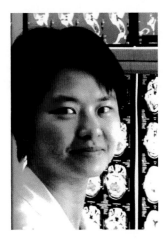

Fig. 10.8 Annie Chan

invasive carcinoma of the breast, status post margin negative resection and negative sentinel node(s) and no evident distant metastatic tumor. The initial strategy was to employ brachytherapy with placement of the catheters during surgery (1997–2001). This treatment was employed on 48 patients. The implant was usually 2–3 planes (1 cm between planes) using ^{192}Ir sources, loaded at ∼3–4 days post-surgery. The dose prescribed was 50, 55, and 60 Gy. The local control rate was similar to that for the standard 6-week whole breast radiation. Morbidity was non-negligible and this program was discontinued [58].

They shifted to external beam techniques and began investigation of accelerated hypofractionated partial breast irradiation (PBI). A recent detailed assessment of the various parameters from patient choice to treatment outcome of PBI vs whole breast irradiation has indicated comparable efficacy and acceptability by patients of 40 and 55 years of age [75]. Macdonald and Taghian have suggested that there is a definite trend to replace whole breast with partial breast irradiation for early-stage disease [60].

A new technique using 3D conformal treatment by two mini-tangents and *en face* electrons was developed and implemented [90]. This was used in a dose-escalation study with the main goal to establish the most clinically effective dose for hypofractionation BID at 4 Gy/fraction PBI. Total doses were 32, 36, and 40 Gy. The study design is to accrue 100 patients for each of the three dose levels (40 Gy dose level expanded to 200 patients). The trial has accrued 330 patients of the 400 planned. The end-points for this study are feasibility, tolerance, efficacy, and cosmesis. This technique has been adopted by several other centers. The dose/fractionation schedule varies slightly between centers.

The use of proton beams in the treatment of the chest wall in patients with locally advanced disease is under study by MacDonald. For patients with left-sided disease and unfavorable cardiac position in the chest, the advantages appear large. Analyses of comparative treatment plans have indicated dramatic decrements in dose to the heart by partial breast irradiation.

Regarding the use of proton beam in PBI, a treatment planning comparison of proton vs photon+electron treatment demonstrated reduced dose to non-target tissues. For treatment based on protons alone vs combined photon + electrons, skin reaction was a problem in a few patients [52, 53].

Intensive studies of the dose distribution and of the magnitude and frequency of set-up errors have been performed. Gierga et al. [30] reported that error can be reduced by imaging of patients in treatment position who have surgically placed clips.

Alm El-Din et al. assessed the rate of breast cancer in 264 women whose treatment at MGH included supra-diaphragmatic irradiation (SDI) for their Hodgkin's lymphoma [1]. The median age of these patients was 26 years and the median follow-up was 15 years. The standard morbidity ratios were 19 and 4.6 for patients ≤30 and >30 years of age at treatment. Importantly the risk increased with length of follow-up observation.

Taghian and Powell were part of an inter-institutional study of tolerance of paclitaxel in addition to RT combined with doxorubicin and cyclophosphamide by patients with stage II or III breast cancer. The finding was that the frequency and severity of pulmonary toxicity was not acceptable [87].

Taghian et al. reported the outcome of 313 patients treated by mastectomy ± chemotherapy for primary lesions ≥5 cm and negative lymph nodes from a very large series of patients in NSABP trials [86]. The finding was low risk of local/regional failure in patients who had chemotherapy and mastectomy for ≥10 nodes removed all being negative. Patients with such tumors do not warrant radiation therapy [89].

Taghian and colleagues have initiated a neoadjuvant chemotherapy trial where tumor physiology and biological markers have been evaluated. They showed that paclitaxel combined with chemotherapy decreases the intra-tumoral pressure and improves oxygenation [88].

A continuing problem in patients undergoing axillary lymph node dissection and breast radiation is non-trivial frequency of arm edema. Taghian has obtained a new high-technology laser device (perometer) to measure the circumference of the arm at several levels prior to and at specified times post-surgery. Taghian was awarded NIH grants (R01 and AVON PFP grants totaling $2.1 M) to fund the lymphedema program. The intent was to screen all patients with breast cancer for lymphedema with multiple measurements at baseline and twice per year after. Patients who develop 5% increase in arm volume are randomly assigned to very early use of a pressure sleeve vs observation. This trial started in September 2009.

Further, Taghian and group are leading a multi-institutional investigation on the effect of irradiation of the heart on the ejection fraction in women who received Herceptin. This is being conducted in collaboration with the Brigham and Women's Hospital, Michigan, Gustave Roussy, and M.D. Anderson.

10.4.1 Biographical Sketches

10.4.1.1 Simon Powell

Simon (Fig. 10.9) was very much oriented toward biology and perhaps medicine upon entering Oxford University. His

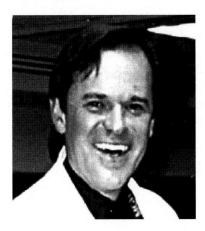

Fig. 10.9 Simon Powell

undergraduate concentration was in physiology or the neurosciences. He did very well and received a first class degree from Oxford University, not a trivial accomplishment. A major career decision for him was graduate studies in biology (he did have an invitation from Cambridge University) or medicine. He opted for medicine with the opportunity for medically related basic research. Simon was admitted to the University College Medical School in London. There he developed a general interest in oncology and was particularly influenced by elective courses at the Royal Marsden Hospital (previously the Royal Cancer Hospital) with Dr. Michael Peckham. This experience had a major impact on his interest in oncology and at that time especially toward medical oncology. Peckham's oncological interest was in radiation and medical oncology and a large fraction of his professional time was directed toward the management of patients with testicular tumors and lymphomas.

Simon elected to enter oncology and at that time there was no separation between radiation oncology and medical oncology. His residency was at the Royal Marsden Hospital in central London and sometimes at the affiliated hospital in Surrey, well outside of London. After some time in the laboratory, he decided to do a research degree, but before that he wished to complete a general medical education, viz., pass the equivalent of our Internal Medical Boards and become a member of the Royal College of Physicians. Subsequently, Simon completed several years as a resident and a senior resident at the Royal Marsden in oncology.

As his career goal was academic medicine the expectation was that one would obtain a Ph.D. degree and he did this. Simon decided to work in the laboratory of Gordon Steele. He commenced this work and after a year he became a formal Ph.D. student and committed for a thesis. His thesis title was *Repair Fidelity in Human Tumors. A Predictor of Radiation Sensitivity*, a study of repair and fidelity of repair of damaged DNA. The experimental method was a novel assay technique for assessment of repair of double-strand breaks in DNA. The interest was not merely a yes-or-no closing of the break, but the quality of the repair in the binding. That is, would the DNA post-repair function normally? He worked on this project for 3 years and received the Ph.D. degree and had several publications. In 1990, he went to the European School of Oncology meeting in Lugano, Switzerland. H. Suit listened to his lecture and was quite impressed and inquired about Simon's coming to the Massachusetts General Hospital. Simon accepted the invitation to come to the MGH and concentrate his clinical work on breast cancer and laboratory research on the repair of radiation-damaged DNA; time was to be allocated on a 50:50 basis between these two. The opportunity to work in breast cancer, as well as the laboratory, was attractive in that breast tumors had been a long-term clinical interest of Simon. This was reflected by one of his clinical papers on the frequency and severity of radiation injury to the brachial plexus. Another area of interest for Simon was the medical justification for a radiation of the entirety of the breast of patients who have relatively small fraction of the breast involved by tumor and particularly after resection with negative margins. This was a treatment approach that he had observed at the Royal Marsden Hospital by John Yarnold using brachytherapy. This is a subject on which Simon and Alphonse Taghian performed a study at the MGH. They concluded that partial breast irradiation was an effective strategy but that the clinical outcome by external beam radiation therapy was superior to that by brachytherapy.

Simon served as the Director of the Breast Cancer Center at the MGH for 4.5 years, ending in 2001. He gave up this position because of the very substantial time commitment required by his expanding laboratory research program.

During his thesis work at the Royal Marsden Hospital he became interested in the role of recombination in the repair of radiation-damaged DNA and now considers it the dominant mechanism in repair of double-strand breaks in DNA. A special emphasis was an examination for a differential in this repair between tumor and normal cells. He investigated the role of p53 and BRCA 1 and 2.

10.4.1.2 Alphonse Taghian

Alphonse (Fig. 10.10) was born in Alexandria, Egypt, in 1955. His education is unusual in that he did his entire pre-university education in a French school, as this was judged by his parents to be the most academically demanding. This was the same education for his two brothers and a sister. He grew up being entirely fluent in French, as well as Arabic. He entered medical school at age 18 in Alexandria University, Egypt.

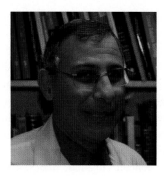

Fig. 10.10 Alphonse Taghian

The stimulus for his deciding on medicine as a career is not clear in his mind. He had pretty much decided by age 15 that he wanted to be a physician and this might have been in part that in his family there were no physicians on his father's side. Further, he knew he had been named after a well-known physician in Alexandria, but one with whom the family had had no contact. An additional factor was that his mother had died, when he was a 14-year-old boy, due to breast cancer at age 36.

Interesting, regarding his academic excellence, is that to achieve admission to the medical school in Egypt one had to rank in the top 2% of the $\sim$ 110,000 taking the final national high school exams, i.e., the Baccalaureate. Thus there were $\sim$ 2000 students admitted to medical schools in Egypt in Alphonse's year.

Medical school was a 7-year program and as the schooling is free there is a requirement that one spend a year working in a small community or village. Alphonse spent his time in upper Egypt in an area close to Luxor, the city famed for the monuments of the Pharaohs. This was followed by 3 years of military service which was obligatory (at least for people who do not have political connections). There was very little for him to do while serving his military assignment, which was in a base near the border with Libya. He began doing extensive reading and he got interested in radiation and the physics of radiation and was reading books from France on this subject. In medical school the courses are taught in English. Accordingly, Alphonse speaks and reads Arabic, French, and English quite readily.

He decided that he definitely wanted to go to France for specialty training. However, he appreciated that getting into a French center would not be easy. Good fortune assisted him in that Professor Daniel Chassagne, who was at that time Chief of the Department of Radiation Therapy at the Institute Gustav Roussy (the French national cancer center), was lecturing in Cairo. There was a very strong and long-standing collaboration between the Egyptians and the French in radiation and medical oncology. Alphonse met Chassagne and gave him a paper that he had written and an unambiguous request that he be given an opportunity to come to France to study radiation therapy.

To his great surprise and delight several months later he received a letter saying that he had been admitted into France to study radiation therapy. He was assigned to Nancy (between Paris and Strasbourg) where he worked with Professor P. Bey. His 3-year period in Nancy was very productive. As required, he passed the written and oral examination with the highest score in France and received the Jean-Pierre Monnier award for best thesis. His thesis was entitled *Endometrial Cancer Treatment by Radiation Alone* and this was published in the *International Radiation, Oncology, Biology, and Physics*. However, his goal was to go to the Institute Gustave Roussy, which Alphonse considered to be the MGH of France.

He was fortunate again in that he met a person on the train from Nancy to Paris to whom he described his intense desire to further his education in the Institute Gustave Roussy. She replied, "That is very interesting because I am having Professor Maurice Tubiana who is President of the Institute for dinner." Evidently, she talked very affectively with Tubiana because he was promptly given an appointment at the Institute Gustave Roussy. There he had a 2-year fellowship in clinical radiation oncology followed by a year in laboratory research. He wrote one important paper during this time, viz., the examination of the incidence sarcomas in the 6919 women following radiation as treatment for their breast cancer. He did the laboratory research with Dr. Malaise. A colleague in the laboratory, Dr. Marcelle Guichard, encouraged him to apply to the MGH to work in the radiation biology laboratory. He was, obviously, accepted and spent 3 years doing full-time research, which was a very busy and productive period resulting in a substantial number of papers. He was then appointed to the clinical group and worked primarily at Boston University from 1993 to 1998 when he was transferred to the MGH.

10.5 Lung

For Specialist clinicians see above

Noah Choi, Head of the unit
Henning Willers

In the early 1970s there was only meager interest in employing radiation in the management of patients with lung cancers of any stage or pathological type. Radiation treatment techniques that permitted high dose levels had not been developed. Further, there were only scant data on sites of failure following surgery or radiation, not even the frequency of death from intra-thoracic tumor with no evident distant metastatic disease. The prevailing perception was that virtually all patients would die of metastatic disease even were the local treatment to be successful. This pertained to non-small cell lung cancer (NSCLC) and to small cell lung cancer (SCLC). Furthermore, chemotherapeutic (CRx) agents available then were of little effect. New technology for imaging, radiation planning, and delivery meant that the accepted wisdom would change progressively with these advances.

None of the staff in 1972 expressed special interest in the challenge to study the potential for improvement in local-regional tumor control and survival for lung cancer patients by radiation therapy. Noah Choi joined the department in 1973 and happily accepted the challenge presented to radiation oncology by lung cancers. An important factor in Noah's interest in this area was that his father had died of lung cancer.

10.5.1 Accelerated Radiation

Accelerated Radiation Therapy. Choi [12] compared two different BID RT schedules with standard QD for acute normal skin reaction and their effectiveness in relief of pain and tumor control in patients with metastatic cancer. Patients were randomized to three groups: schedule A: conventional QD regimen totaling 37.6 Gy/16 fractions/22–23 days; schedule B: BID regimen 34.4 Gy/16 fractions/10–11 days; and schedule C: BID regimen totaling 35.7 Gy/16 fractions/10–11 days. The pattern and magnitude of acute skin reactions in the three schedules were nearly identical but tumor regression and pain relief were achieved faster in the BID fractionation schedules.

They determined that the total dose delivered by QD RT could be administered on a BID schedule in approximately one-half the time, provided the total dose is reduced by ~8%. Were this concept valid, RT on a BID should be more effective than QD for rapidly growing cancers, i.e., small cell lung cancer. These data laid a foundation for subsequent studies and the current use of BID RT for several rapidly growing tumors.

10.5.2 Small Cell Lung

Small Cell Lung Cancer (SCLC). Choi et al. [11, 15] reported that survival was enhanced in patients with locally advanced disease treated by radiation combined with chemotherapy (CRx) than by CRx alone. Choi et al. [13] performed a first of its kind dose–response study of SCLC in 154 patients. Local control rates at 2.5 years increased with dose, viz., 16, 21, 51, 61, and 63% for doses of 30, 35, 40, 45, and 50 Gy, respectively. Then in 1998, Choi et al. [16] reported findings of a dose-escalation study (CALGB 8837) yielding estimates of the maximum tolerated radiation dose (MTD) given with concurrent CRx to SCLC patients. Chemotherapy

consisted of three cycles of cisplatin 33 mg/m^2/day on days 1–3 over 30 min, cyclophosphamide 500 mg/m^2 on day 1 intravenously (IV) over 1 h, and etoposide 80 mg/m^2/day on days 1–3 over 1 h every 3 weeks (PCE), and two cycles of cisplatin 33 mg/m^2/day on days 1–3 over 30 min and etoposide 80 mg/m^2/day on days 1–3 over 1 h every 3 weeks (PE). RT was started at the initiation of the fourth cycle of chemotherapy.

The MTD was ~70 Gy (35 fractions in 7 weeks) for QD and 45 Gy (30 fractions in 3 weeks) for BID fractionation schedules, respectively. The 2- and 3-year survival rates were 54 and 35% for QD (radiation dose ranged from 56 to 70 Gy) and 52 and 25% for BID RT (radiation dose ranged from 45 to 55.5 Gy) schedules.

This study laid a foundation for the current phase III intergroup study (CALGB 30610/RTOG 0538) in which MTD of BID (45 Gy/30 F/3 weeks) is compared with MTD of QD (70 Gy/35 F/7 weeks) and MTD of concomitant boost (61.2 Gy/34 F/5 weeks) schedules in combination with 4 cycles of concurrent chemotherapy. Each cycle of chemotherapy consists of cisplatin 80 mg/m^2 IV over 60 min on day 1, every 21 days, and etoposide 100 mg/m^2 IV over 60 min on days 1, 2, and 3, every 21 days.

10.5.3 Non-small Cell

Non-small Cell Lung Cancer (NSCLC). In 1981, Choi et al. [14] provided data on the radiation dose vs survival of 162 locally advanced and inoperable NSCLC patients; there was no CRx as this was prior to the advent of cisplatin-based protocols. Treatment was in a sequential dose-escalation study and treatment volume expansion to include regional nodes (including bilateral supraclavicular regions). The sequential dose escalation was made from initial 40–45 Gy to a small target volume (2 MV x-ray) to 60–64 Gy to an expanded target volume covering potential microscopic nodal disease with 10 MV x-rays.

Survival results at 3 years were 3% for the low-dose and small volume compared with 28% for the high-dose and large volume groups, respectively. Local control results at ≥ 18 months were 29 and 76% for low-dose and high-dose groups, respectively.

The result of this study led to the subsequent radiation dose-escalation studies in searching for the MTD of radiation in a setting of radiation and concurrent chemotherapy using intensity-modulated radiation therapy (IMXT) (Partners protocol 99-299, PI: Noah Choi) and proton beam therapy (Partners protocol 00-092, PI: Noah Choi) in stage III NSCLC.

10.5.4 Molecular Imaging

Molecular-Imaging Biomarker for Optimized Radiation Therapy. Choi et al. [17] measured tumor glucose metabolic rate (MRglc) using ^{18}F-2-fluoro-2-deoxy-D-glucose (18F-FDG) PET prior to and following pre-operative radiation [45–50 Gy/25–28/5–5.5 weeks) alone or combined with chemotherapy to patients with stage IIIA non-small cell lung cancer (NSCLC). The residual metabolic activity was examined for a correlation with histopathological status in the resected tumor specimen.

They reported that the decrease in FDG uptake post RT or RT + CRx was inversely related to the extent of residual tumor on pathological study of the surgical specimen. From this inverse dose–response relationship, residual MRglc ≤ 0.040 μmol/min/g was found to be correlated with $\geq 95\%$ probability of pathologic complete tumor response (pTCP $\geq 95\%$) (Fig. 10.11). Therefore, residual MRglc > 0.040 μmol/min/g may be a useful surrogate biomarker of tumor response and valuable in defining residual biological target volume (BTV) for planning the patient-specific boost dose and boost PTV. This is to be employed in a study of escalation of the boost dose in non-surgical treatment of both stage III NSCLC and limited stage SCLC. The expectation is that the results will lead to more highly individualized treatment planning and the employment of lower doses to some patients and thus reduce risk of treatment-related morbidity.

However, pathologic complete response may not equal long-term clinical control. To determine the value of residual MRglc after RT that corresponds to $\geq 95\%$ probability of clinical tumor control (MRglc-cTCP $\geq 95\%$), Choi et al. have designed a prospective study in which residual MRglc 10–12 days after RT or RT CC+ chemotherapy will be determined in patients with unresectable stage I–III NSCLC and limited stage SCLC (Partners protocol 03-282). Goals of this study are to determine the dose–response relationship between the residual MRglc at 10–12 days after RT $\pm$ chemotherapy and tumor control at 12 months. From this, the intent is to define the levels of residual MRglc that correspond to cTCP $\geq 95\%$ and TCP 50%.

Once such values are determined, they plan to conduct a phase II study to evaluate the effectiveness of (MRglc-cTCP 95%) surrogate imaging biomarker, after initial dose of 60 Gy/30 F/6 weeks, in guiding biologically targeted patient-specific boost dose and volume of RT to increase tumor control to $\geq 90\%$ from the current level of 40% and improve survival. Choi was awarded an NIH RO1 grant for this new study.

10.5.5 Increased Interstitial Fluid Pressure (IFP) and Altered Pathway of Lymphatic Metastasis

Choi in collaboration with Tim Padera and Rakesh Jain of the Steele Laboratory and Douglas Mathisen, thoracic surgeon, conducted clinical and experimental studies to assess the functional status of lymphatics in mouse tumors expressing normal or elevated levels of vascular endothelial growth

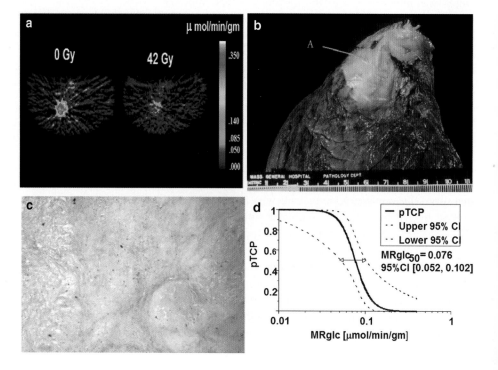
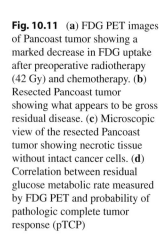

Fig. 10.11 (**a**) FDG PET images of Pancoast tumor showing a marked decrease in FDG uptake after preoperative radiotherapy (42 Gy) and chemotherapy. (**b**) Resected Pancoast tumor showing what appears to be gross residual disease. (**c**) Microscopic view of the resected Pancoast tumor showing necrotic tissue without intact cancer cells. (**d**) Correlation between residual glucose metabolic rate measured by FDG PET and probability of pathologic complete tumor response (pTCP)

factor-C (VEGF-C) and human lung cancer. They measured IFP in lung tumors in 22 patients (at surgical exposure) and stained these tumors for LYVE-1, Prox 1, and CD31. Tumor IFP in these patients was elevated (9.5 ± 1.6 mmHg) but there was no correlation between LYVE-1 staining and IFP, lymph node metastasis, or overall survival [65], suggesting that human lung tumors do not contain functional lymphatics and that LYVE-1 staining is not clinically predictive in this setting.

In both human and mouse tumors, functional lymphatics were present in tumor margins, and no positively identified lymphatic vessels stained with LYVE-1 were noted beyond 500 mμ inward from the tumor margin.

These findings underscore the significance of clinical target volume (CTV) beyond GTV for potential microscopic disease at tumor margin in 3D RT for patients with lung cancer. Without adequate CTV margins, geographic miss may occur. This is the first report on the subject.

10.5.6 Proton Therapy

Proton Therapy. Choi and colleagues have completed a dose-escalation study of IMXT and concurrent chemotherapy for patients with inoperable stage III NSCLC as a part of proton therapy project. The study accrued 12 patients into level 1 of dose escalation, viz., 71.2 Gy/34 F/6.8 weeks. They observed dose-limiting toxicities (DLT) in 2 patients (one with grade 3 esophagitis and the other with grade 3 pneumonitis) and concluded that a total dose of 71.2 Gy/34 F/6.8 weeks was near the MTD. The study was closed and their present intent is to treat 30 additional patients to 72 Gy in 40 fractions over a period of 8 weeks to assess the toxicity and effectiveness.

S. Mori and colleagues completed a quantitative measurement of fluctuation of proton range in lung tissue associated with respiratory motion [62]. This is a critical consideration in estimation of the tolerance of the normal lung to the nominal proton dose because the compensation for density heterogeneity along the path of each voxel will not be constant but varies by up to several cm due to the movement of the solid tumor mass in the planning target volume (PTV) during respiration.

10.5.7 4D CT and 4D IGRT

An important new advance in planning radiation treatment of lung cancers is image-guided radiation therapy (4D IGRT) being developed by G. Chen. See Chapter 5 for details of these developments.

10.5.8 Biographical Sketches

10.5.8.1 Noah Choi

Noah (Fig. 10.12) had his high school education at Inchon, South Korea, 40 miles west of Seoul and housing the Seoul airport. For the historian, Inchon is the site of Mac Arthur's landing in his offensive in the Korean War. For university Noah clearly demonstrated exceptional talents by his acceptance at Seoul National University (SNU), College of Medicine. Admission at SNU is extremely competitive in that only students in the top 5% of students of South Korea are admitted. Noah had the highest score of graduating medical students on the national examination for which he received the very prestigious Chi Suk-Young Gold Medal.

During medical school and internship, he became increasingly interested in the need to develop more effective treatment for cancer patients. While a first year surgical resident at SNU he arranged to come to St. Francis General Hospital in Pittsburgh, PA (1965). By this point he had decided on radiation oncology for his career. Noah then had these residencies and fellowships: 1 year at Victoria General Hospital in Halifax, Nova Scotia, Canada; 2 years at Princess Margaret Hospital in Toronto; and 1 year at Tufts with Fernando Bloedorn. He then applied to and was accepted for a staff position at the MGH in 1973.

He was recommended to concentrate on pulmonary tumors as they had and were receiving little serious attention in radiation oncology and provided real opportunities. In addition to heavy clinical responsibilities at the MGH, Noah worked half time at the Mt. Auburn Hospital managing their radiation oncology program until it was acquired by the Beth Israel-Deaconess system. Further, he managed to complete several clinically relevant experiments on laboratory mice. Definitely, Noah was a fully busy and well-organized physician. He combined this with being an effective and admired teacher of residents. Noah was promoted to the rank of professor in 2007 at HMS. In the celebration ceremony in the Trustee's room, Bulfinch Building, there was a moving series

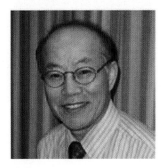

Fig. 10.12 Noah Choi

of statements of most generous praise by faculty within and beyond the department.

Notation is made here of experiments on laboratory animals in the Steele Laboratory that he performed as a young and extremely busy faculty member. One of his experiments is described in Chapter 8.

Noah and Jae-Eun have four children. Three have graduated from Harvard College, two of whom are also graduates from Harvard Medical School. One graduated from both Harvard Law School and Graduate School of Harvard University with Ph.D. in economics. He was appointed the youngest professor in the history of the Law School of the University of California, Berkeley.

10.5.8.2 Henning Willers

Henning (Fig. 10.13) started life in Würzburg in Bavaria. As we know, Conrad Roentgen was the Professor of Physics at the Würzburg University when he discovered x-rays in 1895.

Young Henning had his childhood in a very strong medical family. His mother is a retired anesthesiologist, and an additional ∼15 family members are/have been physicians. He enjoyed many conversations at home regarding medicine and observations of his mother at the hospital. He entered medical school at age 18 in Hamburg, in the far north of Germany. As his course was nearing completion, he had to consider a topic for his thesis, a requirement for the title Doctor in the German system. At a student function, he sat next to Prof. Hans-Peter Beck-Bornholdt and had no appreciation of his status as an internationally renowned radiation biologist. Henning mentioned his interest in a thesis, the conversation expanded, and he became a student of Beck-Bornholdt. The title of Henning's thesis was *The Influence of the Time Factor on the Results of X-ray Therapy of Malignant Tumors* and focused on the historical origins of fractionation and timing of radiation therapy in Germany

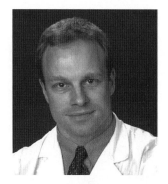

Fig. 10.13 Henning Willers

and Austria. Part of this work was published later as a paper in English in the journal *Radiotherapy and Oncology* "Origins of Radiotherapy and Radiobiology: Separation of the Influence of Dose per Fraction and Overall Treatment Time on Normal Tissue Damage by Reisner and Miescher in the 1930s" [101]. Henning combined this thesis project with an elective in radiation oncology at the University of Hamburg. These events led to his decision to enter radiation oncology for his career.

In 1993, Henning decided that he had to know much more of the science of the actions of radiation on tissues and cells. He applied to the MGH and was accepted for a rotation while a medical student. As he was leaving in 1994, Suit suggested that he return for a fellowship. After completing some time in radiation oncology residency in Hamburg, he applied for a scholarship from the German Cancer Aid Foundation, was accepted, and did come back for a laboratory research fellowship with Simon Powell. This was quite productive. He had enormous respect and regard for Simon as a very talented leader and mentor. Henning clearly had a thoroughly good time in the science and socially as well. His research was principally in radiation and molecular biology and resulted in a fine series of papers. Incidentally, he learned from a peer about the potential of obtaining a medical license to practice medicine in the USA. He quickly applied, took and passed the USMLE steps 1–3. He then applied for residency training at MGH and was accepted. He did a 1-year internship and then the 4-year residency, finishing in 2005. As reflection of his performance, he was given a staff appointment and laboratory space and support. For 3 years, his clinical practice was at Boston Medical Center with a focus on the treatment of patients with lung cancer while continuing as a principal investigator in the former laboratory of Simon Powell who had left in 2004 to become the Chair of Radiation Oncology at Washington University. Henning continued the study of the genetics and molecular mechanisms of DNA double-strand break repair. Due to his clinical interest in lung cancer, he also turned his attention toward the study of aberrant signal transduction pathways in these tumors and their impact on radiation sensitivity and DNA repair. Through a collaborative effort with Jeffrey Settleman, Ph.D. (Director of Molecular Therapeutics at the MGH Cancer Center), Henning became an investigator within the Dana-Farber/Harvard Cancer Center Lung Cancer SPORE (Specialized Program Of Research Excellence) to study the effects of epidermal growth factor receptor signaling on radiation resistance of lung cancers. In 2008, his clinical practice transferred back to the MGH to work with Noah Choi in the thoracic oncology program. Fortunately, the arrangement includes half time in the laboratory. The many challenges and opportunities in thoracic oncology are being energetically approached by Henning.

A most happy note is that he has recently married an exceptionally attractive and talented gynecologist, Shruthi Mahalingaiah, M.D., who is pursuing a successful career in reproductive endocrinology and infertility at the Brigham and Woman's Hospital.

10.6 GI

Specialist clinicians:

Ted Hong, Head of the unit
Earlier Heads of the GI Unit:
Len Gunderson, Joel Tepper, and Chris Willett

10.6.1 Len Gunderson

In the USA in 1970 there were no radiation oncologists specializing in GI oncology. Suit's plan was that the department would be based on sub-specialists. There was a potential for a major GI radiation oncology program based on the many GI cancer patients at the MGH and the exceptional quality of the MGH surgeons with special interest in GI oncology. Suit was quite aware of the innovative work of Len Gunderson, met him, was highly impressed of his potential to develop a highly productive GI radiation oncology unit and decided to recruit him.

Len Gunderson as a radiation oncology resident at the Hospital of the Latter Day Saints in Salt Lake City applied to and was accepted by the Department of Surgery of the University of Minnesota to analyze the sites of failure following surgical resection of rectal cancer at their center. The U Minnesota had one of the very largest and best organized patient records system for surgically treated rectal cancer patients in the USA, making the study feasible. This was a clearly remarkable event, viz., a radiation oncology resident at a non-university hospital being permitted to perform an outcome analysis of an obviously important and large group of patients at one of the world's leading GI surgical units and then publishing the results as the first author. This was the mark of an exceptional, young physician who could bring a concept for a clinical study to detailed planning, execution, and data analysis to publication. Len accepted the invitation to join our faculty and specialize exclusively on GI oncology. Thus, in 1976 Len became the first GI radiation oncologist in the USA.

He promptly commenced collaborative work with the surgeons and medical oncologists to develop a GI oncology clinic that has evolved into a GI Oncology Center.

An important component of the developmental work of our GI radiation oncologists and physicists has been directed to implementation and assessing the efficacy of IOERT as reviewed in Chapter 7. For an early paper on IOERT as the boost dose see Gunderson, 1982 [36].

Gunderson et al. [37] described tumor control and toxicity in 36 patients with stage NoMo carcinoma of the stomach treated by surgery and considered for post-operative irradiation and chemotherapy. He employed tightly contoured radiation fields and was able to administer 45–52 Gy in 5–6 weeks. The 3-year survival and local control rate was viewed as an improvement over that by surgery alone. Hoskins et al. in 1985 [42] reported the local control results in 95 patients with rectosigmoid and rectal cancer given 50.4–52 Gy post-operatively and 103 patients treated by surgery alone. At the MGH, local failure rates in the surgery alone and surgery + radiation patients were 39 and 9%, respectively.

Len moved to the Mayo clinic and was shortly advanced to Chief of Radiation Oncology and then Director of the Mayo Cancer program.

10.6.2 Joel Tepper

The new leader of our program in GI radiation oncology was Joel Tepper, an early graduate of our residency program. Following 2 years in the army and a productive time at the NCI with Eli Glatstein, we recruited him back to the MGH in 1981. Joel was experienced and led the MGH program very effectively. An early study by Tepper et al. was the exploration of efficacy of intra-arterial infusion of misonidazole to reduce the negative impact of hypoxic cell population just prior to IOERT of cancers of the pancreas [92]. There was no evident gain and this was not pursued. Landry et al. [57] continued the determination of sites of failure among gastric cancer patients treated at the MGH by curative resection. The local regional failure rate in 130 patients was 38% (49/130). The most common sites of local regional failure were in the anastomosis or stump. They suggested that including radiation in the treatment might well reduce this category of failure.

Of great pride for the department is the writing and editing by Gunderson and Tepper of the text book *Clinical Radiation Oncology* [34]. Both Tepper and Gunderson have been elected presidents of ASTRO. In addition, Gunderson and Willett with Harrison and Calvo are authors of the book *Intra-operative Irradiation* [35].

10.6.3 Chris Willett

Joel was recruited to be the Chief of Radiation Oncology at University of North Carolina in 1987. Chris Willett was appointed the third Head of GI radiation oncology. Chris is also a graduate of our residency program. He had worked closely with Joel as a resident and as a young staff on the GI program. Further, he had been productively involved in the GI clinical studies for several years.

Chakravarti and Willett et al. [7] found that the 5-year local control rates in patients treated for rectal cancers by local excision alone or excision and radiation were 72 and 90% with survival rates 66 and 74%, respectively. Willett et al. [105] examined the frequency of acute and late toxicity in 28 patients who had inflammatory bowel disease and were treated by abdominal and pelvic irradiation. The incidence of severe reactions was 46%. Further, 29% developed late toxicity so severe as to require hospitalization. Their findings require the employment of innovative techniques to confine radiation dose to carefully defined targets in these patients.

An extremely impressive and innovative advance was the clinical finding of a phase 1 clinical study by Willett, Jain, and team that pre-operative anti-angiogenic agent bevicizumab with radiation (50.4 Gy in 5.5 weeks) and chemotherapy for patients with locally advanced rectal carcinoma (T3–4) yielded very large gains in local control [106]. This work had been preceded by a series of brilliant laboratory studies by R. Jain and team, see Chapter 8. Their initial report was based on six consecutive patients. As of 2008, 22 of 22 patients have sustained local control (C. Willett, personal communication, 2008). This work has been a major factor in a large expansion of interest in a significant clinical role of anti-angiogenic agents in the treatment of cancer patients. Another advance found by Willett et al. [104] for IOERT was in the treatment for retroperitoneal sarcoma.

10.6.4 Ted Hong

Ted Hong was recruited as the fourth and present Head of the GI radiation oncology program, shortly after Chris moved to Duke as the Chief of Radiation Oncology in 2002. Ted participated in the 2008 analysis by Hoffman et al. [39] of the SEER data: 1574 patients treated for rectal carcinoma by external beam radiation and sphincter sparing surgery; 3114 patients treated for rectal cancer by surgery alone; and 24,578 patients with colon cancer treated by surgery alone. The incidence of prostate cancer was compared to that in the general population There was a significant reduction in frequency of prostate cancer in the irradiated patients, viz., the observed/expected ratio was 0.28 (95% CL 0.17, 0.43). For surgery alone, this ratio was 0.94 for rectal and 1.02 for colon cancer patients. The implication is that the incidental irradiation of the prostate significantly lowers the risk of later development of cancer.

Hong et al. have assessed the utility of multi-criteria optimized IMXT treatment plans for 10 patients with advanced pancreatic cancer [41]. Dose constraints on sensitive adjacent organs were specified and reference was made to a Pareto analysis system to display the dose to the organs at risk (OARs). This generates estimates of the importance of variation in the weight of the different fields, field arrangement, and number of fields. This provides a quick means for selecting the best feasible IMXT plan in terms of the dose to each of the OARs for a constant dose and dose distribution to the target. This method of data analysis is expected to augment the gains from patient outcome data.

Kozak et al. completed an analysis of comparative treatment planning of IMXT and proton therapy for irradiation of cancer of the pancreas [54]. The proton plan provided significant reductions in dose to the kidneys, small bowel, and liver.

10.6.5 Biographical Sketches

10.6.5.1 Ted Hong

Ted Hong (Fig. 10.14) has his origins in Cheshire Connecticut where he developed a very early interest in science. He comes from a science-oriented family and that almost certainly had a significant impact on his career ambitions. His father is a chemical engineer who had served as the project leader on the Royal Seal tire which was the first self-sealant tire. A grandfather had been a professor of electrical engineering at Seoul National University. His father was also a graduate of Seoul National University, which is perhaps one of the most competitive universities on this planet in terms of gaining admission. His father's uncle was a former President of Seoul National University.

At Harvard, Ted majored in chemistry and sub-specialized in physical chemistry. He had a particularly strong teacher in chemistry, Dr. Dudley Hershbach, a winner of the Nobel Prize in Chemistry in 1986. Ted's research dealt with "stringing together a carbon polymer through a novel molecular beam technique where there was a supersonic expansion out of a nozzle of simple carbon molecules which came out as strings." This was analyzed by a mass spectrometer technique. He was also positively influenced by Professor Bill Klemperer, a physical chemist. Ted considered entering chemistry graduate school because of

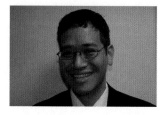

Fig. 10.14 Ted Hong

the impact of these two superstar teachers. One significant work was that of participating with Klemperer in organizing a course in spectrometry and that course is still given at Harvard.

As an additional activity Ted served as a volunteer at the Cambridge Hospice, one of the oldest in the country. This had an important impact on his career plans and his decision to change from chemistry to medicine. His brother had gone to medical school and that was another factor in Ted's career choice of medicine. His brother became a medical oncologist.

Ted graduated from Harvard in 1996 and attended medical school at the University of Connecticut; the cost in Connecticut was one-fourth of that of Harvard. During his third year he had an opportunity to be involved with several cancer patients who were receiving radiation. Ted met the oncologist there, Dr. Robert Dowsett.

Upon deciding on radiation oncology he went to the University of Wisconsin for his residency. Drs. Paul Harari and Minesh Meht at the University of Wisconsin similarly had a very positive impact on Hong's development. He became familiar with TOMO therapy and had very good interactions with Rock Mackie, Head of Physics.

Ted became facile with the LQ modeling, α/β values, and more, from his interactions with Jack Fowler, the famous radiation biologist from the Gray Lab at the Mt. Vernon Hospital, London. He became particularly interested in head and neck cancer and thought he would pursue that in his post-residency work. However, Ted had married and by that time had one child and thought it would be an advantage for his family to be in the northeast and closer to their families. He learned of a position at the MGH from L. Kachnik and was interested. He applied and was accepted for a staff position. Chris Willett had recently left to be Chief at Duke, so Ted was invited and accepted to be Head of the GI Radiation Oncology Service. He has performed most impressively. Ted has enjoyed working with the physicists in IMXT as he is sensitive to the yet undefined impact of the dose bath to large volumes of normal tissues. Additionally, he initiated and commenced a program of proton therapy in the treatment of patients with hepatic tumors. Another major interest is the use of IOERT. He also is very impressed with the exceptional quality and innovations in MGH imaging studies (MRI, CT, etc.).

Ted's interests while a resident was the combination of radiation with some of the biological agents. He was, of course, fascinated by the MGH experience of Willett and Jain in the treatment of patients with locally advanced rectal carcinoma by bevacizumab, chemotherapy, and radiation prior to surgery, viz., a 100% local control result in 22 patients up to the present. This line of study is continuing. Further, he has initiated a discussion with Dr. Fernandez regarding administering one of the biological agents intra-arterially immediately before IOERT.

Currently, he is developing protocols for the use of hypofractionated proton irradiation (5 Gy RBE×5) for locally advanced pancreatic cancer.

10.6.5.2 Len Gunderson

Biographical sketch of Len (Fig. 10.15) is given in large part in the first portion of this section. Len is the current President of ASTRO.

10.6.5.3 Joel Tepper

Joel (Fig. 10.16) received his undergraduate degree in electrical engineering in 1968 from MIT and decided on a career in medicine and went to Washington University School of Medicine in St. Louis, graduating in 1972. He was advised by a diagnostic radiologist, after explaining his subject preferences, that radiation oncology might be a good field for him. He then met and talked with Carlos Perez, a young faculty at Wash U. He also met with Dr. Lauren Ackerman. He was a senior surgical pathologist whose book *Cancer Diagnosis and Treatment* co-authored with Juan del Regato is still on many shelves. Dr. Ackerman advised that were he interested

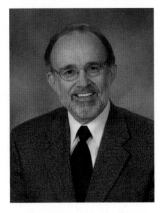

Fig. 10.15 Len Gunderson

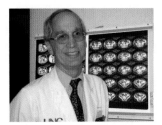

Fig. 10.16 Joel Tepper

in radiation oncology he should consider the MGH and talk with Suit.

This was attractive as he knew the Boston area (MIT). In his fourth year in medical school, he visited Boston and discussed the residency for about $1\frac{1}{2}$ h with Suit in his office in the old Temp 2 building, now long gone. He was offered and accepted a position in the residency program. The MGH was the only program to which he applied and he does not recall completing an application form. Joel started his residency in the old unit on White 2. As a resident, Joel was an important member of the team preparing for the initiation of proton therapy. Also of significance he led the determination of RBE of the mid-point of a SOBP with single dose or 20 equal dose fractions with mouse jejunal crypt cell survival as the end-point. RBE was independent of dose over the range $\sim$ 15 to 1 Gy.

After his residency, Joel spent 2 years in the Air Force and then worked as a Senior Investigator at the NCI with Eli Glatstein. There he developed the IOERT program and was heavily involved in clinical trials on patients with soft tissue sarcoma. When Len Gunderson left the MGH, Joel was recruited to Head the GI radiation oncology unit and to care for a few sarcoma patients. A major investigation was the assessment of the efficacy of IOERT. The study was extended to include a series of pancreatic cancers. Additionally, he ran an RTOG study of hypoxic cell sensitization with IORT.

Then in 1987, he was recruited to be the Chair of the department at the University of North Carolina in Chapel Hill. He was the first chair of a new department and had a new building. Joel worked as Vice-Chair of the GI committee in the CALGB for 15 years. More recently he is serving as Co-Chair of the NCI GI Intergroup (now the GI Steering Committee). He also developed a more direct involvement in translational research, and served as principal investigator of the UNC GI SPORE (specialized program of research excellence) grant.

An additional national distinction was his election as President and then Chairman of the Board of ASTRO. A major effort was to enhance biological research by radiation oncologists and the educational opportunities in the field. He has spent a substantial amount of time working in ASCO activities and with surgical colleagues.

Joel has kept close ties with the MGH. His daughter completed her residency in psychiatry at MGH/McLean. In 2005 Joel received the MGH Radiation Oncology Distinguished Alumnus Award. That occasion provided him the opportunity to give his first lecture in the Ether Dome.

10.6.5.4 Chris Willett

Chris (Fig. 10.17) is the son of a quite special radiation oncologist who had completed a surgical residency at

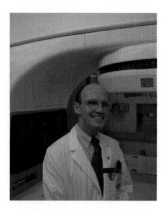

Fig. 10.17 Christopher Willett

Memorial Sloan Kettering and then decided to employ radiation rather than the scalpel. After a residency, he became a full-time radiation oncologist at the Boston, VA hospital. Chris matured in the Boston area and graduated from Tufts medical school in 1981. He had developed a special interest in GI malignancies and won an American Cancer Society fellowship to study rectal cancer patients treated by pre-operative radiation. After a year in general surgery at Vanderbilt, he entered the MGH residency, being especially attracted to Len Gunderson and the GI surgeons of the MGH, judged by Chris to be the world's finest. To Chris's great disappointment, Len moved to the Mayo in 1981, shortly before he started his residency. Chris was indeed fortunate as the successor to Len was Joel Tepper, with whom he had several informative rotations, worked well with as a young staff, and shared interest in IOERT.

As a young staff, Chris was asked to concentrate initially on the proton program with John Munzenrider and Mary Austin-Seymour. He was particularly interested in the technical and medical aspects of treatment of small children with retinoblastoma, but wished to concentrate on GI tumors. In 1987, Joel accepted the position of Chief at U North Carolina and Chris was made Head of the GI radiation oncology program. Chris was particularly proud of the installation of the Linac in OR 43 for the IOERT program. There was expansion of the use of IOERT well beyond the GI tract, viz., GYN, sarcomas, and to a lesser extent head/neck and thoracic lesions. An important success of Chris is the improved outcomes of patients with retroperitoneal sarcomas.

Chris has greatly enjoyed the interaction with George Chen and clinical physicists for the implementation of 4D IGRT, especially for hepatic tumors. He was interested in correcting motion of the target during irradiation. This is being pursued by Ted Hong, present Head of GI radiation oncology. In 2002, Chris was invited by Duke to be their Chief of Radiation Oncology. He accepted and has led a really successful program there. Chris serves as Chair of the

GI section of RTOG and has participated in several clinical trials.

Chris has a happy and talented family. His wife, Mary Sunday, is a research scientist in pathology and has enjoyed many years of uninterrupted RO1 funding.

10.7 GYN

Specialist clinician:

Tim Russell, Head of the unit at MGH and BMC

Radiation oncologists who have had a major interest in the gynecological cancer patients were initially Milford Schulz and C.C. Wang. Subsequently we have had Daniel Flynn, James McIntyre, and Thomas DeLaney as full-time specialists in this area. Since April 2003, Tim Russell has concentrated exclusively on gynecological oncology. He was initially responsible for GYN patients at MGH and at BMC, but when additional full-time faculty were recruited at BMC, Ariel Hirsch assumed responsibility for GYN patients at that facility.

The incidence of carcinoma of the uterine cervix in the USA has declined steeply in the recent 25 years from ~18,000 to 11,500. This reflects the impact of screening procedures. Of the patients diagnosed at present, 50% have never had a Pap smear and an additional 10% have not been screened in 5 years or longer. Patients with invasive disease are derived, to a large extent, from socially disadvantaged populations and recent immigrant populations. The indications are that further decline over the coming 25 years will largely depend on how new screening modalities and strategies (exfoliative cytology combined with screening for high-risk papilloma virus serotypes) are implemented as well as efforts at prevention including recent development of poly-valent human papilloma virus (HPV) vaccines. How broadly vaccination becomes available and how effective this strategy will ultimately prove remain the subject of conjecture.

Holmes and Schulz discuss the use of radiation against uterine cervical cancer in their 1950 book. The policy that had developed at the MGH over some time had been for all patients other than small stage 1 disease to be treated by external beam therapy, i.e., 250 kVp x-rays, followed by intra-cavitary radium. In some instances there were residual tumors accessible for interstitial therapy, and small masses were implanted. Radium insertions were usually accomplished in two or three sessions. This had the advantage of smaller volumes of tumor at the time of the second or third application. The dose gradient across the cancer improved with tumor regression. At the MGH there was an impressive variety of applicators for the placement of radium in the uterine canal and in the vaginal fornices. An additional option was the use of a trans-vaginal cone to apply radiation directly to the cervix. The success rate of intracavitary radium therapy alone or combined with EBRT was quite high but decreased rather steeply with increases in tumor volume.

In 1973, afterloading Fletcher Suit applicators were brought into service after modification to accommodate ^{137}Cs sources. The new applicators were made in our machine shop. In 1992, the department commenced the use of a high dose rate remote afterloading system for intracavitary radiation of patients with cervix cancer. This provided several advantages: (1) virtual elimination of radiation exposure to any member of the hospital staff; (2) performance as out-patient procedures (no immobilization in bed with the applicators in place); (3) avoidance of the infrequent complications of the prolonged 24–72 h in bed (thromboembolic events, labial suture abscesses, aspiration pneumonias); (4) immobilization prior to imaging-based dosimetry and treatment decreasing motion effects; and (5) increasing flexibility in planning, improving (individualized) dose distributions by varying source dwell times in both the tandem and ovoids. This latter capability is further improved by the adoption of CT and MRI-compatible plastic and titanium applicators. The total dose and fractionation used in these high dose rate treatments appears to have been well chosen prior to our adoption of this approach, as the late normal tissue tolerance of these patients is judged to be equivalent to the low dose rate method used historically. Since 2003, all MGH intracavitary GYN radiation treatment has been by the high dose rate technique. This is usually administered on an out-patient basis. For cancer of the cervix patients, this is customarily accomplished in five fractions. In 2007, two titanium tandem and ovoid sets were obtained. Their advantage is greatly improved CT and MRI imaging capability with the applicators in situ. This makes feasible planning of treatment based on the position of the applicator system in the patient at the time of radiation and more accurate calculation of dose administered both to tumor and to vulnerable, adjacent normal tissues (small and large bowel, urinary bladder).

There had been a rather marked increase in the number of brachytherapy patients treated at MGH up to ~ 2004. Referrals for this treatment have recently declined consequent to the installation of four of these high dose rate units elsewhere in eastern Massachusetts.

C.C. Wang was among the first to employ hyperfractionated accelerated radiation therapy for pelvic cancer to reduce the impact of tumor cell proliferation between fractions. He concluded that 1.5 Gy BID and ≥4 h between fractions in treatment of pelvic lesions were well tolerated provided the total dose was reduced by ~ 15%. For abdominal treatment he judged that the dose should be 1 Gy BID with similar total dose modification [97]. He reckoned that the results warranted a clinical trial. This accelerated dose fractionation is now commonly used for treatment of vulvar and select vaginal cancer; for these patients the radiation is usually combined with chemotherapy. Also, BID radiation and chemotherapy are used in several clinics for patients with small cell hypercalcemic ovarian cancer.

In an outcome analysis of the prognostic importance of endometriosis in 84 patients with clear cell ovarian cancer, Orezzoli et al. [64] concluded that endometriosis concurrent with ovarian clear cell cancer was associated with better prognosis despite no difference in resectability.

Adjuvant IMXT following hysterectomy for uterine malignancies commenced in 2004. The volume of normal tissue in the PTV was decreased by the planned bladder distension program. For this, the patient is CT planned with the bladder empty and with the bladder distended to a specified volume. Patients have a catheter in place Monday through Friday and just prior to irradiation the empty bladder is filled to the planned volume.

The first intra-operative electron therapy (IOERT) was performed in 1978 on a patient with a pelvic wall soft tissue metastatic lesion from a squamous cell carcinoma of the uterine cervix. This was the start of this program and the first to employ IOERT as the boost dose. IOERT continues to be employed for gynecological cancer patients, but less commonly with the current enthusiasm for proton therapy, IMXT, etc. The paper by del Carmen et al. in 2000 is an account of IOERT for patients with gynecology lesions [20]. They emphasize the negative prognostic effect of only partial resection.

Proton beams have been available on a very restricted basis due to very heavy demand on the quite limited beam time. There are plans for starting some proton protocols for the gynecological patients as extended hours of operation of the proton center become a reality. These efforts are intended reduce steeply dose to the GI track compared to 3D or IMXT photon plans.

Consequent to more comprehensive surgical evaluation of disease extent (staging) fewer patients with endometrial cancers have radiation as part of their treatment. Currently, many patients receiving adjuvant radiotherapy following hysterectomy for endometrial cancer have such treatment limited to vaginal brachytherapy without teletherapy. However, for patients found to have spread to regional lymph nodes, "consolidative" radiotherapy is frequently administered following hysterectomy, lymphadenectomy, and four to six cycles of poly agent chemotherapy. Commonly such patients are treated to extended volumes which can include both pelvic soft tissues (parametria) as well as pelvic and para-aortic lymph nodes. Preliminary observations from multiple centers suggest the efficacy of this tri-modality approach for selected, high-risk patients. Proton therapy is anticipated to show meaningful reductions in both acute and late toxicities when such large volumes require radiation treatment.

Increasingly, management of gynecological cancers has become multimodal. Patients with cancers of the cervix, vulva, and vagina are routinely administered cytotoxic chemotherapy synchronously with radiation therapy as the prime therapeutic intervention. Selected patients with cancers of the cervix and vulva will have surgery prior to, or after, chemoradiation. Because of the involvement of multiple physicians in the care of individual patients, and the increasing complexity of the care administered, communication and coordination of care become essential for patient safety and quality assurance.

There are combined multi-disciplinary GYN clinics three times/week. GYN pathology and GYN medical oncology conferences are held weekly. A multidisciplinary presurgical conference is held twice monthly, and a multidisciplinary conference with diagnostic imaging (radiology) is held monthly.

10.7.1 Biographical Sketch

10.7.1.1 Tim Russell

Tim (Fig. 10.18) is an enthusiastic fisherman and travels widely to explore a variety of spots for a fine catch. Here he is with a large brown trout at 4 lbs caught and released on a light fly line on the Big Horn River in southwest Montana in the summer of 2004.

Tim completed his MGH residency in 1979 and returned to the department to head the Gynecologic Radiation Oncology Unit in 2003.

Tim originated in the West Bronx section of New York City in 1948. He attended private school and had a highly enjoyable time. As he describes those years, he was active

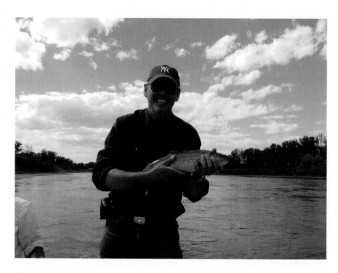

Fig. 10.18 Tim (Anthony) Russell

in "soccer, chasing girls, poker and other" but managed to have a few minutes for studies, as a minimum sufficient to be admitted to Columbia. There he performed well in his major, liberal arts, and several science courses. These science courses interested him rather seriously as he transferred to MIT for the third and fourth years. There he was exposed to serious science and had to take study more seriously. To get started he took two calculus courses over the summer before entering MIT. He adapted much better than he realized. In one math course while a formal MIT student, the final exam was quite difficult. Tim judged that he had only attempted answers to 6 questions of a total of 10. He was enormously surprised and delighted when the instructor later told him that he had done reasonably well. Specifically, Tim had gotten 64 of 200 points but that was the second highest in the class. His introductory course in biology was given by Salvatore Luria (Nobel Prize winner). Also while at MIT he had lectures by David Baltimore (Nobel Prize) and many other stars in science. His time there was one sustained with intellectual pleasure. The institution was an undisguised meritocracy in that one's performance was essentially the sole measure of status, viz., social origin, geographic origin, ethnicity, religion were negligible factors.

During this phase, he decided on medicine for his career. Tim attributes this decision to his relations with the obstetrician who delivered him and his four siblings. The family connection was even deeper, as this physician was the father of an aunt. This physician was a professor at Columbia who had left Vienna because of its Nazi regime. Relevant to Tim's interest in oncology was his definite awareness that a large fraction of deaths in his parent's generation were due to cancer.

Tim was accepted into Harvard Medical School and had the general aim of specializing in internal medicine. Entirely unexpected was his rotation on radiology at MGH and a brief 2-day exposure to radiation oncology on White 2. Resident Warren Sewall showed him many of the departmental activities. He was extremely impressed by a patient who had been treated by C.C. Wang for extensive laryngeal cancer. The patient was doing very nicely, i.e., with a good speaking voice. Tim followed this experience with an elective at the JCRT which was also very positive. During an internship at the University of Virginia he realized that he really liked the potential of curing cancer patients by non-surgical methods and the employment of high and getting higher technology. He did have some important but quite negative advice contra the plan to enter radiation oncology. Namely, his friend, the obstetrician, commented that there was no future as the very rapid developments in drugs would eliminate any need for radiation therapy within only 10 years. Tim listened politely but thought it to be in error.

Tim had been invited to be a resident in internal medicine but was given only 48 h to decide. He called several centers regarding a residency position. Sam Hellman had no

openings and suggested that he try the MGH. By an odd turn of events, one of those accepted to become residents at MGH had just cancelled (this has happened twice between 1970 and 2000). This slot was offered during phone conversation and Tim accepted, i.e., there was no interview. A graduate of MIT and HMS with internship at U Virginia was an automatic acceptance at any program in that early era for radiation oncology in the USA. This surely does not apply in 2008, when radiation oncology is one of the very top choices of medical students. During his residency he had a special interest in the gynecological patients and also participated in IOERT treatments.

Tim then worked for 7 years in radiation oncology at the University of Washington in Seattle. During that period he published 24 papers; 16 were co-authored with residents. For 1 year he was the resident program director. Then he transferred to a very large practice group in Sacramento that was affiliated with the University of California at Davis. He worked there for 17 years and concentrated on GYN oncology. During this period, Tim gave substantial time to mentoring young physicians. Two are now departmental chairs. Dr. Lloyd Smith is Chief of Ob/Gyn at UC Davis and Dr. Leiserowitz the Head of Gyn Oncology. His teaching activities included seven lectures at the Los Angeles Radiological Society, one refresher course at ASTRO, and four courses to the Gynecologic Oncologists Society. Further, he has lectured at Memorial Hospital, NY, and the NCI, Bethesda. An additional and clinically important activity, Tim was a leader in regional and national co-operative trial groups. He completed studies on the combination of chemotherapy and radiation in the management of patients with gynecological cancer, with special gains for patients with vulva carcinoma.

He was invited to return to the MGH and lead the program in radiation gynecological oncology. He has responsibility for these patients at the MGH and at BUMC. Tim quickly began use of high dose rate unit for essentially all intracavitary therapy. We had employed this system since 1991 and Tim sharply increased its utilization. His treatments used five fractions for tandem/ovoid and three fractions for cylinder techniques. Tim obtained a new and computer-operated unit in 2006. He employs five fractions for most patients and is able to plan the dose distributions by use of variable dwell times. The BUMC patients come to MGH for these treatments.

10.8 Genitourinary

Clinician specialists:

William Shipley, Head of the GU unit
Anthony Zietman
John Coen
Jason Efstathiou

10.8.1 Urinary Bladder

Carcinoma of the urinary bladder is a relatively frequent cancer in the USA. The estimate for 2007 is ~67,160 new cases and a fatality of 20.5% of patients [44]. The male:female ratio is 3:1 for incidence and 2.3:1 for mortality. This implies a higher frequency of superficial cancers in men. The standard of care for patients with bladder cancers has been and is surgery, viz., transurethral resection of bladder tumor (TURBT) for superficial lesions and cystectomy for muscle-invading lesions. Radiation alone as the definitive treatment has been employed for medically inoperable patients or for patients who declined surgery. Local control and survival results have been significantly lower for radiation than for radical cystectomy. The latter does carry an important frequency of complications in addition to the loss of the bladder and a surgical mortality of 1–2%. These facts have been the basis for sustained efforts to improve efficacy of radiation treatment alone or combined with systemic agents to achieve survival results comparable to those by radical surgery and to preserve a near normally functioning bladder.

Starting in the early 1970s, Shipley has led the effort in the USA to achieve that goal. After demonstrating that local control was higher in radiation-treated patients who had had the gross tumor removed by TUBRT, he extended the treatment strategy to include cisplatin chemotherapy [78]. For this effort he has enjoyed effective and productive collaboration with radiation oncologists A. Zietman and J. Coen, medical oncologist D. Kaufman, and urologic surgeons George Prout, Niall Heney, and others.[3] They have established multi-disciplinary GU tumor clinics that provide convenient access of patients to a highly talented and comprehensive team of GU oncology specialists. Significantly, these GU oncologists have worked with colleagues in other centers in the USA and abroad. This work has been greatly facilitated by Shipley's long service as Chair of the RTOG Committee on GU Oncology, 1987–1997.

Shipley et al. [80] published 10-year results in 190 patients treated for invasive bladder carcinoma by TURBT and radiation + cisplatin and other chemotherapeutic agents. Treatment protocol was (1) grossly complete TURBT, (2) 40 Gy (QD or BID), and (3) cisplatin-based chemotherapy during the irradiation. If assessment after this treatment indicated a complete response, the additional treatment was 24 Gy, i.e., a total of 64–65 Gy, and further chemotherapy. Patients who were judged to have had less than a complete response were recommended for cystectomy. The

median follow-up was 6.7 years for all surviving patients. The 10-year disease-specific survival (DSS) results for the 66 patients who had cystectomy for T2 and T3–4 lesions were 39 and 42%, respectively. For the patients who had bladder conservation treatment, the 10-year DSS results were 50 and 24% for T2 and T3–4 staged lesions, respectively. These positive results for the conservative treatment of bladder cancer patients are being confirmed in more recent experience here and by reports from other centers and by clinical trials [38, 81].

Efstathiou et al. [27] reviewed the status of these bladder conservative treatment strategies for invasive cancer and found the yield to be high bladder retention rates and that those bladders had good functional status. Tsai [95] reported on 286 patients treated at MGH, 1986–2003, by TURBT, radiation, and chemotherapy. Statins were taken with other modalities in 12% of patients There was a suggestion of improved local control in patients who received a statin, indicating a potential clinical gain by including biological agents in the treatment protocol for patients with invasive bladder cancer.

In summary, Shipley and team have largely achieved their goal in selected patients, viz., radiation given to patients who have a complete response after the first phase of the treatment. The outlook for patients with invasive bladder cancer has clearly been enhanced. Local control and disease-free survival results have been demonstrated to be comparable to that by radical cystectomy at ~50–55% but with the truly important advantage of retained bladder with near-normal function.

This program in bladder carcinoma constitutes a major contribution by this department to oncology.

10.8.2 Prostate Cancer

Prostate cancer is the most common cancer in men in the USA, the estimated incidence for 2007 being ~ 219,000, viz., approximately twice as common as lung cancer in men at 115,000. In sharp contrast, the mortality figures were estimated at 27,000 and 89,500 for prostate and lung (men), respectively [44].

W. Shipley led the RTOG GU Group from 1987 to 1997 in a "golden age" of GU research with the initiation of many randomized trials examining the role and duration of androgen deprivation when given with radiation. These continuing studies have and are defining the role of radiation alone or combined with hormone therapy in the management of patients with prostate cancer throughout North America and Europe.

Accurate definition of the target is a critical step in successful radiation treatment of cancer patients by radiation. In a highly innovative study, Shih et al. [76] injected

---

[3] The surgical members of his team have varied with time.

nanoparticles of a ferric iron material intravenously. These particles are taken up by the normal nodal tissue in nearly 100% of normal nodes at all body sites. On MRI imaging, the nanoparticles are distributed almost uniformly throughout normal nodes. A nanoparticle "cold spot" in the node indicates presence of disease. In prostate cancer patients, the defect is in nearly all instances a metastatic focus. This provides quite accurate detection of metastatic foci of ≥ 0.6 mm in lymph nodes and the anatomic distribution of the positive pelvic nodes. Their finding was that virtually all of the positive nodes were clustered around the major vessels and that a 2 cm radial expansion of the CTV would include $\sim 95\%$ of the pelvic nodes judged to be at risk. This procedure was not approved for use in the USA until early 2010.

There was concern that the available radiation treatment method yielded a substantial local failure rate and alternate methods were sought. Coen et al. examined the incidence of distant failure among patients who achieved local control and those who developed distant metastasis alone. The data indicated a higher distant failure rate in those with local failure [19].

There was a serious interest in the use of proton beam therapy for prostate cancer patients due to the clearly dose distribution gains relative to conventional x-ray techniques. Shipley et al. were the first to employ proton beams in the treatment of prostate cancer patients. The 17 patients had locally advanced disease and were given 50.4 Gy by 4 field x-ray technique and 25.2 Gy (RBE) by a perineal proton field, viz., a total dose of 75.6 Gy (RBE). This experience was reported in 1979 [77]. Toxicity was judged to be acceptable. This led to a phase III trial of radiation dose escalation on 202 T3–4 prostate cancer patients using protons for the high boost dose arm. All patients were administered 50.4 Gy by photon therapy to the pelvis and were then randomly assigned to receive a 17.2 Gy photon boost or a 27.2 Gy (RBE) proton boost by perineal field. Local control was higher in the proton arm (73 vs 59% at 8 years, $p>0.05$), but for the Gleason 7–10, the gain was significant [79]. Overall survival was unchanged because of the high risk of distant metastases in these men with advanced disease.

This was followed by a phase III trial led by A. Zietman of dose escalation on 393 patients with T1b–T2b prostate cancer (PSA <15 ng/ml). This was a combined investigation with Loma Linda University. Patients were treated at MGH and Loma Linda from January 1996 through December 1999. All patients were treated by photons and protons with total doses of 70.2 vs 79.2 Gy (RBE). The 10-year biochemical control rates were 68 and 82% for the 70.2 and the 79.2 Gy (RBE) groups, respectively, $p<0.001$. Grade 3 RTOG rectal and bladder morbidity rates were similar for the two dose groups [91].

A study by A. Trofimov et al. [94] demonstrated that the dose distribution by parallel opposed lateral proton fields using passive energy modulated beams did not yield a dose conformation to the defined GTV as close as did the complex multiple field intensity-modulated x-ray beam technology. There is the expectation that the proton dose distribution will be sharply improved and superior to that of IMXT by the soon-to-be-available pencil beam scanning technology. However, for both proton beam technologies, there is the significantly lower dose lateral to the beam paths and the use of far fewer beams. The result is that the total body integral dose is lower by a factor of ~ 2.

Zietman et al. reported in 2004 the local control and biochemical control of 205 patients with T1–2 prostate cancer treated by photon radiation alone to 68.4 Gy (no chemotherapy or hormonal therapy) [117]. The 10-year clinical local control rate was 82% but the biochemical relapse-free rate was lower at 49%. This was an important database for the move to biochemical relapse-free rate as the end-point of treatment success rate in prostate cancer patients. This yielded a much quicker and more reliable indicator of success or lack thereof. Several MGH studies formed the basis of the ASTRO criteria of failure that have been widely employed since 1997 [112].

Zietman presented very strong evidence that many, perhaps the majority, of older men with early stage prostate cancer do not require curative treatment. They can be safely followed and treatment given only to the disease that has progressed [111, 116].

Laboratory research includes several important results. Using a nude mouse model, a synergistic time and sequence-dependent relationship between androgen deprivation and radiation effect was demonstrated. The TCD50 is greatly reduced when androgen deprivation precedes radiation and when radiation is delayed until maximal tumor regression has occurred [113, 114]. The ability of androgen deprivation to cause tumor regression through changes in tumor blood flow was first demonstrated by Jain in the same model.

Survivin, an inhibitor of apoptosis (IAP), is associated with both cancer progression and drug resistance. A laboratory study found that the inhibition by survivin sensitizes prostate cancer cells to paclitaxel-induced apoptosis through a caspase-dependent mechanism in vitro and in vivo [110].

An interesting clinical finding was that non-prostate cancer patients receiving intermediate dose levels to the prostate had an appreciably lower risk of subsequent primary prostate cancer [115].

10.8.3 Biographical Sketches

10.8.3.1 John Coen

John (Fig. 10.19) was a first generation Irish American born in the Boston Lying-In Hospital (now incorporated into the Brigham Hospital). His home was in Westwood, MA, where

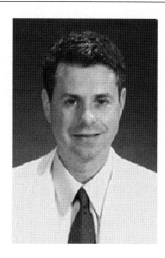

Fig. 10.19 John Coen

he attended public schools. His family spent a lot of time on the Cape with John working with children and as a life guard. John demonstrated talent in math and science. His father attended Northeastern University and had graduated in electrical engineering. He developed a business as an electrical contractor. This home contact with science and technology facilitated young John's enthusiasm for the sciences and math. An additional factor in his final career choice was a physician neighbor, a pediatric radiologist at Boston University Medical Center.

The next educational step was as an engineering student at Dartmouth College. This he enjoyed but after graduation, he understood that he definitely wanted a more humanistic career and decided on medicine. However, he had not been a pre-med student but knew that he should get some serious exposure to medicine in a hospital setting. He circulated his resume to medical programs in the Boston area. Anthony Zietman invited him for an interview. This went well and he commenced work in the department building databases, learning biostatistics, and using his considerable computer skills to analyze outcome data. John worked primarily with Zietman and Shipley for 2 years in the early 1990s, concentrating his studies on PSA and prostate cancer patients, a field in its infancy at that time. He along with them was disappointed that the treatment outcomes for the prostate cancer patients were substantially less satisfactory than assumed. These results stimulated new and more aggressive radiation treatment strategies, viz., IMXT and proton beam therapy. John later decided on radiation oncology for his specialty.

While a medical student he was inclined to pediatrics, due in large part to his happy summers on the Cape working as a life guard and teaching sailing to children. John returned to the MGH for an elective in radiation oncology. This was the critical experience. His engineering and math

background combined with the positive time in the department and especially with Anthony led him to apply to our residency program. He ranks his residency as really an excellent educational experience. One resident project was an analysis of prostate cancer patient outcome data which indicated that patients who achieved long-term local control had a lower frequency of distant metastasis.

Upon finishing the residency, John joined the GU group. He is responsible for the GU patients at BUMC and is part-time member of GU radiation oncology team at the MGH.

John is engaged to marry Melissa Good in September 2008. She works with Matt Smith in Medical Oncology.

10.8.3.2 Jason Efstathiou

To a Greek engineer and his German wife living in Sri Lanka a healthy son was born in 1973. As a child he lived for 4 years in the Middle East and then brief periods in Germany and England. From ages 5 to 16, Jason (Fig. 10.20) was near Toronto, Canada. He was a superb student, graduating with many honors at 16, followed by an additional year on a scholarship in a high school in Cheltenham, England. By age 17 he entered Yale with a concentration in biology and science. He won the McKeown Scholarship for his D.Phil. studies at Trinity College, Oxford. There he had the special good fortune to be in the Oxford laboratory of Sir Walter Bodmer, and his doctoral studies examined the role of adhesion molecules in colorectal carcinoma. His next step was 5 years at Harvard Medical School, including a quite useful year in the laboratory of Judah Folkman. He had decided on a career in oncology and more specifically radiation oncology. Before his residency he had 1 year in medicine at the Brigham Hospital. To no surprise, he was accepted at his first choice for a residency, viz., the Harvard residency in radiation oncology. He completed

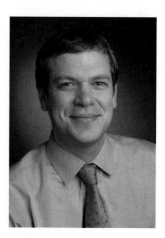

Fig. 10.20 Jason Efstathiou

several significant projects and was invited to join our faculty, effective July 2008, and has recently been promoted to Assistant Professor at Harvard Medical School. His clinical practice focuses on the treatment of men with prostate cancer and other urologic malignancies. Currently, his clinical research concentrates on technology assessment and he has led a consortium to perform a randomized trial looking at the comparative effectiveness of proton beam therapy vs IMRT for prostate cancer, as well as developing a national radiation oncology registry for prostate cancer treatments. Other researches include investigations into the adverse effects of hormonal therapy for prostate cancer, long-term outcomes and late toxicities with bladder-sparing chemoradiation, and the effects of obesity and lifestyle modification on cancer control. Dr. Efstathiou is actively involved in clinical trial design and with the RTOG, where he serves as the lead for proton evaluation in the translational research program.

10.8.3.3 William U. Shipley

Bill Shipley (Fig. 10.21) had from his youth aspired to become an academic scientist. He had an uncommonly strong family tradition of academic careers and medicine. The Ph.D.s were on his father's side and M.D.s on his mother's side. Bill completed his undergraduate education at Yale with a major in biophysics from Yale in 1962, magma cum laude. Richard Setlow was his academic advisor. Despite this basic science education, Bill decided that medicine was to be his career. He performed at a sufficiently high level that he won acceptance into the MGH surgical residency, one of the most sought after US residencies of all specialties at that period. After completion of 2 years in surgery (1966–1968), Shipley had to commence his mandatory 2 years of military service. He was admitted

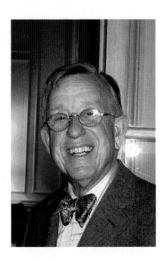

Fig. 10.21 William U. Shipley

to a program in the US Navy and managed to be assigned to the NCI at Bethesda. There he worked in the laboratory of Mort Elkind, one of the very top cell radiation biologists. He learned much quantitative biology and met many highly regarded biophysicists who visited the laboratory. Bill published four papers.

Bill returned to his MGH surgical residency. On the completion of 2 years, he decided to transfer to radiation oncology at the JCRT program, whose chief was Sam Hellman. Before completing the residency, Hellman encouraged Bill to have a year in a "Finishing School" in a European center. Bill judged that a sound proposal and was in any case favorably inclined to learn from European scientists. He received a Harvard Mosley Fellowship and had a productive year in the laboratory of Len Lamerton at the Royal Marsden Cancer Hospital, London. Most of the work was in fact with Gordon Steele. There he employed micro-metastasis systems to investigate potential lethal damage repair. These experiments resulted in several papers. Bill's time in London was an important factor in his long-term interest in international radiation oncology. From this period he published four additional papers in referred journals.

Shipley accepted an invitation to join the MGH radiation oncology faculty and develop a GU a multidisciplinary program in 1974. This was anticipated to be a difficult assignment as GU surgeons were perceived as the least likely to be receptive to seriously consider the potential of radiation for their patients. However, with 2 years as an MGH surgical resident and credentials in lab research, he was the person to succeed. The only GU radiation therapy specialists in the country, at that time, were Malcolm Bagshaw at Stanford and Lowell Miller at the M.D. Anderson Cancer Hospital in Houston.

A highly important credit to Shipley is his almost immediate establishment of an effective rapport with George Prout, Chief of Urology, and the other urologists. George was keen to know data and rationale for new strategies of patient management. These were enthusiastically provided by Bill. A strategy that Bill found effective was to avoid discussion of an alternate treatment method for a specific patient at conferences or rounds. Rather, new methods were discussed privately with the staff surgeon. This avoided difficulty for the surgeon of changing a planned treatment because of evidence presented by a non-surgeon.

One of Bill's most important contributions to oncology was to lead the development of bladder conservation treatment for invasive cancer by combining chemotherapy, moderate dose radiation, and TURBT. Shipley, Prout, and Kaufman supported by pathologists and diagnostic radiologists soon developed weekly GU oncology conferences. They progressively modified the treatment protocol yielding gradually improving outcome results. There were related clinical studies starting in Europe. This conservative strategy is now adopted by many centers.

During the period 1975–1986 Bill was a member of the NCI National Bladder Cancer Group chairing the Radiation Oncology Protocol Development. He also was Chair of the RTOG GU Site Committee, 1978–1997. In that capacity he was a leader in an impressive series of clinical trials that have greatly clarified the place of bladder conservative management. Bill has been very active in the rapidly evolving role of radiation for prostate cancer patients. This dealt with the value of PSA as a prognostic indicator, need for radiation dose increments, and initial testing of brachytherapy and proton radiation therapy.

Bill has had major appointments to ASTRO committees and board, national oncology groups, and served on editorial boards of seven journals. He has been awarded the ASRO Gold Medal in 2009. Another major plus for Bill has been his highly effective support and encouragement of the career of Anthony Zietman. The GU program has grown quite substantially under his leadership. Recently, there has been the addition of John Coen and Jason Efstathiou to the GU team.

A moment of special pride for the Shipleys and the department was the appointment of Anthony as the first William and Jenzy Shipley Professor of Radiation Oncology at the Harvard Medical School and MGH in October 2007.

10.8.3.4   Anthony Zietman

A Londoner by heritage, birth, and education, Anthony (Fig. 10.22) went to a science-oriented school that was located quite close to his home. Earlier, he had no special interest in science. In that science environment, he found himself enthusiastic about science, so that by age 16, he was specializing in chemistry and especially biology, most particularly human biology. The young lad was not focused on human biology exclusively, but had a parallel fascination in European history. This excitement for modern history actually became dominant such that on entering Oxford he chose to major in politics, philosophy, and economics (PPE), but with a commitment to make a pass in chemistry, zoology, and botany. At Oxford, he was admitted to Hartford College, the first of the Oxford colleges to be co-ed. It emphasized science and law. Anthony was clearly not free of ambition, viz., his aim was to become prime minister. However, upon realizing that there were 250 very bright students studying PPE with precisely the same goal, he began to reconsider. AZ judged that medicine was the career that he would enormously enjoy and also contribute to humanity in a clearly positive manner. Accordingly, at the end of his first year, he changed to pre-med. He did this for 3 years, with a concentration on developmental biology. This is the basis for his long-time serious and productive interest in embryology. Before entering medical school, he went to Nigeria on a Commonwealth Scholarship to teach and to provide some care for the really disadvantaged. There were political disturbances and he had less positive impact than expected. He does judge that his time teaching at the medical school was of value to himself and of real educational value to the students, whom he rated as extremely bright.

For clinical medicine, Anthony went to the famous Middlesex Hospital, i.e., back to London and near his family. At school, he met and interacted with Roger Berry, Tony Geloff, and Margaret Spittle, but especially Berry.[4] Not long after graduation, Anthony decided to become an oncologist. He knew that he wanted to do some time in a research laboratory. To consider the potentials of such an option, he discussed his career plans with Roger Berry. After a brief conversation, Berry called his friend Suit and arranged for Anthony to move to Boston in 1985 for a year or two in the tumor biology research laboratory. Anthony had never considered spending time in the USA and had had no knowledge of any cancer program in Boston, i.e., this was a big and quite unexpected turn of events. Despite this apprehension, Roger had it "fixed up" so he came. Anthony was married to Allison, a very attractive young physician, who had also had a year in Africa.

The two laboratory years were especially productive, viz., 14 papers. He was especially interested in quantitation of the effect of genetic differences between mice and the acceptance tumor transplants. On a different question, he found that doxorubicin at dose levels that resulted in no acute

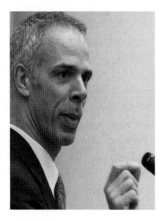

Fig. 10.22   Anthony Zietman

[4] Berry was an American who had spent some time in Oxford and married an English woman. After a period back in the USA for his 2 years of military duty, actually at the NCI, he returned to Oxford as Head of the Radiation Biology unit. He so enjoyed his time that he became a UK citizen. He did join the Royal Navy and had several long tours as the physician on an attack submarine. He later was appointed Prof of Oncology at the Middlesex Medical School. This was an early example of the "Reverse Brain Drain."

mortality, viz., deaths before 30 days, significantly shortened life span of his laboratory mice.

While in Boston, his wife had a premature baby boy, viz., 2 lbs and 13 oz. He has done extremely well and has won admission to Columbia University. When they returned to England, they had another premature boy; this one had a birth weight of 1 lb and 12 oz. This was delivered at the Radcliffe Hospital in Oxford. This lad has grown into a normal looking and very active teenager who clearly is far above average in intelligence. His major interest is art and is now preparing application to universities.

Anthony and Allison returned to London, where he completed his general medical training. An opening developed at the MGH and Suit was again on the phone for him to work part time in GU and part time at BUMC. Anthony really wanted a position in head/neck with CC but there was no opening. He did accept and returned. He was pleased that at BUMC he had many head/neck patients. He began assessing the new field in GU with the advent of PSA and Shipley's innovative work on bladder cancer. Anthony and Bill Shipley became close colleagues and promptly made a highly productive team. They have worked closely with G. Prout and several of the urologists and with medical oncologists, Don Kaufman.

Anthony has been exceptionally organized and productive in GU radiation oncology with special emphasis on not only prostate cancer but also bladder cancer. Anthony had been promoted rapidly at Harvard Medical School, viz., research fellow in 1986 to professor in 2003. Then in 2007, he was named to the Jensie W. and William U. Shipley Professorship in Radiation Oncology.

Zietman has been very active in ASTRO, serving as Program Committee Chair and a member of the Board of Directors. He became the ASTRO President at the 2009 meeting. Further, he has served as an Oral Board Examiner for the American Board of Radiology. Additionally he has been Co-Chair of the National Patterns of Care in Radiation Oncology, GU, and the NCI Kidney/Bladder Cancer Progress Review Group.

10.9 Pediatric Radiation Oncology

Clinician specialists:

Torunn Yock, Head of the unit
Nancy J Tarbell
Shannon MacDonald

Linggood started this program in 1976 and continued to 1993. She worked with Chris Willett on the allowances needed for target motion in radiation treatment of mediastinal lymphoma in 1987 and 1988 [102, 103]. This commenced a

growing and sustained interest in proton beams for pediatric patients.

MacDonald et al. [61] evaluated the outcome of 17 pediatric patients with intracranial ependymomas treated by proton beams to 55 Gy (RBE). They obtained local control and progression-free survival rates at 26 months of 86 and 80%. Complete resection combined with the proton radiation vs sub-total resection and proton radiation yielded local control results of 14/14 vs 2/4, respectively.

They compared treatment plans that delivered the same target dose using intensity-modulated x-ray beams (IMXT), passive energy modulated proton beams, and intensity-modulated proton beam therapy by pencil beam scanning (IMPT). The dose constraints for the several normal tissues or organs at risk were constant. The doses to the normal tissues were clearly and markedly lesser by proton beam therapy. The advantage was greatest for IMPT. The implication from this small series is that 55 Gy (RBE) is sufficient to achieve a high TCP.

Krejcarek et al. [55] evaluated the dose distribution in the vertebral bodies by proton irradiation of the cranial spinal axis in young patients still in active bone growth phase. There were two groups of patients. For one, the proton dose covered the entire vertebral body; for the second group, the proton range was just sufficient to include the entire dural sac and stop in the posterior third of the vertebral body. The distribution of delivered dose was clearly demonstrated by sagittal MRI imaging, i.e., the radiation changes were distributed exactly as planned. That such elegant dose distributions are achievable in patients is indeed impressive.

In a related study, Kozak et al. [51] performed a comparative treatment-planning study of proton therapy vs IMXT for a series of 10 pediatric patients treated for parameningeal rhabdomyosarcoma. The dose to the target volume was the same for proton therapy and IMXT. There was significantly lower dose to normal tissues except for the ipsilateral cochlea and mastoid and that for the ipsilateral parotid was significant at only 0.05.

Cochran et al. performed comparative treatment plan analysis to determine dose to the lens in 39 patients undergoing craniospinal irradiation [18]. They analyzed one photon and two proton plans. The protons delivered to the lens on average less than 50% of dose given by photons. This effect was much greater for children less than 10 years of age.

A comparative treatment-planning study by Krengli et al. [56] (2007) of proton treatment of retinoblastomas to 46 Gy RBE to the grossly evident lesion at several sites within the globe demonstrated an important decrease in radiation dose to orbital and near orbital structures by proton beam techniques. Yock et al. reported a study of seven children treated for rhabdomyosarcoma of the orbit by proton beam therapy and chemotherapy with a median follow-up of 6.3 years [107]. The treatment plan was to deliver no increase in dose to tumor but a major reduction in dose to non-target structures in the orbit, skull, and intracranial contents. Patient evaluations to date confirm their predictions. Observations for 10–20 years on a larger number of patients are required for a more definitive statement on the magnitude of the clinical gains achieved. Their conclusion was that local control was as anticipated but the decreased dose to normal tissues was significant and will result in lesser late radiation morbidity. These several studies document the obvious that there is a lesser dose to normal tissues by proton beam therapy than IMXT.

Yock et al. [109] reviewed the outcome data on 75 patients treated for non-metastatic pelvic Ewing's sarcoma on Children's Oncology Group protocol INT-0091. The median follow-up was 4.4 years (0.6–11.4 years). All patients received chemotherapy, viz., doxorubicin, vincristine, cyclophosphamide, and dactinomycin ± ifosamide and etoposide (VACA or VACA + IE). Local treatment was surgery for 12, radiation therapy for 44, and surgery combined with radiation for 19 patients. The local control outcome was 75% for surgery alone, 75% for radiation alone, but 89.5% for radiation and surgery. Interestingly, they did not detect significant differences in event-free survival by treatment, viz., 42, 51, and 47%, respectively. Further event-free survival was the same for lesions ≤8 and >8 cm. There was an indication of a gain in local control in the VACA + IE vs VACA for treatment by either surgery alone or radiation alone.

Fung et al. [29] found that of 98 consecutive patients treated by radiation for orbital adnexal lymphoma at a mean follow-up of 82 months, the actuarial 5-year local control result was 98%. In the MALT lymphoma patients the local control rates were 81 and 100% for dose <30 Gy but 100% for dose ≥30 Gy.

Tarbell participated in an MGH study of transplantation of bone marrow vs peripheral blood stem cells (PBSC) in the treatment of 54 patients with hematological malignancies. Their finding was that patients treated with PBSCs achieved full donor chimerism, 83 vs 48%, but at the cost of higher rate of severe graft vs host disease [26]. Tarbell has served as Co-Editor of the standard text in Pediatric Radiation Oncology throughout its five editions, the most recent being 2005.

Yock and Tarbell published a broad review of proton beam irradiation of pediatric tumors of the brain in *Nature Clinical Practice Oncology* [108].

10.9.1 Biographical Sketches

10.9.1.1 Shannon MacDonald

Shannon (Fig. 10.23) is a first generation American; her father came from Canada and her mother from Ireland. Shannon had her childhood in Billerica, a town close to

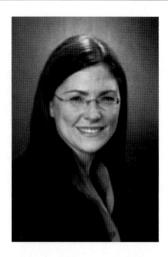

Fig. 10.23 Shannon MacDonald

Boston. As a youngster, she was enthusiastic in science courses and reading in general. She is a graduate of the local public high school. For the next phase of her education she went to Boston College as biology major and was a general pre-med student. This was largely an independent decision as there were no physicians or scientists in her family. While an undergraduate student she did an elective in a genetics lab at the Brigham Hospital. An extremely good turn of fortune was her 2 years in lab work (one as an elective and for one she was full time) in research on the retina.

For her choice of medical school, she had several friends who were at Loyola in Chicago and recommended it quite highly, especially for clinical education. She accepted their advice and attended Loyola. As a student, Shannon was interested in surgical and medical oncology but became acquainted with radiation oncology. She liked the role of anatomy and the intensive use of imaging and the much closer relationship between the radiation oncologist and patient than obtains for the surgeon. Namely, the radiation oncologist sees the patient at least weekly during treatment and for very long term follow-up. She decided on radiation oncology during her third year in medical school and took her residency at NYU. There she learned of the MGH pediatric radiation oncology, especially to use of proton beam therapy, and was involved in sending several patients to Drs. Tarbell and Yock.

Shannon was appointed to the MGH staff to work 50:50 at MGH on pediatric and breast and then at Newton-Wellesley Hospital. There she saw patients and arranged for many of them to come to MGH for actual treatment. She is now full time at the MGH and working on the pediatric and breast services.

Shannon is a competitive runner, especially the marathon. She plans to run for the MGH children's program in the coming race.

10.9.1.2 Nancy Tarbell

Nancy (Fig. 10.24) was one of six girls, the fourth in an Irish Catholic family in Hudson, MA. That there were no boys to do some of the heavy tasks, e.g., trash, lawn mowing, contributed to a spirit of independence and "Can Do" in Nancy. With six children, her family was not affluent. Her mom wrote for a newspaper and her father was a mechanical engineer. Nancy reckons that she inherited her math/science interests from her father. As a child she recalls being "in love" with science. Serious interest in medicine came at the age of 14 when she had to be hospitalized briefly. Her roommate had leukemia and died rather quickly. This tragic exposure to a child with a fatal cancer has had a large influence on her career.

Nancy did not expect that there were opportunities for women in medicine and so planned to be a kindergarten teacher. While a senior at the University of Rhode Island (*summa cum laude* graduate), a roommate with a quite strong personality called the Dean of Columbia School of General Studies and made an appointment for an interview for June 14 using Nancy's name. She informed Nancy and gave her "instructions" to go and to apply to complete her pre-med studies and then apply for admission to medical school. This was a rather dramatic development. This friend went to law school. Nancy accepted the advice and commenced taking more science courses, including organic chemistry. The images of the girl with leukemia were a constant reminder that she must do well and get into medical school.

Nancy performed at a high level at Columbia. Significantly, Nancy was accepted at all eight of the medical schools to which she applied. However, her family moved to upstate NY and she had to go to Up-State Medical Center in Syracuse (this has proved fortunate for radiation oncology) as the cost differential was substantial. In her fourth year she encountered Robert Sagerman, Chief of radiation oncology there. He was a pioneer in the radiation treatment of pediatric cancer patients, especially those with retinoblastoma.

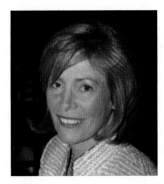

Fig. 10.24 Nancy Tarbell

Nancy had a 1 month elective in radiation oncology in her fourth year and found it to be exceptionally informative. This made a decisive impact. This was her clear favorite of all of the clinical rotations. Almost by co-incidence, Sagerman had trained Bob Cassidy who later was the pediatric radiation oncologist at Boston Children's Hospital and for the Joint Center for Radiation Oncology. This connection between Sagerman and Cassidy was decisive in her selection of the JCRT for her residency, starting in 1979. Near completion of the residency, the faculty did not encourage a sub-specialization in pediatrics as the prospects were limited and Cassidy was likely to be at the Children's for quite a number of years. Even so, she elected to work in pediatrics.

Life offers many unexpected twists in its path. A year later, Cassidy moved to be the Chief of radiation oncology at Lahey Clinic. Nancy became the head of the pediatric oncology program for the JCRT. Cassidy was immediately available for consult by phone. She had a highly productive 14 years in that position (1983–1997).

In 1996–1997, Suit was recruiting for a head of the proton program. The search committee ranked Jay Loeffler the top candidate. Then news leaked that Nancy and Jay had accepted positions at U Maryland as Vice-President for Medical Affairs and Chair of the Department of Radiation Oncology, respectively. This immediately raised the possibility that Nancy might be recruited here, were we to act speedily. HDS had never considered that there was any possibility of getting Nancy to the MGH. As she had decided to leave the Children's hospital, Suit went into full throttle to make highly attractive offers to both Nancy and Jay. There could be little doubt that the proton program would be a very large factor in the near future in pediatric oncology. Hence, there was realism in an intense effort to recruit Nancy to lead the pediatric radiation oncology program.

A very large credit must be given to Jane Claflin for our success in this recruitment, viz., Nancy and Jay. Jane was a former trustee and an exceptionally influential person at the hospital. A common impression is that an institution as famous and old with myriad traditions as was the MGH could not create new positions within a mere few days. In fact, this was accomplished, viz., Nancy was offered the opportunity to develop a major program around proton radiation therapy for pediatric patients and to participate in an important growth of pediatric oncology at the MGH and the position of Director of the Partner's Office for Women's Careers at MGH. Our offers were accepted to the enormous relief of many at this hospital. Jay and Nancy were able to obtain a release from the house they had signed to purchase in Maryland.

In 2004, Nancy's office was expanded to be the Center for Faculty Development, viz., serve the needs of the entire faculty. There are two branch offices: the Office for Women's Careers and the Office for Research Career Development that addresses issues unique to the researchers. Nancy proudly notes that there is now a Native American woman who is a full professor of psychiatry.

Nancy has enjoyed her work in the department and has definite success in improving the care of children with cancer. She immediately commenced working closely with the pediatric oncologist and pediatric surgeons. Principally due to Nancy and the proton program, there was a definite contribution to growth of the pediatric oncology patient numbers. Within the department, Nancy had an extremely good working relationship with C.C. Wang and greatly admired him for his clinical acumen and splendid sense of humor, gingerly flavored with Chinese proverbs. Another favorite has been Eve Malkin, social worker for the pediatric patients. Nancy has been a favorite staff for the residents. She has published more than 200 papers and book chapters.

In 2007, Nancy was appointed the CC Wang Professor of Radiation Oncology at the MGH. In 2008, her work received special recognition in being named the Dean for Academic and Clinical Affairs at the Harvard Medical School. This is a major expansion of her administrative role, viz., she has "responsibility for promoting, co-coordinating and supporting the academic and clinical activities of the MGH faculty, with an emphasis on faculty development and diversity." Additionally, she is to oversee the "Office of Faculty Affairs, Office of Faculty and Research Integrity, Office for Diversity and Community Partnership, the Department of Ambulatory Care and Prevention." These activities are only a part of total responsibilities as she does carry a patient load at the MGH.

In 1999, Nancy was given the Distinguished Alumnae Award of SUNY Upstate Medical Center in Syracuse, NY. Nancy was elected to the Institute of Medicine of the National Academy of Sciences in 2002.

The leadership of the Pediatric Radiation Oncology has passed to Torunn Yock.

10.9.1.3 Torunn Yock, M.D.

Torunn (Fig. 10.25) became fascinated with science primarily as a result of childhood reading of books given to her by her parents that were oriented toward microscopes and microbes, etc. As young student, she found herself to be very fortunate in that close to her home was the newly built Thomas Jefferson High School of Science and Technology. Torunn was a member of the first graduating class. This school achieved a very high reputation and was rated in 2007 by the US World and News as the number one high school in the USA. She remembers her school teachers with great fondness and comments that despite the fact that she was not particularly oriented toward English her English teacher was her favorite.

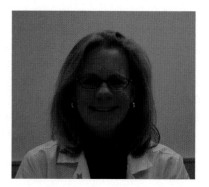

Fig. 10.25 Torunn Yock

Clearly, she had an excellent time in high school and was well prepared and enthusiastic to enter Duke. As evidence of her academic achievements at high school, she won an academic scholarship "The Angier Biddle Duke Scholarship" and this covered her entire tuition cost and summer session at New College, at Oxford University. For her studies at Duke, her major interest was in bio-ethics, but there was no major in that particular field so she put together an assortment of courses that had an acceptable plan. She did this by using ethics, religion, and various independent studies into one package. There was only one genetics class and she of course took that and in addition, there were all of the general chemistry and biology classes. With the growing interest in bio-ethics, several years after she graduated, Duke did establish a bio-ethics program. Her interest in bio-ethics was provoked by her fascination with the genome, which was just beginning to unfold in a relatively comprehensive manner. Namely, what was the impact of genetics on the behavior of people and their health care? This is a highly complex and difficult question to investigate, but definitely of exceptional interest.

Her senior thesis while at Duke considered the problem of a collective risk for society and how insurance companies and society will deal with individuals who as a result of their genetic make-up are at high risk of developing serious "costly" diseases. Aside from her course work, while at Duke, she served as a volunteer in the education program of disadvantaged children in that area. She was very much involved by the fact that a child to whom she was assigned was not learning very much at all and it was soon evident that the child could not see the page. This was despite the fact that the child had passed from first into second grade. Torunn simply arranged for her to get a pair of glass, but she does not know how the child faired because she soon went to Australia.

She went to the university near South Wales with the intent of obtaining a degree in public health. She did concentrate most of her time on science, but was particularly fascinated by the study and evaluation of the healthcare system in Australia, i.e., an universal healthcare system that was about 20 years old when she arrived.

After graduating from Duke and a year in Australia she returned to the USA to enter medical school; however, between her first and second year she returned to Australia and completed her thesis *A Comparison of Doctor Satisfaction in Boston and Sydney Australia with Their Two Health Systems*. She discovered unexpectedly that there were very many access issues and waiting lists in Boston's medical practices.

Torunn entered Harvard Medical School and completed her work at the University of South Wales while a medical student. However, during her third year of medical school on an elective in radiology at the MGH, lectures by Jim McIntyre and by Ira Spiro introduced her to the field of radiation oncology. Prior to that point she had considered going into emergency medicine. She then spent a short elective with McIntyre and Spiro and decided that this was much more interesting. In 1997, she did her fourth year elective at the MGH and during this time she encountered protons. Both Nancy Tarbell and Jay Loeffler described their excitement about the field. She had very much planned on going to California for the advantage in the weather, but she decided to apply to the program at the MGH, and she was accepted. During her residency she worked on problems associated with prostate cancer, breast cancer, and CNS neoplasms. She was particularly intrigued and interested in pediatrics after dealing with children and of course the attractiveness of the proton beams particularly for pediatric patients.

Torunn has married Tim Padera, a staff scientist working in the Rakesh Jain group, and they have a 2-year-old daughter and an infant son.

10.10 Mesenchymal Tumors

Clinician specialists:

Thomas DeLaney, Head of the unit
Yen Lin Chen, N. Liebsch, H. Suit, Ira Spiro

10.10.1 Soft Tissue Sarcomas (STS)

These constitute a highly diverse group of tumors, viz., ~ 50 pathological sub-types, but in toto comprise $\leq 1\%$ of all cancers in the USA. STS arise at virtually all anatomic sites, vary in grade and volume, and occur predominantly in patients at ≥ 50 years of age. Etiological factors include several genetic diseases, chronic trauma, and an array of chemicals, ionization radiation, and other agents.

Sarcomas had been traditionally judged to be highly radiation resistant and radiation of little clinical value. The finding Puck et al. in the 1950s of a narrow range of in vitro radiation sensitivity for a wide spectrum of mammalian cells made Suit skeptical of the then standard opinion that sarcoma cells were exceptionally radiation resistant.[5] He considered that the low success rate of radiation therapy might well be due to hypoxia or the large volume of sarcomas at treatment. This was the basis for the initial studies of his treatment of patients with extremity sarcoma at the start of the 1960s at the M.D. Anderson Cancer Center. The strategy was to minimize the role of hypoxia by application of tourniquet to induce hypoxia of normal and tumor tissue, i.e., no differential sensitivity based on pO_2 and to employ very large doses per fraction, viz., 10 Gy. The patients had had inadequate surgery, i.e., treated post-operatively. Due to the high success rate, the combined surgery and radiation treatment was extended to non-extremity sites (i.e., tourniquet not applicable) and 2 Gy/fraction. The tourniquet treatment was discontinued.

The result was that radiation in well-tolerated doses at standard fractionation combined with conservative surgery yielded local control rates comparable to those by radical surgery [84]. Importantly, the result was preservation of a useful limb in a high proportion of patients. These findings have been confirmed in other centers and contributed to the acceptance of this "limb conservation" strategy. The data from those studies were accepted as indicating that the dominant indicators of outcome for a specified treatment were tumor size and grade and not pathological type for sarcomas in adult patients [74, 85]. Myxoid liposarcomas are more responsive and more readily controlled by radiation than other sarcoma types.

The start of a multi-disciplinary management of mesenchymal tumors at the MGH occurred in 1972 with Henry Mankin arriving as the Chief of Orthopedic Surgery, an orthopedic oncologist. There immediately developed a close interaction and friendship between Mankin and Suit. This team expanded with sub-specialists in connective tissue tumors: David Harmon in medical oncology, Dan Rosenthal in diagnostic radiology, Al Schiller in pathology, and on a less formal basis, John Raker of General Surgery (there was not a sub-specialist for sarcomas among the general surgeons at that time), as most sarcomas were seen by the orthopedic surgeons.

This team grew to include Mark Gebhardt,[6] Dempsey Springfield, Fran Hornicek, Candice Jennings,[6] Kevin

---

[5] A later study, 1996, of the cellular radiation sensitivity, by Ruka, a research fellow in the Steele laboratory, showed that the SF_2s for soft tissue sarcoma cell lines were not different from those derived from breast carcinomas [73].

Raskin, and J. Schwab in Orthopaedic Oncology; Ira Spiro,[7] Thomas DeLaney, and Yen Lin Chen in Radiation Oncology; Sam Yoon in Oncologic Surgery; Andrew Rosenberg, Pietr Nielsen, and Al Schiller in Pathology.[6] We operate as a Sarcoma Center with patients being evaluated by representatives of the involved specialists in a single visit.

See the section on pediatric tumors for consideration of sarcomas in children.

One of the first questions examined was the timing of the surgery and radiation. Initially, radiation was administered post-operatively or as the sole modality. There has been a steady move to administered radiation, often combined with chemotherapy, prior to resection. The rationale is (1) treatment volume is planned exclusively on the anatomic site and local extent of tumor; and (2) sarcoma cells spilled into the wound or extravasated into the blood vascular system had been irradiated and, hence, less likely to autotransplant in the wound or to establish metastasis. The pre-operative dose is ~50 Gy (9–10 Gy/week). For microscopic positive margins 15 Gy is given post-operatively. For patients treated only by post-operative irradiation, the dose is 60 Gy for margin- negative and 65–70 for margin-positive resections. That is for pre-operative irradiation, the treatment volume is smaller, the dose is lower, and cells exfoliated into the circulatory system have been irradiated. The results from pre-operative irradiation were expected to be improved and appear to be so. There is, however, the requirement of more gentle handling of the irradiated tissues and more liberal use of grafts.

Ira Spiro and David Harmon initiated a study of pre-operative radiation (44 Gy) and MAID chemotherapy for large (≥8 cm diameter) and G II-III soft tissue sarcomas. The radiation dose was 44 Gy at 2 Gy/fraction with 11 fractions given between MAID courses 1 and 2 and between courses 3 and 4. This was followed by surgery and then two additional cycles of MAID. Post-operative irradiation was used only for margin-positive resections. MAID is mensa, doxorubicin, ifosfamide, and dacarbazine. They performed a matched pair analysis of MGH patients treated by radiation and surgery and there was evidence of a modest gain from the chemotherapy.

DeLaney et al. [23] reported the 5-year local control in 48 patients managed by this MAID + radiation pre-operative protocol to be 92 as compared to 86% in historical matched control patients managed by surgery and radiation, $p=0.1$. Disease-free and overall survival was significantly higher in the MAID-treated patients. Pervaiz et al. have completed a comprehensive meta-analysis of 18 trials of chemotherapy combined with surgery ± radiation and reported small gains

in local control and survival for the chemotherapy-treated patients [69].

Spiro et al. [83] judged that the dominant factor in local control was margin status and that higher doses are required for patients whose resection was margin positive.

Currently, DeLaney and team are participating in a neo-adjuvant chemotherapy combined with the anti-angiogenesis agent Avastin. There is at present a non-negligible increment in toxicity.

Radiation as the sole modality is an effective curative option to surgery in the medically or technically inoperable patient provided radical dose irradiation is feasible as reported by Kepka et al. [47]. Of 112 patients treated by radiation alone for gross disease, the 5-year local control rates were 60 and 22% for total dose of ≥63 vs ≤63 Gy. Complication rates were 27 vs 8% for doses of ≥68 vs <68 Gy; median follow-up was 11 years. She and colleagues also assessed local control of 78 patients treated by radiation alone (median dose was 66 Gy) after an "unplanned resection." The 10-year local control was 86%, indicating that repeat resection is not required for a high local control result [46]. DeLaney et al. determined local control in 154 patients who had positive surgical margins (ink of tumor cells). Local control results for doses of >64 and <64 Gy were 85 and 66%, respectively [25].

Desmoid tumors are non-metastasizing fibroblastic lesions that are locally destructive or fatal in some patients if not treated successfully. In the MGH series, radiation alone has been effective for both primary and recurrent lesions, viz., local control of 100 and 90% in 5 and 10 patients, respectively, as reported by Spear et al. [82]. In this small series, higher rates of local control have been obtained than by surgery. Also, radiation alone or combined with surgery was equally effective in a small series of patients with dermatofibrosarcoma protuberans.

10.10.2 Bone Sarcoma

The advance by the MGH Radiation Oncology in this area has been the use of proton beams alone or combined with surgery for chordoma and chondrosarcoma of the skull base and spinal column. In addition, high control rates have been reported for proton treatment of other categories of tumors in the spine.

The 15-year local control of chondrosarcoma of the skull base by proton and photon irradiation is reported at 95% in the series of 200 patients [72]. The results were substantially less good for the chordomas, viz., 59% at 5 years [93]. Further, the control rate declined further out to 10 years, viz., appearing to plateau at 42%.

For patients treated by radiation (proton and photon) for primary sacral chordomas at doses of 77 Gy RBE, local

---

[6] Moved to another center.

[7] Deceased.

Fig. 10.26 (**a**) Exposed dura and (**b**) with a yttrium plaque positioned over the dura to which sarcoma was attached

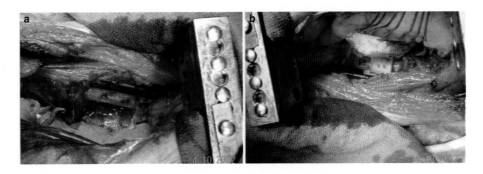

control was achieved in 8 of 9 patients, with a 5-year actuarial rate of 87% [21]. These, quite aggressive does levels, are associated with a significant frequency of late morbidity, viz., one each with sacral neuropathy and erectile dysfunction. For results in patients with sacral chordoma treated with surgery combined with radiation [67]. Among those patients, results were much less satisfactory for recurrent chordomas at treatment.

Radiation at high dose levels combined with chemotherapy is yielding substantial local control rates of osteosarcoma. DeLaney et al. have examined results in the MGH series of 41 patients treated by chemotherapy and post gross total resection irradiation, sub-total resection, and radiation alone [24]. Chemotherapy was administered to 35 of these patients. Local control was achieved in 78, 78, and 40% for the three groups, respectively [24]. These findings indicate a significant clinical role for radiation in treatment of some categories of OGS.

DeLaney et al. introduced selective irradiation of the dura for patients whose sarcoma (bone or soft tissue origin) were in contact with the dura. Irradiation of the dura to a high dose while respecting cord tolerance is not feasible by external beam techniques. The technique developed at the MGH is to design and fabricate (by an outside firm) a customized plaque impregnated with ^{90}yttrium and then applied to the exposed dura for delivery of 10–15 Gy in ~10 min to the region of the dura judged to be at risk [22]. This is illustrated in Fig. 10.26. The early results are a very low failure rate.

10.10.3 Connective Tissue Oncology Society (CTOS)

The MGH radiation oncology sarcoma group has been active in collaborating with other centers. As an example note that the formation of the Connective Tissue Oncology Society was initiated by the actions of Suit and colleagues. The first meeting was held at the MGH; he served as president for the initial 2 years. Tom DeLaney and Mark Gebhardt have been very active and have served as officers. This is an international society and is fully interdisciplinary, with heavy interest on research. CTOS meets annually and alternates between the USA, Europe, and Asia.

10.10.4 Biographical Sketches

10.10.4.1 Thomas F. DeLaney

Tom (Fig. 10.27) was born into a medical family; his father was an internist, in Morristown, NJ. Tom quite early developed an interest in patients and efforts to improve their health status. Performance at school was a clear success as evidenced by his admission to Harvard College. To develop a broad knowledge base, he majored in history and remains a "history buff" to this day, with special attention to the events that led to WWI and WWII. His plan prior to his start at Harvard was a career in medicine and he did gain admission to Harvard Medical School in 1978. During his third year his mother developed colo-rectal carcinoma and ultimately died of metastatic tumor. This was an important factor in directing his talent to oncology.

He took a course on basic oncology at the school run by H. Suit. They met after the course and he was invited to take an elective laboratory period in the department at MGH. For this, he worked with Leo Gerweck. He was invited to spend a few mornings in the clinic. This was quite impressive in demonstrating several long-term follow-up patients with excellent results. These patient outcomes were interpreted as powerful evidence that radiation was effective as a curative treatment modality, especially when combined with less than radical surgery.

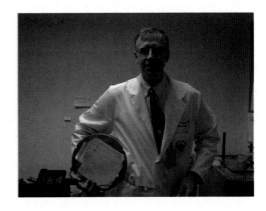

Fig. 10.27 Thomas F. DeLaney

For his PG 1, he had a year as a surgical resident at Yale. There he saw a substantial number of cancer patients and interacted with the radiation oncology staff at Yale. The next phase was his residency in radiation oncology at the MGH. His co-residents were Paul Busse and Paul Okunieff. The close work with other residents both senior and junior to him was highly valuable to learning. This was in addition to positive interactions with the several faculty members. He was particularly impressed by the course in physics. Another experience was work with Len Gunderson and learning of the clear importance of analysis of patterns of failure. Another was the use of interstitial brachytherapy of the prostate by Bill Shipley. He was quite impressed by the book allowance and the encouragement from HDS to subscribe to *Science* or *Nature*. He has continued his subscription of *Science* to the present.

For his first staff position, he went to the NCI and worked with Eli Glatstein. There he participated in IOERT and clinical trials on sarcoma patients. Next he was recruited back to Boston to be Chief of the BUMC (recently merged Boston University Medical Center and Boston City Hospital). As the MGH department had accepted responsibility for the operation of the radiation oncology program at BUMC, he had appointments at MGH and HMS. Tom rapidly and efficiently improved the program there. MGH staff A. Taghian, Anthony Zietman, Bruce Borgelt, and Claire Fung were at BUMC on a part-time basis or for special patients. Quite importantly, our residency program was modified to include a rotation at BUMC. This has proved to be highly popular with our residents.

Tom worked to enhance the affiliation with Jordan Hospital in Plymouth and attended Oncology Rounds at Carney and the Shattuck Hospitals. Tom worked with the Southwest Oncology Group.

Upon the tragic death of Ira Spiro, Tom was recruited to the sarcoma and the gynecological units in 2000 and became involved in the proton program. He continued the development of the dural plaque technique for tumors abutting the dura. He also became intensively involved in clinical trials for soft tissue sarcoma organized by RTOG. When Jay Loeffler was appointed Chief of the department, Tom became the Director of the proton program and PI of the NCI program project grant. Clinical research in proton therapy under his leadership has been strongly positive with protocols for skull base sarcoma, paranasal sinus, nasopharynx, lung, partial breast irradiation, pediatric tumor, and prostate tumor. The number of patients treated per day has progressively increased to ~ 60. This work load includes an average of 14 pediatric patients per day, with 6 requiring general anesthesia.

Tom has developed a close collaboration with the proton therapy center at M.D. Anderson Hospital. They have submitted a combined application to the NCI for continued support for the clinical and physics research in proton radiation therapy. This application has been approved and funded, a major achievement at any time but especially at present with large cuts in new grants being funded.

10.10.4.2 Yen Lin Chen

Yen Lin (Fig. 10.28) came with her parents from Taipei, Taiwan, to San Antonio, TX, at age 13. Her father entered an MBA program and her mother worked very heavy hours as a seamstress to support the family, viz., a husband in graduate, Yen Lin, and her two younger sisters. They lived in a very low income area and she had to pass metal detectors to enter school. Only ~ 10% of the students at her school ever attended university. Despite these factors, Yen Lin judges that the school had some impressive science teachers. Their courses strongly stimulated her interest in chemistry. She did very well on exams and was admitted to Harvard on a Coca Cola scholarship as a major in chemistry. The concentration on biochemistry extended into molecular biology as an important experience for her was a project with Dr. P. Hynes in basic cancer biology. Additionally, she had a positive experience working at the Ronald McDonald House and interacting with the children. These were two large factors in her decision to enter medical school. Again, her high level of performance was recognized and she received a full scholarship for the 4 years at Vanderbilt medical school. She had become engaged to a student while an undergraduate and they wished to have the residency in the same city. This was achieved with her acceptance into the MGH residency in radiation oncology.

Her young man was an immigrant from Vietnam when his parents fled to the USA when he was a baby of 2 years. In this country he was also a star performer, winning scholarships to

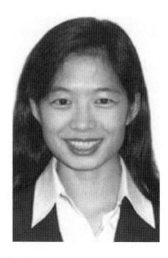

Fig. 10.28   Yen Lin Chen

a science high school and then Harvard College and Medical School. Yen Lin continued to perform at an exceptional level as a resident and was invited to continue at the MGH as a staff radiation oncologist. She accepted and works on the sarcoma team of Tom DeLaney. Her husband is on the staff at Beth Israel in Dermatologic Surgery.

10.10.4.3 Ira J. Spiro 1954–2001

Ira Spiro (Fig. 10.29) was the close collaborator with Suit for several years in the radiation management of mesenchymal tumor patients. The plan was for him to assume leadership of that program. In addition he became very keen in assessing the clinical potential of proton beams in radiation oncology. Ira was appointed the Associate Medical Director of the proton therapy program. He contributed quite importantly to both clinical areas. He was also very strongly supported by Jay Loeffler. No surprise to those who knew Ira was his continued productivity in laboratory research.

Ira started life in 1954 and as a very young lad displayed remarkable interest combined with knowledge, enthusiasm, and skills in science. This was made quite clear at the age of 7 by winning the first prize at the Franklin Institute Science Fair (in Philadelphia). This keenness toward science was sustained and after graduation from La Salle College of Philadelphia, Ira went to Colorado State as a graduate student with Bill Dewey as his mentor. Ira was a highly effective student not only in his own work but also in his positive impact on the progress of fellow students. He made one of the first studies of genetic factors determining cell injury by hyperthermia. During this period, his interest extended to medicine and he moved to George Washington University for medical school combined with further laboratory research in the Clift Ling group. The latter was in part directed to analysis of genes involved in repair of radiation-damaged DNA.

His medical interest naturally focused on radiation oncology from his many years in radiation biology laboratory programs. He came to the MGH for residency and was clearly an outstanding young radiation oncologist. Ira was viewed by all as a superb human being. His area of specialization was mesenchymal tissue tumors and was being prepared to lead the radiation oncology program for that group of patients.

One major study that he initiated with David Harmon was an assessment of the clinical efficacy of pre-operative radiation and MAID chemotherapy to patients with G11/111 soft tissue sarcomas of ≥ 8 cm diameter. Post-operatively, the treatment was three additional cycles of MAID.[8] These patients were matched in detail for grade and size with earlier patients treated pre-operatively by radiation alone. Analysis of patient outcome indicated a positive result, though not a large gain. This study has been the basis for several later clinical trials.

The discovery in Ira of bilateral renal cell carcinoma with bony metastases was a profound shock to all of the many who had interacted with him. Ira was highly respected for his exceptional qualities as a human being. He was an extraordinarily fine friend and physician. He accepted the rigorous treatment calmly but to little avail. He died on February 1, 2001. He is survived by his wife Jan and two young sons who are ripe with high promise.

The talents and enterprise of Ira were fully appreciated well beyond the department. The exceptional esteem with which he was held is reflected in the annual Ira J. Spiro Lectures organized by Jay Loeffler. These are listed in Chapter 11 "Special Lectures."

References

1. Alm El-Din MA, Hughes KS, Finkelstein DM, et al. Breast cancer after treatment of Hodgkin's lymphoma: risk factors that really matter. Int J Radiat Oncol Biol Phys. 2009;73(1):69–74.
2. Arvold ND, Lessell S, Bussiere M, et al. Visual outcomes and tumor control after conformal radiotherapy for patients with optic nerve sheath meningioma. Int J Radiat Oncol Biol Phys. 2009;75(4):1166–72.
3. Barker FG 2nd, Butler WE, Lyons S, et al. Dose-volume prediction of radiation-related complications after proton beam radiosurgery for cerebral arteriovenous malformations. J Neurosurg. 2003;99(2):254–63.
4. Batchelor TT, Sorenson AG, di Tomaso E, et al. AZD2171, a pan-VEGF receptor tyrosine kinase inhibitor, normalizes tumor vasculature and alleviates edema in glioblastoma patients. Cancer Cell. 2007;11(1):83–95.
5. Batchelor TT, Duda DG, di Tomaso E, et al. Phase II study of cediranib, an oral pan-vascular endothelial growth factor receptor tyrosine kinase inhibitor, in patients with recurrent glioblastoma. J Clin Oncol. 2010;28(17):2817–23.

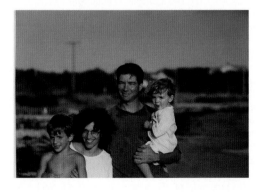

Fig. 10.29 Ira J. Spiro

---

[8] Were the surgical margins positive, additional radiation was administered.

6. Biggs PJ, Wang CC. An intra-oral cone for an 18 MeV linear accelerator. Int J Radiat Oncol Biol Phys. 1982; 8(7):1251–6.

7. Chakravarti A, Compton CC, Shellito PC, et al. Long-term follow-up of patients with rectal cancer managed by local excision with and without adjuvant irradiation. Ann Surg. 1999;230(1):49–54.

8. Chan AW, Liebsch NJ. Proton radiation therapy for head and neck cancer. J Surg Oncol. 2008;97(8):697–700.

9. Chan AW, Tarbell NJ, Black PM, et al. Adult medulloblastoma: prognostic factors and patterns of relapse. Neurosurgery. 2000;47(3):623–31.

10. Chan AW, Black P, Ojemann RG, et al. Stereotactic radiotherapy for vestibular schwannomas: favorable outcome with minimal toxicity. Neurosurgery. 2005; 57(1):60–70.

11. Choi C, Carey R. Small cell anaplastic carcinoma of lung. Reappraisal of current management. Cancer. 1976;37(6):2651–7.

12. Choi CH, Suit HD. Evaluation of rapid radiation treatment schedules utilizing two treatment sessions per day. Radiology. l975;116(3):703–7.

13. Choi NC, Carey RW. Importance of radiation dose in achieving improved loco-regional tumor control in limited stage small-cell lung carcinoma: an update. Int J Radiat Oncol Biol Phys. 1989;17(2):307–10.

14. Choi NC, Doucette JA. Improved survival of patients with unresectable non-small-cell bronchogenic carcinoma by an innovated high-dose en-bloc radiotherapeutic approach. Cancer. 1981;48(1):101–9.

15. Choi NC, Carey RW, Kaufman SD, et al. Small cell carcinoma of the lung. A progress report of 15 years' experience. Cancer. 1987;59(1):6–14.

16. Choi NC, Herndon JE 2nd, Rosenman J, et al. Phase I study to determine the maximum-tolerated dose of radiation in standard daily and hyperfractionated-accelerated twice-daily radiation schedules with concurrent chemotherapy for limited-stage small-cell lung cancer. J Clin Oncol. 1998;16(11):3528–36.

17. Choi NC, Fischman AJ, Niemierko A, et al. Dose-response relationship between probability of pathologic tumor control and glucose metabolic rate measured with FDG PET after preoperative chemoradiotherapy in locally advanced non-small-cell lung cancer. Int J Radiat Oncol Biol Phys. 2002;54(4):1024–35.

18. Cochran DM, Yock TI, Adams JA Radiation dose to the lens during craniospinal irradiation-an improvement in proton radiotherapy technique. Int J Radiat Oncol Biol Phys. 2008;70(5):1336–42.

19. Coen JJ, Zietman AL, Thakral H et al. Radical radiation for localized prostate cancer: local persistence of disease results in a late wave of metastases. J Clin Oncol. 2002;20(15):3199–205.

20. del Carmen MG, McIntyre JF, Fuller AF, et al. Intraoperative radiation therapy in the treatment of pelvic gynecologic malignancies: a review of fifteen cases. Gynecol Oncol. 2000;79(3):457–62.

21. DeLaney T, Liebsch N, Pedlow F, et al. Phase II study of high-dose photon/proton radiotherapy in the management of spine sarcomas. Int J Radiat Oncol Biol Phys. 2009;74(3):732–9.

22. DeLaney TF, Chen GT, Mauceri TC, et al. Intraoperative dural irradiation by customized 192iridium and 90yttrium brachytherapy plaques. Int J Radiat Oncol Biol Phys. 2003;57(1):239–45.

23. DeLaney TF, Spiro IJ, Suit HD, et al. Neoadjuvant chemotherapy and radiotherapy for large extremity soft-tissue sarcomas. Int J Radiat Oncol Biol Phys. 2003;56(4):1117–27.

24. DeLaney TF, Park L, Goldberg SI, et al. Radiotherapy for local control of osteosarcoma. Int J Radiat Oncol Biol Phys. 2005;61(2):492–8.

25. DeLaney TF, Kepka L, Goldberg SI, et al. Radiation therapy for control of soft-tissue sarcomas resected with positive margins. Int J Radiat Oncol Biol Phys. 2007;67(5):1460–9.

26. Dey BR, Shaffer J, Yee AJ, et al. Comparison of outcomes after transplantation of peripheral blood stem cells versus bone marrow following an identical nonmyeloablative conditioning regimen. Bone Marrow Transplant. 2007;40(1):19–27.

27. Efstathiou JA, Zietman AL, Kaufman DS, et al. Bladder-sparing approaches to invasive disease. World J Urol. 2006;24(5):517–29.

28. Fitzek MM, Thornton AF, Rabinov JD, et al. Accelerated fractionated proton/photon irradiation to 90 cobalt gray equivalent for glioblastoma multiforme: results of a phase II prospective trial. J Neurosurg. 1999;91(2):251–60.

29. Fung CY, Tarbell NJ, Lucarelli MJ, et al. Ocular adnexal lymphoma: clinical behavior of distinct World Health Organization classification subtypes. Int J Radiat Oncol Biol Phys. 2003;57(5):1382–91.

30. Gierga DP, Riboldi M, Turcotte JC, et al. Comparison of target registration errors for multiple image-guided techniques in accelerated partial breast irradiation. Int J Radiat Oncol Biol Phys. 2008;70(4):1239–46.

31. Goitein M, Miller T. Planning proton therapy of the eye. Med Phys. 1983;10(3):275–83.

32. Gragoudas E, Li W, Goitein M, Lane AM, et al. Evidence-based estimates of outcome in patients irradiated for intraocular melanoma. Arch Ophthalmol. 2002;120(12):1665–71.

33. Gragoudas ES, Lane AM, Regan S, et al. A randomized controlled trial of varying radiation doses in the treatment of choroidal melanoma. Arch Ophthalmol. 2000;118(6):773–8.

34. Gunderson L, Tepper J. Clinical radiation oncology. Philadelphia, PA: Churchill Livingstone; 2000.

35. Gunderson L, Willett C, Harrison L, et al. Intraoperative Irradiation: techniques and results. Totowa, NJ: Humana; 1999.

36. Gunderson LL, Shipley WU, Suit HD, et al. Intraoperative irradiation: a pilot study combining external beam photons with "boost" dose intraoperative electrons. Cancer. 1982;49(11):2259–66.

37. Gunderson LL, Hoskins RB, Cohen AC, et al. Combined modality treatment of gastric cancer. Int J Radiat Oncol Biol Phys. 1983;9(7):965–75.

38. Hagan MP, Winter KA, Kaufman DS, et al. RTOG 97-06: initial report of a phase I-II trial of selective bladder conservation using TURBT, twice-daily accelerated irradiation sensitized with cisplatin, and adjuvant MCV combination chemotherapy. Int J Radiat Oncol Biol Phys. 2003;57(3):665–72

39. Hoffman KE, Hong TS, Zietman AL, Russell AH. External beam radiation treatment for rectal cancer is associated with a decrease in subsequent prostate cancer diagnosis. Cancer. 2008;112(4):943–9.

40. Holmes G, Schulz M. Therapeutic radiology. Philadelphia, PA: Lea and Febiger; 1950.

41. Hong TS, Craft DL, Carlsson F, et al. Multicriteria optimization in intensity-modulated radiation therapy treatment planning for locally advanced cancer of the pancreatic head. Int J Radiat Oncol Biol Phys. 2008;72(4):1208–14.

42. Hoskins RB, Gunderson LL, Dosoretz DE, et al. Adjuvant postoperative radiotherapy in carcinoma of the rectum and rectosigmoid. Cancer. 1985;55(1):61–71.

43. Hug EB, Devries A, Thornton AF, et al. Management of atypical and malignant meningiomas: role of high-dose, 3D-conformal radiation therapy. J Neurooncol. 2000;48(2):151–60.

44. Jemal A, Siegel R, Ward E, et al. Cancer statistics, 2007. CA Cancer J Clin. 2007;57(1):43–66.

45. Karakoyun-Celik O, Norris CM Jr, Tishler R, et al. Definitive radiotherapy with interstitial implant boost for squamous cell carcinoma of the tongue base. Head Neck. 2005;27(5):353–61.

46. Kepka L, Suit HD, Goldberg SI, et al. Results of radiation therapy performed after unplanned surgery (without re-excision) for soft tissue sarcomas. J Surg Oncol. 2005;92(1):39–45.

47. Kepka L, DeLaney TF, Suit HD, et al. Results of radiation therapy for unresected soft-tissue sarcomas. Int J Radiat Oncol Biol Phys. 2005;63(3):852–9.

48. Kjellberg RN, Kliman B. Bragg peak proton treatment for pituitary-related conditions. Proc R Soc Med. 1974;67(1):32–2.

49. Kjellberg RN, Shintani A, Franz AG, et al. Proton-beam therapy in acromegaly. N Engl J Med. 1968;278(13):689–95.

50. Kjellberg RN, Hanamura T, Davis KR, et al. Bragg-peak proton-beam therapy for arteriovenous malformations of the brain. N Engl J Med. 1983;309(5):269–74.

51. Kozak K, Adams J, Krejcarek S, et al. A dosimetric comparison of proton and intensity modulated photon radiation therapy for pediatric parameningeal rhabdomyosarcomas. Int J Radiat Oncol Biol Phys. 2009;74(1):179–86.

52. Kozak KR, Katz A, Adams J, et al. Dosimetric comparison of proton and photon three-dimensional, conformal, external beam accelerated partial breast irradiation techniques. Int J Radiat Oncol Biol Phys. 2006;65(5):1572–8.

53. Kozak KR, Smith BL, Adams J, et al. Accelerated partial-breast irradiation using proton beams: initial clinical experience. Int J Radiat Oncol Biol Phys. 2006;66(3):691–8.

54. Kozak KR, Kachnic LA, Adams J, et al. Dosimetric feasibility of hypofractionated proton radiotherapy for neoadjuvant pancreatic cancer treatment. Int J Radiat Oncol Biol Phys. 2007;68(5):1557–66.

55. Krejcarek SC, Grant PE, Henson JW, et al. Physiologic and radiographic evidence of the distal edge of the proton beam in craniospinal irradiation. Int J Radiat Oncol Biol Phys. 2007;68(3):646–9.

56. Krengli M, Hug EB, Adams JA, et al. Proton radiation therapy for retinoblastoma: comparison of various intraocular tumor locations and beam arrangements. Int J Radiat Oncol Biol Phys. 2005;61(2):583–93.

57. Landry J, Tepper JE, Wood WC, et al. Patterns of failure following curative resection of gastric carcinoma. Int J Radiat Oncol Biol Phys. 1990;19(6):1357–62.

58. Lawenda BD, Taghian AG, Kachnic LA, et al. Dose-volume analysis of radiotherapy for T1N0 invasive breast cancer treated by local excision and partial breast irradiation by low-dose-rate interstitial implant. Int J Radiat Oncol Biol Phys. 2003;56(3):671–80.

59. Lawenda BD, Gagne HM, Gierga DP, et al. Permanent alopecia after cranial irradiation: dose-response relationship. Int J Radiat Oncol Biol Phys. 2004;60(3):879–87.

60. Macdonald SM, Taghian AG. Partial-breast irradiation: towards a replacement for whole-breast Irradiation? Expert Rev Anticancer Ther. 2007;7(2):123–34.

61. MacDonald SM, Safai S, Trofimov A, et al. Proton radiotherapy for childhood ependymoma: initial clinical outcomes and dose comparisons. Int J Radiat Oncol Biol Phys. 2008;71(4):979–86.

62. Mori S, Wolfgang J, Lu HM, Schneider R, et al. Quantitative assessment of range fluctuations in charged particle lung irradiation. Int J Radiat Oncol Biol Phys. 2008;70(1):253–61.

63. Nguyen PL, Chakravarti A, Finkelstein DM, et al. Results of whole-brain radiation as salvage of methotrexate failure for immunocompetent patients with primary CNS lymphoma. J Clin Oncol. 2005;23(7):1507–13.

64. Orezzoli JP, Russell AH, Oliva E, et al. Prognostic implication of endometriosis in clear cell carcinoma of the ovary. Gynecol Oncol. 2008;110(3):336–44.

65. Padera TP, Kadambi A, di Tomaso E, et al. Lymphatic metastasis in the absence of functional intratumor lymphatics. Science. 2002;296(5574):1883–6.

66. Pai HH, Thornton A, Katznelson L, et al. Hypothalamic/pituitary function following high-dose conformal radiotherapy to the base of skull: demonstration of a dose-effect relationship using dose-volume histogram analysis. Int J Radiat Oncol Biol Phys. 2001;49(4):1079–92.

67. Park L, DeLaney TF, Liebsch NJ, et al. Sacral chordomas: impact of high-dose proton/photon-beam radiation therapy combined with or without surgery for primary versus recurrent tumor. Int J Radiat Oncol Biol Phys. 2006;65(5):1514–21.

68. Patel S, Adams JA, Chan AW. Nasopharynx. In: DeLaney T, Kooy H, eds. Proton and heavier charged particle radiotherapy. Philadelphia, PA: Lippincott, Williams and Wilkins; 2008: 197–205.

69. Pervaiz N, Colterjohn N, Farrokhyar F, et al. A systematic meta-analysis of randomized controlled trials of adjuvant chemotherapy for localized resectable soft-tissue sarcoma. Cancer. 2008;113(3):573–81.

70. Pommier P, Liebsch NJ, Deschler DG, et al. Proton beam radiation therapy for skull base adenoid cystic carcinoma. Arch Otolaryngol Head Neck Surg. 2006;132(11):1242–9.

71. Pommier P, Krengli M, Thornton A, et al. Paranasal sinus and nasal cavity. In: DeLaney T, Kooy H, eds. Proton and heavier charged particle radiotherapy. Philadelphia, PA: Lippincott, Williams and Wilkins; 2008:187–97.

72. Rosenberg A, Nielsen G, Keel S, et al. Chondrosarcoma of the base of the skull: a clinicopathological study of 200 cases with emphasis on it's distinction from chordoma. Am J Surg Pathol. 1999;23:1370–8.

73. Ruka W, Taghian A, Gioioso D, et al. Comparison between the in vitro intrinsic radiation sensitivity of human soft tissue sarcoma and breast cancer cell lines. J Surg Oncol. 1996;61(4):290–4.

74. Russell WO, Cohen J, Enzinger F, et al. A clinical and pathological staging system for soft tissue sarcomas. Cancer. 1977;40(4):1562–70.

75. Sher DJ, Wittenberg E, Taghian AG, et al. Partial breast irradiation versus whole breast radiotherapy for early-stage breast cancer: a decision analysis. Int J Radiat Oncol Biol Phys. 2008;70(2):469–76.

76. Shih HA, Harisinghani M, Zietman AL, et al. Mapping of nodal disease in locally advanced prostate cancer: rethinking the clinical target volume for pelvic nodal irradiation based on vascular rather than bony anatomy. Int J Radiat Oncol Biol Phys. 2005;63(4):1262–9.

77. Shipley WU, Tepper JE, Prout GR Jr, et al. Proton radiation as boost therapy for localized prostatic carcinoma. JAMA. 1979;241(18):1912–5.

78. Shipley WU, Coombs LJ, Einstein AB Jr, et al. Cisplatin and full dose irradiation for patients with invasive bladder carcinoma: a preliminary report of tolerance and local response. J Urol. 1984;132(5):899–903.

79. Shipley WU, Verhey LJ, Munzenrider JE, et al. Advanced prostate cancer: the results of a randomized comparative trial of high dose irradiation boosting with conformal protons compared with conventional dose irradiation using photons alone. Int J Radiat Oncol Biol Phys. 1995;32(1):3–12.

80. Shipley WU, Kaufman DS, Zehr E, et al. Selective bladder preservation by combined modality protocol treatment: long-term outcomes of 190 patients with invasive bladder cancer. Urology. 2002;60(1):62–7.

81. Shipley WU, Zietman AL, Kaufman DS, et al. Selective bladder preservation by trimodality therapy for patients with

muscularis propria-invasive bladder cancer and who are cystectomy candidates – the Massachusetts General Hospital and Radiation Therapy Oncology Group experiences. Semin Radiat Oncol. 2005;15(1):36–41, 290–4.

82. Spear MA, Jennings LC, Mankin HJ, et al. Individualizing management of aggressive fibromatoses. Int J Radiat Oncol Biol Phys. 1998;40(3):637–45.

83. Spiro IJ, Gebhardt MC, Jennings LC, et al. Prognostic factors for local control of sarcomas of the soft tissues managed by radiation and surgery. Semin Oncol. 1997;24(5):540–6.

84. Suit HD, Russell WO, Martin RG. Management of patients with sarcoma of soft tissue in an extremity. Cancer. 1973;31(5): 1247–55.

85. Suit HD, Russell WO, Martin RG. Sarcoma of soft tissue: clinical and histopathologic parameters and response to treatment. Cancer. 1975;35(5):1478–83.

86. Taghian A, Jeong JH, Mamounas E, et al. Patterns of locoregional failure in patients with operable breast cancer treated by mastectomy and adjuvant chemotherapy with or without tamoxifen and without radiotherapy: results from five National Surgical Adjuvant Breast and Bowel Project randomized clinical trials. J Clin Oncol. 2004;22(21):4247–54.

87. Taghian AG, Assaad SI, Niemierko A, et al. Risk of pneumonitis in breast cancer patients treated with radiation therapy and combination chemotherapy with paclitaxel. J Natl Cancer Inst. 2001;93(23):1806–11.

88. Taghian AG, Abi-Raad R, Assaad SI, et al. Paclitaxel decreases the interstitial fluid pressure and improves oxygenation in breast cancers in patients treated with neoadjuvant chemotherapy: clinical implications. J Clin Oncol. 2005;23(9): 1951–61.

89. Taghian AG, Jeong JH, Mamounas EP, et al. Low locoregional recurrence rate among node-negative breast cancer patients with tumors 5 cm or larger treated by mastectomy, with or without adjuvant systemic therapy and without radiotherapy: results from five national surgical adjuvant breast and bowel project randomized clinical trials. J Clin Oncol. 2006;24(24): 3927–32.

90. Taghian AG, Kozak KR, Doppke K, et al. Initial dosimetric experience using simple three-dimensional conformal external-beam accelerated partial breast irradiation. Int J Radiat Oncol Biol Phys. 2006;64(4):1092–9.

91. Talcott JA, Rossi C, Shipley WU, et al. Patient-reported long-term outcomes after conventional and high-dose combined proton and photon radiation for early prostate cancer. JAMA. 2010;303(11):1046–53.

92. Tepper JE, Shipley WU, Warshaw AL, et al. The role of misonidazole combined with Intraoperative radiation therapy in the treatment of pancreatic carcinoma. J Clin Oncol. 1987;5(4): 579–84.

93. Terahara A, Niemierko A, Goitein M, et al. Analysis of the relationship between tumor dose inhomogeneity and local control in patients with skull base chordoma. Int J Radiat Oncol Biol Phys. 1999;45:351–8.

94. Trofimov A, Nguyen PL, Coen JJ, et al. Radiotherapy treatment of early-stage prostate cancer with IMRT and protons: a treatment planning comparison. Int J Radiat Oncol Biol Phys. 2007;69(2):444–53.

95. Tsai HK, Katz MS, Coen JJ, et al. Association of statin use with improved local control in patients treated with selective bladder preservation for muscle-invasive bladder cancer. Urology. 2006;68(6):1188–92.

96. Wang C. Radiation therapy for head and neck neoplasms. 3rd ed. New York, NY: Wiley-Liss; 1997.

97. Wang CC. Altered fractionation of radiation therapy for gynecologic cancers. Cancer. 1987; 60(8 suppl):2064–7.

98. Wang CC, Doppke KP, Biggs PJ. Intra-oral cone radiation therapy for selected carcinomas of the oral cavity. Int J Radiat Oncol Biol Phys. 1983;9(8):1185–9.

99. Weber DC, Chan AW, Lessell S, et al. Visual outcome of accelerated fractionated radiation for advanced sinonasal malignancies employing photons/protons. Radiother Oncol. 2006; 81(3): 243–9.

100. Wenkel E, Thornton AF, Finkelstein D, et al. Benign meningioma: partially resected, biopsied, and recurrent intracranial tumors treated with combined proton and photon radiotherapy. Int J Radiat Oncol Biol Phys. 2000;48(5):1363–70.

101. Willers H, Beck-Bornholdt HP. Origins of radiotherapy and radiobiology: separation of the influence of dose per fraction and overall treatment time on normal tissue damage by Reisner and Miescher in the 1930s. Radiother Oncol. 1996;38(2): 171–3.

102. Willett CG, Linggood RM, Stracher MA, et al. The effect of the respiratory cycle on mediastinal and lung dimensions in Hodgkin's disease. Implications for radiotherapy gated to respiration. Cancer. 1987;60(6):1232–7.

103. Willett CG, Linggood RM, Leong JC, et al. Stage IA to IIB mediastinal Hodgkin's disease: three-dimensional volumetric assessment of response to treatment. J Clin Oncol. 1988;6(5): 819–24

104. Willett CG, Suit HD, Tepper JE, et al. Intraoperative electron beam radiation therapy for retroperitoneal soft tissue sarcoma. Cancer. 1991;68(2):278–83.

105. Willett CG, Ooi CJ, Zietman AL, et al. Acute and late toxicity of patients with inflammatory bowel disease undergoing irradiation for abdominal and pelvic neoplasms. Int J Radiat Oncol Biol Phys. 2000;46(4):995–8.

106. Willett CG, Boucher Y, di Tomaso E, et al. Direct evidence that the VEGF-specific antibody bevacizumab has antivascular effects in human rectal cancer. Nat Med. 2004;10(2): 145–7.

107. Yock T, Schneider R, Friedmann A, et al. Proton radiotherapy for orbital rhabdomyosarcoma: clinical outcome and a dosimetric comparison with photons. Int J Radiat Oncol Biol Phys. 2005;63(4):1161–8.

108. Yock TI, Tarbell NJ. Technology insight: proton beam radiotherapy for treatment in pediatric brain tumors. Nat Clin Pract Oncol. 2004;1(2):97–103; quiz 1 p following 111. Erratum in: Nat Clin Pract Oncol. 2005;2(4):222.

109. Yock TI, Krailo M, Fryer CJ, et al. Local control in pelvic Ewing sarcoma: analysis from INT-0091 – a report from the Children's Oncology Group. J Clin Oncol. 2006;24(24):3838–43. Erratum in: J Clin Oncol. 2006;24(30):4947.

110. Zhang M, Mukherjee N, Bermudez RS, et al. Adenovirus-mediated inhibition of survivin expression sensitizes human prostate cancer cells to paclitaxel in vitro and in vivo. Prostate. 2005;64(3):293–302.

111. Zietman AL. Evidence-based medicine, conscience-based medicine, and the management of low-risk prostate cancer. J Clin Oncol. 2009;27(30):4935–6.

112. Zietman AL, Dallow K, McManus P, et al. Time to second prostate-specific antigen failure is a surrogate endpoint for prostate cancer death in a prospective trial of therapy for localized disease. Urology. 1996;47(2):236–9.

113. Zietman AL, Nakfoor BM, Prince EA, et al. The effect of androgen deprivation and radiation therapy on an androgen-sensitive murine tumor: an in vitro and in vivo study. Cancer J Sci Am. 1997;3(1):31–6.

114. Zietman AL, Prince E, Nakfoor BEAM, et al. Androgen deprivation and radiation therapy: sequencing studies using the Shionogi in vivo tumor system. Int J Radiat Oncol Biol Phys. 1997;38(5):1067–70.

115. Zietman AL, Zehr EM, Shipley WU. The long-term effect on PSA values of incidental prostatic irradiation in patients with pelvic malignancies other than prostate cancer. Int J Radiat Oncol Biol Phys. 1999;43(4):715–8.

116. Zietman AL, Thakral HJ, Wilson L, et al. Conservative management of prostate cancer in the prostate specific antigen era: the incidence and time course of subsequent therapy. J Urol. 2001;166(5):1702–6.

117. Zietman AL, Chung CS, Coen JJ, et al. 10-year outcome for men with localized prostate cancer treated with external radiation therapy: results of a cohort study. J Urol. 2004;171(1): 210–4.

Chapter 11

Education Programs

11.1 MGH Radiation Oncology Residency Program

11.1.1 Residency in Radiology

The first residency in radiology in the USA was in 1915 and at MGH. The first resident was appointed for 12 months. This initiative was primarily due to the interest and enthusiasm for teaching by Holmes. That first resident was Dr. A. S. Merrill. On completion of the 1-year residency he was appointed to the staff and was given primary responsibility for the therapy section. His interest was not in therapy and he was soon transferred to diagnosis. In 1939 the American Board of Radiology increased the residency requirement to 3 years. The result was a gain from one resident for 1 year in 1915 to three residents in 1939 (one new resident/year and to thirty by 1970 for the 3-year residency). Education of young physicians in radiology explicitly included time in both diagnosis and therapy, i.e., the goal was that the radiologist be competent in all aspects of radiology.

Additionally, from 1917 onwards, the MGH department was very active in the organization and teaching of radiology to students at Harvard Medical School under G. Holmes. Although one could sub-specialize in diagnostic or therapeutic radiology and be credentialed by the American Board of Radiology as of 1939, the first to do so from the MGH program was not until 1968.

MGH graduates in radiology who became especially active in radiation oncology included Richard Dresser (Huntington Memorial Hospital), Charles Martin (Baylor, Dallas), Oscar Peterson (U Vermont), Y. Maruyama (U Kentucky), Martin Levene (Beth Israel, and Joint Center for Radiation Therapy). Researchers in the area of radiation biology were Stafford Warren (U Rochester, UCLA, Manhattan Project) and Jack Little (Harvard School of Public Health).

11.2 MGH Radiation Oncology Residency

The MGH Department of Radiation Oncology residency program has had clinical and science education from its inception in 1970. This has included residents, post-doctoral fellows, and graduate students in radiation biophysics and radiation biology of normal and tumor tissues. The concept has been that these programs should be designed to maximize the yield of innovators and leaders in this area of medicine and science combined with the production of first-rank clinicians.

Additionally, we are very active participants in programs with the University of Vermont, Laboure College and Suffolk University at both the college/university and the MGH, in the education of young people to be radiation therapists. We serve as the site of the clinical training and our staff presents lectures at the parent institution. This has resulted in a steady inflow of highly talented young radiation therapists at a time when there has been and continues to be a significant shortfall regionally and nationally.

Immediately upon formation of the Department of Radiation Oncology, the program of residency in general radiology was discontinued and one in radiation oncology initiated. The three radiology residents in 1970 who had selected radiation oncology were Sidney Kadish (1968), Susan Pittman (1970), and Warren Sewall (1970).

The first director of the residency program was Len Gunderson, 1976–1980. John Munzenrider was given this responsibility in 1980 and continued in this capacity until 1998. At that point, Anthony Zietman took over that position and he is continuing in that role to the present.

During the years 1970–2002, our residency program was exclusively an MGH program. The number of residents increased during this time from 6 to 11 and the total number was 99. In 2003, the separate residency programs of the MGH, BWH, and BID were restructured by the Dean of HMS to be components of a newly formed Harvard

H.D. Suit, J.S. Loeffler, *Evolution of Radiation Oncology at Massachusetts General Hospital*, DOI 10.1007/978-1-4419-6744-2_11, © Springer Science+Business Media, LLC 2011

Residency in Radiation Oncology with residents rotating through each of the BID, BWH, and MGH. There are 28 residents in this program. Residents on their rotation to the MGH spend a portion of their time at Boston Medical Center while those on rotation to BWH spend some of their time at the Dana Farber and the Children's Hospital.

Over this period 1970–2008, radiation oncology moved nationally from being one of the least sought after to one of the most sought after specialties. One result is that the academic record of the applicants has definitely become more impressive. The basis for the change is not clear as radiation oncology has had minimal formal coverage in the curriculum of US medical schools. Interestingly, only in the recent past have there been lecture courses in oncology in most medical schools. Oncology was taught as portions of other courses, e.g., general medicine, general surgery plus some coverage in neurology/neurosurgery, GU, and Gyn.

11.3 The MGH Radiation Oncology Residency Program: 1970–2002, i.e., 32 years

Residents in Radiation Oncology were educated in a 4-year program: 3 years on clinical rotations and 1 year for research/special academic activity. The options for the research have been, with few exceptions, in biology, physics, or a major clinical outcome analysis. Several residents used that time as part of their studies for an M.Sc. at the Harvard School of Public Health, in either biostatistics or studying a specific public health issue. The sites for laboratory research year have been in our department, other MGH laboratories or HMS laboratories, and in institutions other than MGH or HMS, viz., MIT and centers beyond Boston, one resident at the Gray Laboratory in London.

The 36 months of education in patient care are structured as a series of 3-month rotations with sub-specialist faculty members. This provides periods of intense concentration on specific categories of tumors, e.g., CNS, Head and Neck, breast, thoracic, GI, GU, pediatric, and mesenchymal tumors. In addition, there is a rotation to BUMC for general practice radiation oncology. The remaining three 3-month periods are elective for additional time with the sub-specialist of interest or with medical or surgical oncology, radiology, or pathology. The staff of each of the oncological multi-disciplinary clinics are sub-specialists in the tumor patient category seen at that clinic, e.g., a CNS clinic would have one or more surgeon, medical oncologist, radiation oncologist, and direct communication with a radiologist and a pathologist; each of these limits their practice to the CNS tumors. General radiation oncology is now largely history.

In this department, there were no "House Cases" in that each patient is the legal and medical responsibility of the staff physician. The resident actively participates in each step of the management of the patient. This policy commenced in 1970. During clinical rotations, the resident is a member of the oncology team at the respective multi-disciplinary clinic and participates in the examination and evaluation of new patients. For patients referred for radiation oncology, the resident takes the history, examines the patient, and reviews the imaging studies and pathological material. Then the findings, impressions, and recommendations are assessed with the attending radiation oncologist and other staff of the clinic. For patients accepted for radiation treatment, the resident participates in determining the treatment intent, defining the target, performing simulation, evaluation of treatment plans, and seeing the patient at the first treatment and at the weekly status check examinations. Additionally, the resident participates in follow-up examinations to observe the status of patients at varying times post-treatment.

As part of their education, residents (1) present the management rationale and treatment plan for each patient who started treatment in the previous week, (2) case presentations with review of the most relevant literature on two mornings per week with faculty attending, and (3) special lectures or conferences the other three mornings. These activities are heavily complimented by lecture courses. For the first 2 weeks of the residency, there is an intensive lecture course in physics. All residents and many fellows and visiting physicians/scientists from other MGH departments and outside institutions attend. Residents and research fellows make presentations in the monthly departmental Journal Club meetings. For the early years, the Journal Club was a dinner program at the Harvard Faculty Club, which later moved to the MIT faculty Club and then in the 1990s to the MGH[1]. Recently, the Journal Club has met from 12:15 to 1:15 PM for a luncheon session on the first Friday of the month.[1] The general plan is for three papers to be presented: one each on clinical radiation oncology, physics, and biology topic. The presenters are a resident, a graduate student, or post-doctoral fellow in biology and one in physics. These sessions are well attended, with some 40–50 staff, residents, students, and fellows.

Each resident is informed that they are expected to produce ≥ 1 first-authored paper in a referred journal during their 4-year residency. There have been only the extremely rare residents who did not meet that expectation. Most resident have ≥ 2 papers.

---

[1] These changes were made to reduce pressure on resident's time and their important non medical responsibilities, viz. many are raising young families.

Residents are invited to attend the weekly scientific sessions of the physics and biology research groups. Residents also are expected to deliver papers at regional and national meetings (ASTRO, ASCO, Radiation Research, American Radium Society, and others) and at international meetings, principally ESTRO. Additionally, there are many lectures during the year presented by visiting clinicians and scientists, *vide infra*. Further, the residents and research fellows have access to Teleconference lectures on a spectrum of topics.

Each resident has access to many journals and books at the MGH Treadwell library and the Harvard Countway Medical Library. The Treadwell library is the largest hospital library in the USA, and the Countway is the largest medical library in the USA outside of the National library of Medicine.

Our department was the first MGH department to provide each resident with a PC. Virtually all of the radiation oncology, radiation physics, tumor and radiation biology, medical and surgical oncology journals are available online. The total number of journals online at the Countway is ~1800. Further, the resident has online access to 59 major reference books, e.g., *Handbook of Chemistry and Physics*, *Oxford English Dictionary*, encyclopedias. All of this is in addition to the vast information on virtually all subjects on the many public online search engines. Of significant value is the resident's access to the Widener Library of Harvard University. Not only the residents can check out books from the Widener but also they can use the stacks. The Harvard University Library is one of the five great libraries of the world at ~15,000,000 volumes and is the only one in which students and faculties have access to the stacks.

Also, the residents have been provided a yearly allowance for purchase of books or other educational material from the start of the department to the present. This stipend, initially $200, has risen to $800/year at present.

11.4 Harvard Residency in Radiation Oncology 2003–Present

The residents on rotation to the MGH have virtually the same educational program as described above. Many of the residents take their research year at the MGH biology laboratories of R. Jain, K. Held, and L. Gerweck or the physics units with T. Bortfeld, G. Chen, and others.

There are increasing formal requirements for recording of patients seen by residents and the work performed. For instance, the resident must record in some detail the clinical activity during each rotation. Thus, the resident has a comprehensive log book (kept online at the ACGME Website) and this log is reviewed with the program director annually. Tables 11.1, 11.2, 11.3, and 11.4 giving the residents and clinical and proton fellows were kindly prepared by Dominique Jeudy.

Table 11.1 MGH radiation oncology residents starting 1970–2002

Willett	Christopher	1982–1986	Kachnic	Lisa	1992–1996
Busse[a]	Paul	1983–1986	Lewis	Anne	1992–1996
DeLaney	Thomas	1983–1986	Nakfoor	Bruce	1992–1996
Okunieff	Paul	1983–1986	Colvett	Kyle	1993–1996
Landry	Jerome	1985–1988	Hartford[a]	Alan	1993–1998
Sailer	Scott	1985–1988	Kanady	Kirk	1993–1996
Westgate	Steven	1985–1988	Proulx	Gary	1993–1997
Becht	James	1985–1988	Tibbs	Martha	1993–1997
Burton	Noreen	1986–1989	Douglas	Robert	1994–1998
Konchan	Donald	1986–1989	Morris	Monica	1994–1998
Marks	Lawrence	1986–1969	Spear	Matthew	1994–1998
Pardo	Francisco	1986–1990	Morris	Astrid	1995–1999
Walsh	Christopher	1986–1989	Surgery	Catherine	1995–1998
Dugan	Thomas	1987–1990	Chakravarti	Arnab	1996–2000
Jones	Christopher	1987–1990	Chan	Wai Fong	1996–2000
Dunbar	Susan	1988–1992	Gardner	Barry	1996–2000
Hug	Eugen	1988–1992	Sharis	Christine	1996–2000
McAnaw	Robert	1988–1992	Czito	Brian	1997–2001
Schwartz	Laurent	1988–1991	Kiggundu	Edward	1997–2001
Zietman	Anthony	1988–1991	Lane	Steven	1997–2000
Sobczak	Mark	1989–1991	St.Clair[a]	William	1997–2001
Fung	Claire	1989–1993	Ceilley-Hyslop	Elizabeth	1998–2002
Spiro[a]	Ira	1989–1992	Chawla	Ashish	1999–2003
Zlotecki[a]	Robert	1989–1993	Chon	Brian	1999–2003
Abraham	Edward	1989–1993	Coen	John	1999–2003
Garner	Daniel	1989–1992	Brown	Alan	2000–2004
McIntyre	James	1990–1993	Lawenda	Brian	2000–2004
Hagan[a]	Michael	1990–1993	Yock	Torunn	2000–2004
Tamler	Bradley	1990–1993	Kirsch[a]	David	2001–2005
Hahn	Carol	1991–1994	Roof	Kevin	2001–2005
Anne'	Pramila	1991–1995	Shih	Helen	2001–2005
Chen[a]	Yuhchyau	1991–1994	Willers	Henning	2001–2005
Fitzek	Markus	1992–1996			
Huncharek	Michael	1992–1996			

[a]M.D. and Ph.D.

Table 11.2 Harvard radiation oncology residency 2002–present

Chen	Yen-Lin	2002–2006	Kozono	David	2005
Jagsi	Reshma	2002–2006	Lee	Larissa	2005
Mohiuddin	Majid	2002–2006	Nguyen	Paul	2005
Balboni	Tracy	2003–2007	Wang	Zhuang	2005
Chen	Aileen	2003–2007	Elia	Andrew	2006
Liu	Arthur	2003–2007	Martin	Neil	2006
Petit	Joshua	2003–2007	Nanda	Akash	2006
Rodrigues	Neesha	2003–2007	Winkfield	Karen	2006
Tsai	Henry	2003–2007	Wo	Jennifer	2006
Chung	Christine	2003–2007	Cotter	Shane	2007
Efstathiou	Jason	2004–2008	Halasz	Lia	2007
Floyd	Scott	2004–2008	Khandekar	Melin	2007
Kimmelman	Alec	2004–2008	Mak	Raymond	2007
Kozak	Kevin	2004–2008	Margalit	Danielle	2007
Patel	Abhijit	2004–2008	Miyamoto	David	2007
Sher	David	2004–2008	Wang	Victoria	2007
Tuamokumo	Nimi	2004–2008	Arvold	Nils	2008
Alexander	Brian	2005	Hattangadi	Jona	2008
Chen	Ronald	2005	Krejcarek	Stephanie	2008
Dosoretz	Amy	2005	Mittin	Timur	2008
Gabeau-Lact	Darlene	2005	Pacold	Michael	2008
Haglund	Karl	2005	Westover	Ken	2008

Table 11.3 MGH radiation biophysics graduate students

Last name	First name	Degree granting university	Year	Faculty supervisor
Current Ph.D. students				
Daartz	Juliane	U Heidelberg	2009	Kooy
Cui	Ying	N.E. University	2008	Jiang
Kanoulas	Evangelos	N.E. University	2010	Jiang
Kurugol	Sila	N.E. University	2010	Sharp
Knopf	Antje	U Heidelberg	2009	Bortfeld, Paganetti
Graduates of Ph.D. program				
Thieke	Christian	U Heidelberg	2004	Bortfeld
Chan	Timothy	MIT	2007	Bortfeld
Halabi	Tarek	U MA	2007	Bortfeld, Craft
Aljarrah	Khalid	U MA – Lowell	2005	Jiang
Wu	Huanmei	N.E. University	2005	Jiang
Boldea	Vlad	U Lumier 2 Lyon	2007	Sharp
Riboldi	Marco	Politecnico di Milano	2006	Chen
Scherrer	Alexander	U Kaiserslautern	2006	Bortfeld
Martin	Ben	Boston University	2008	Bortfeld
Current M.Sc. student				
Eram	Burak	N.E. University	2009	Sharp
Graduates of M.Sc. program				
Chu	Alan	MIT	2007	Chen
Book	Lynn	MIT	2007	Gierga
Birkenfeld	Judith	U Mannheim-Heidelberg	2006	Paganetti
Fleckenstein	Jens	U Mannheim-Heidelberg	2006	Paganetti
Vrancic	Christian	U Mannheim-Heidelberg	2007	Trofimov
Büttner	Florian		2007	Paganetti
Bangert	Mark	U Heidelberg	2007	Kooy
Knopf	Antje	U Mannheim-Heidelberg	2005	Paganetti, Trofimov
Daartz	Juliane	U Mannheim-Heidelberg	2005	Kooy
Gansemer	Cornelia	U Mannheim-Heidelberg	2008	Trofimov
Hoyer	Patrick	U Mannheim-Heidelberg	2008	Sharp

Residents: Mark Langer; Helen Shih; Larissa Lee.
Medical students: Michael Folkert (Harvard–MIT); Michael Gensheimer (Vanderbilt).
Radiation Physics: Ph.D. students 6; M.Sc. student 2; Undergraduate students 2; Residents 3; Ph.D. graduates 9; M.Sc. graduates 14; AAPM fellows 2.

Clinical Fellows at the MGH. Several physicians at the resident and post-resident levels have come to the MGH for special experience with selected staff clinicians for 4- to 24-month periods. Often, these individuals are powerfully motivated and commence immediately on seeing specific patient populations *and* initiate clinical studies. Many of these have completed a project and published their findings in peer reviewed. A high proportion of the clinical fellows have come from European, Canadian, and Asian centers.

Clinical Photon Fellows			
K. Bujko	Warsaw	J. Mazeron	Paris
R. Miralbell	Barcelona	D. Weber	Zurich
Clinical Proton Fellows			
V. Benk	Paris	M. Krengli	Italy
D. Cole	Oxford	Anita Mahajin	Montreal
J. Debus	Heidelberg	T. Nakano	Tokyo
W. DuBois	Netherlands	H. Pai	Canada
S. Graffman	Uppsala	R. Santoni	Florence
P. Henssens	Belgium	H. Tatsuzki	Tokyo
June Kim	Eastern VA	H. Terahara	Japan

11.5 Graduate Students and Post-doctoral Fellows

Education of young scientists and physicians has been a central goal for the department. The graduate students are in our labs for their thesis work with their course work at a university. We also have a very large program of post-doctoral fellowships. Each student and post-doctoral fellow has a faculty person formally assigned as a mentor. Our track record has been highly positive as each student

Table 11.4 MGH radiation tumor and normal tissue biology graduate students

Current Ph.D. students

Last name	First name	
These	Janet	
Poh	Ming-Zer	
Chauhan	Vikash	
Diopfrimpong	Benjamin	
Lanning	Ryan	

Ph.D. graduates

Last name	First name	End date
Zhu	Hui	1996
Gazit	Yuval	1996
Hobbs	Susan	1998
Koenig	David	1998
Swartz	Melody	1998
Stoll	Brian	2003
Mckee	Trevor	2005
Cochran	David	2005
Tong	Ricky	2005
Mok	Wilson	2007
Junker	Nanna	2003
Padera	Timothy	2003
Au	Patrick	2008
Tam	Joshua	2008

Residents

Chen	Yen-lin	2002–2006
Dull (Anesthesia)	Randall	
Hartford	Alan	1993–1998
Kozak	Kevin	2004–2008
Lawenda	Brian	2000–2004
Snuder (Pathology)	Matija	
Zlotecki	Robert	1989–1993

Medical students

Last name	First name	End date
Demhartner	Thomas	1992
Salehi	Hassan	1994
Witwer	Brian	1995
Greif	Daniel	1995
Loskin	Albert	1996
Safabakhsh	Nina	1996
Ang	Jennifer	1999
Alt	Amy	2001
Awd	Michael	2003
Finn	Aloke	2006

Steele Laboratory Summary: Ph.D. Students 7; Ph.D. Graduates 15; Residents 2; Medical Students 10.

K Held Laboratory– M.Sc. Graduates (MIT): Vered Anzenberg; Nicole Larrier.

Post-doctoral fellows: Nesrin Asaad; Elena Rusyn; Asima Chakraborty; Laurence Tartier; Wei Han; Hongying Yang; Aruna Karkala Dr.; Zhixiang Zho; Martin Purschke; Zhixiang Zho.

Residents: Majid Mohuiddin.

Simon Powell Laboratory – Post-doctoral fellows: Robert Delsite; Zhihui Feng; Larissa Romanova; Alejandro Treszezamsky; Danielle Taghian; Henning Willers; Wei Tang; Fen Xia; Junran Zhang.

Residents: Rani Anne; Robert Delsite; Lisa Kachnic.

L. Gerweck Laboratory–Post-doctoral fellows: Rolf Issels; Sergey Kozin; Hideyuki Majima; Kazuhiko Ogaw; Kala Seetharaman; Susan Stocks; Shashirekha Vijayappa.

Medical students: Thomas DeLaney[2]

H. Suit Laboratory– Residents: P. Bitzer; D. Dosoretz; A. Elman; L. Fagundes; A. Hartford; O. Mendiondo; P. Okunieff; J. Overgaard; T. Rich; J. Tepper; C. Willett; A. Zietman.

Fellows: A. Azinovic; T. Todoroki; M. Baumann; Gill Tozer, W. Budach; Y. Yamashita; P. Huang; T. Hwang; Kozin; S. Suzanne Lauk; Jane Maher; R. Miralbell; L. Perez; J. Ramsay; A. Ruka; V. Silobrcic.

---

[2] Tom later was a resident and is now Associate Professor and Head of the Sarcoma Team and director of the MGH proton therapy program.

and fellow has been contributors to research creativity and productivity. In addition, there are medical and other students in the laboratories on elective periods.

Radiation Biophysics. Physics has had a very productive program for graduate students. For the period to ~2000, the policy of the physicists was to have post-doctoral fellows. This changed in ~2000 and there has been a highly successful graduate student program in physics. As of early 2008, the biophysics division has had nine students receive their Ph.D. and there are five Ph.D. students at present. In addition, 11 students have received their M.Sc. and there is one M.Sc. student at present.

T. Bortfeld gives a course in Medical Physics for MIT. Several members of the group jointly teach a course on *Heavy Charged Particles for Cancer Radiation Therapy* for Harvard and MIT, through the health sciences and technology (HST) program.

11.6 Molecular, Cellular, Tissue, and Organism Radiation Biology

Graduate students have been a prominent aspect of the R. Jain tumor biology research laboratory. Since the start of his program, 15 students have received the Ph.D. degree. Three have been M.D.–Ph.D. students via the doctoral program between Harvard Medical School and MIT.

Jain is the lecturer in MIT course *Tumor Pathophysiology*, HST-5255. This has proven popular and has been given on yearly basis for many years. An important yield of this course has been graduate students for the Steele Lab.

11.7 Residents Had Laboratory Research Project in Facilities Outside of the Department

E. Abraham	MGH
E. Halperin	MGH
D. Kirsch	MIT
M. Fitzek	HSPH
T. Rich	Gray Laboratory, London
M. Huncharek	HSPH

11.8 Formal Lecture Courses for Residents

On alternate years the department provides year long lecture courses on Radiation Biophysics and on Molecular, Cellular, and Tissue Radiation Biology.

A. Radiation Biophysics Lecture Course Organized and directed by Peter Biggs
    42 Lectures covering atomic structure to radiation protection.
B. Molecular, Cellular, Tissue, and Organism Radiation Biology lecture course. Organized and directed by Kathy Held
    31 lectures covering material and radiation chemistry to photodynamics therapy

Prior to the establishment of the Harvard wide residency program in radiation oncology, the course was an MGH function. Since 2002, the lectures are presented live to the three hospitals (MGH, BWH, and BID) by Teleconference. All residents participate in the question and discussion periods.

Chapter 12

Special Lecture Series

12.1 The Milford D. Schulz Lecturers

These were held as a tribute to the first radiologist at the MGH to limit his practice almost exclusively to therapeutic radiology. Many interest facets of the life and career of Milford were illuminated in this series. These were held on a yearly and then on a bi-annual basis and the event was designated the department Science Festivity Day.

The lecturer had time with residents and interested staff. Following the lecture, the department had a celebration of science at the Harvard Fogg Museum of Art or on a few years at other Harvard facilities and 1 year at the Boston Museum of Science. After the dinner, Suit gave a 30 min talk with images of one of the diverse academic treasures of Harvard to increase appreciation of the exceptional privilege to be part of this extraordinary university. These subjects for the talks included the Widener Library, the Fogg Museum, the Villa I. Tatti (Harvard Center for Italian Renaissance Studies on a hill outside of Florence), Houghton Rare Books library, Museum of Natural History, Harvard Smithsonian Center for Astrophysics, Dumbarton Oaks in Washington, DC, Harvard Yenching Institute. The talk was usually followed by a solo musical performance, often by a resident, fellow, or student or alumnus and then dancing and viewing of the art collection of the museum.

The lecturers and their lecture titles are below. There is a broad spectrum of material covered. Two of these lecturers were radiation oncologists, H. Kaplan and H.R. Withers. Two of the lecturers spoke here before they received their Nobel prize, viz., E. Donnall Thomas, and D. Baltimore. There were notables in several areas: genetics R. Weinberg, B. Seed, D. Livingston; biologists L. Liotta, J. Folkman, J. Kerr; physicists H. Johns; radiation biologists G. Adams, D. Chapman M. Elkind, R. Sutherland; and medical oncologist B. Chabner.

12.2 Milford D. Schulz Lecturers

Year	Lecturer	Title
1978	Henry S. Kaplan	*Biology and Virology of Human Malignant Lymphomas*
1979	G.E. Adams	*Development of Sensitizers of Hypoxic Cells*
1980	Harold E. Johns	*The Physicist in Cancer Detection and Treatment*
1981	E. Donnall Thomas	*The Use and Potential of Bone Marrow Allograft and Whole Body Irradiation in the Treatment of Leukemia*
1982	Robert A. Weinberg	*Oncogenes of Human Tumors*
1983	J. Donald Chapman	*The Detection and Measurement of Viable Hypoxic Cells in Solid Tumors*
1984	Mortimer Elkind	*DNA Damage and Cell Killing, Cause and Effect*
1985	Robert Sutherland	*Importance of Critical Metabolites and Cellular Interactions in the Biology of Micro-Regions of Tumors*
1986	David Baltimore	*Modulation of Oncogene Products and/or Suppression of Oncogenes as a Therapeutic Strategy*
1989	H. Rodney Withers	*Dose Fractionation and Standard Radiation Therapy Practice*
1991	Lance Liotta	*Cancer Invasion and Metastasis*
1993	John Kerr	*Apoptosis: Its Significance in Cancer and Cancer Therapy*
1995	Bruce Chabner	*Drug Resistance in Patients with Malignant Lymphoma – The Role of MDR*
1997	Judah Folkman	*Endogenous Angiogenesis Inhibitors: Do They Have a Role in Radiotherapy*
1999	David Livingstone	*Functional Analysis of the BRCA-1 and 2 Gene Products*
2001	Brian Seed	*Tumor Necrosis Factor Alpha in Death and Immune Cell Activation*

H.D. Suit, J.S. Loeffler, *Evolution of Radiation Oncology at Massachusetts General Hospital*, DOI 10.1007/978-1-4419-6744-2_12, © Springer Science+Business Media, LLC 2011

12.3 Ira J. Spiro Visiting Professorships This Series Was Established to Honor Our Colleague and Friend

2002:   Clifton C. Ling   *From Oxygen and Dose-Rate Effects to Biological Imaging*: In Tribute to Ira J. Spiro, M.D., Ph.D.

2003:   Dennis Shrieve   *Stereotactic Radiotherapy: Advances in the First Decade*

2004:   Mary Gospodarowicz   *Future of Radiation Therapy in Localized Lymphomas*

2005:   Sarah Donaldson   *Perspectives on Pediatric Hodgkin's Disease – Progress and Issues*

2006:   Christopher Willett   *Technique & Translation: Twins of Radiation Oncology – A Tribute to Ira J. Spiro, M.D.*

2007:   Brian O'Sullivan   *Soft Tissue Sarcoma: No Longer One Disease Scenario*

2008:   Thomas DeLaney   *Integration of Advanced Technology Radiation Therapy into the Multidisciplinary Management of Sarcomas*

2009:   Andrew Rosenberg   *A Pathologist's Perspective*

12.4 Distinguished Alumni Lecturers

2005:   Joel Tepper   *The Integration of Physics & Biology in Radiation Oncology: Lessons Learned from the MGH*

2006:   Leonard Gunderson   *Gastric Cancer – Indications for and Results of Chemoradiation as a Component of Treatment*

2007:   Edward Halperin   *The Poor, the Black, and Marginalized Women in US Anatomical Education*

2008   *Cancelled due to a Health Problem*

2009   Daniel Dosoretz   *Radiation Therapy: Our Path to the Future*

12.5 Collins Lectures Series

This lecture series is supported by funds from the estate of Robert D. Collins, a New Jersey business consultant who was prominent after the Second World War in the development of profit sharing, group insurance, and pension plans for major American companies. He died in 2000 at the age of 90 having spent his retirement years initiating and supporting major additions to his local hospital, library, and church. The support for this lecture series is provided by the son David and Holiday Collins

2006	Biography of the Proton	
March 29	Andrew Cohen	Physics. Boston U
		The Early Universe and the Origin of Matter
April 5	Richard Wilson	Physics. Harvard U
		The Size and Shape of the Proton
April 12	Michael Goitein	HMS
		The Interactions of Protons within the Patient
April 19	Herman D. Suit	MGH
		Discovery of the Proton
April 26	Kenneth Gall	Stillwater, Inc.
		New Particle Accelerator Designs for Radiation Therapy
		Protons and Heavy Ion
May 3	Thomas Delaney	MGH
		Future Prospects for Proton Therapy
May 10	Larry Sulak	Physics Boston U
		The Demise of the Proton
2007	**Basic Tumor and Radiation Biology**	
March 20	Robert Weinberg	Whitehead Inst. MIT
		Mechanisms of Malignant Progression
March 27	Umar Mhmood	Radiology, MGH
		Optical and MR Molecular Imaging Approaches
April 3	Michael Baumann	Dresden U.
		Molecular Targeting Combined with Radiation
April 10	David Scadden	HMS, MGH
		Prospects for Stem Cell-Based Medicine
April 24	Rakesh Jain	MGH
		Normalization of Tumor Vasculature and Micro-Environment by Anti-Angiogenic Therapies: From the Bench to the Bedside and Back
May 1	Eric Hall	Columbia U
		Some Characteristics of Biological Damage Induced by Ionizing Radiations
May 8	David Kirsch	MGH
		Endothelial and Epithelial Cell Apoptosis in the Acute Radiation Syndrome and During Radiation Therapy
May 15	Eric Lander	Broad Inst. MIT
		Biology as Information: Genomics and Medicine in the 21st century
2008	**Basic Biology and Radiation Oncology**	
Feb 5	M. Swamy	MGH
		siRNA Delivery to the CNS to Suppress Flavivira Encephalitis and Potentially Other CNS Diseases
March 5	Takashi Nakano	Gunma University
		^{12}C Ion Radiation Therapy Rationale and Technical Aspects of ^{12}C vs. Proton Therapy
March 11	William Crowley	*MGH Department Medicine*
		Changing Models of Bedside to Bench
Research		
April 1	Michael Goitein	HMS
	Title	*Protonic Concerns*
May 23	Herman Suit	MGH
		Potential Clinical Gains by Proton and Carbon Ion Beam Therapy
June 3	Marcia Angel	HMS
		Pharma: Marketing and Profits
Sept 9	Randy Jirtle	Duke U
		The New Genetics of Cancer Susceptibility
Dec 9	Soren Bentzen	U Wisconsin
		Radiation Therapy in the Era of Molecular Biology

Chapter 13

Radiation Therapists, Nurses, Medical Records, Receptionists and Cox Front Door Welcoming Team

13.1 Radiation Therapists (RTTs)

Kathy Bruce (Fig. 13.1) was recruited from Maine in 1980 to be Head of the MGH RTT unit. She continued very effectively in that role until 2008 when she accepted a senior administrative position.

Christine Cerrato (Fig. 13.2) was appointed at the start of 2009 as Technical Director of the complex of 65 RTTs at the MGH plus those at the Emerson, Newton Wellesley, and North Shore hospitals. Part of the goal is to increase quality and safety of care and lead to an integration of staff in the photon–electron with the proton therapy programs. She has appointed Kelly Seybolt as the Assistant Technical Director of Cox and Jim Matthews as the Assistant Technical Director at the FHBPTC (protons therapy).

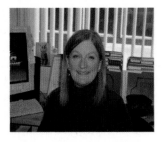

Fig. 13.1 Kathy Bruce

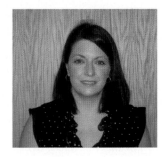

Fig. 13.2 Christine Cerrato

At the start of the department in 1970, the RTT staff with Milford and CC were dual qualified, viz., RTT and RN. Although a radiation therapist staff with the dual qualification was desirable, it could not be continued as virtually the entire talent pool by that time had been trained in RTT alone. In accord with this reality, we changed policy and new staff was trained as RTT alone.

In 1975, the department moved *in toto* to Cox ground floor. This involved new technology and the recruitment of many new therapists, not only from the USA but also from Canada, Europe, India, and South Africa. This yielded much serious talent, viz., Elizabeth Haining from Scotland, Paul Van Ocken from Belgium, J.C. Thakral from India (he continues and is a star), Katrina Keefe from England, a second RTT from India was excellent but shortly moved to Florida and has become a clinical physicist, and a recruit from South Africa who also performed well but moved in short order to California. This talent inflow from abroad greatly eased our staffing needs. RTTs from the USA during that transition period to Cox ground were Tom Eggleston, Linda Gillies, Christine Michelinie, and Phil Litch. The Mould Room Artiste was Josh Camblos. Phil has been a loyal and effective member and is continuing to work at a high level.

This section was prepared by Kathy Bruce. "Our lives in Cox Ground were relatively quiet and enjoyed a good spirit of camaraderie. We went for runs on the Charles at lunchtime. Patient care was the number 1 interest. Non-urgent patients came back 2 days after simulation to start their treatments, viz., those who could not be started the same day as simulation. The department policy was that there be concentration of patients with a defined group of tumors to be managed on a designated machine, viz., tumor type-machine specialization. This was in accord with sub-specialization of the clinicians.

We have some excellent treatment techniques that made the MGH an especially interesting place to be a therapist viz., IOC, IOERT, protons, stereotactic radiosurgery, fractionated stereotactic radiation therapy, 4D imaging, 4D image-guided radiation therapy, BID for most H&N patients, chemotherapy combined with radiation for bladder preservation, BWID

H.D. Suit, J.S. Loeffler, *Evolution of Radiation Oncology at Massachusetts General Hospital*, DOI 10.1007/978-1-4419-6744-2_13, © Springer Science+Business Media, LLC 2011

beam flattening filters for prostate treatment, chemo/RT for limb sparing for sarcoma patients.

In 2000 the department installed its own CT scanner. We wanted to get the most out of this high-end scanner and sought a CT technologist. Nancy Ditullio was recruited from Radiology in March, 2000 to operate the CT unit.

We worked with Dr. Walter Johnston, Chair of physics and Engineering at Suffolk University to move to establishment of an RTT school. This quickly was achieved and has been highly important to us. The University of Vermont extended their program to 4 years and the awarding of B.Sc. degrees. Laboure decided against expanding their program to 4 years and our relationship was discontinued.

Radiation Therapy Technologists fought to go by another name. The ASRT worked with ASTRO to change our designation to Radiation Therapist. Previously the radiation oncology physicians had gone by this title. The change took hold. The attitude of the RTTs is "Please don't call us technicians; it's as dated as parallel-opposed treatment for lung cancer" At present, the department has 42 RTs.

The proton therapy program moved in 2001 from the Harvard Cyclotron Laboratory to the new Francis H Burr Proton Therapy Center. Currently 10 RTTs provide proton treatments and commonly treat 60 patients in a day, more than double the peak at HCL. The first IMRT treatments were delivered in the fall of 2002 and it is the standard of care for many of our patients".

13.2 Radiation Oncology Nursing

In 1970, the nursing staff of radiation oncology consisted of Alice MacManus, RN, and Joanne Benjamin, nursing assistant. Their primary responsibilities included assisting Schultz, Wang and new staff with exams and procedures, facilitating the clinical activities of patients undergoing treatment, scheduling related studies or tests and more. Ena Chang joined the staff in the 1970s as Head Nurse with Mac's retirement and the department relocation to the Cox B.

Katie Mannix (Fig. 13.3) has served with high effectiveness as Nursing Director, Radiation Oncology Nursing Unit. 1995–2000. Clinical Manager 2000–present.

Katie prepared this section. "The nursing staff expanded, became more specialized, and participated in multidisciplinary clinics on Cox 1 with colleagues from medical oncology. Pat McManus joined the staff as a clinical research nurse and worked principally at the HCL and later at FHBPTC.

Oncology treatment options for patients became more complex, and multimodality treatment demanded a solid oncology foundation to understand the impact that surgery and chemotherapy had on a patient's tolerance of radiation

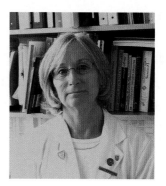

Fig. 13.3 Katie Mannix

treatment. Nursing responsibilities were direct care of patients, coordination of care to individual patients, patient/family education of the disease, course of treatment, potential side effects, symptom management, procedures, explanation of clinical trials, and referral to support services. Nursing care extended to participation in brachytherapy procedures, HDR applications, transrectal ultrasounds, neurosurgical frame placement for SRS, and others. Age-specific care was required for the increasing number of pediatric patients, many of whom required daily anesthesia for treatment. As the role of radiation oncology nursing expanded, there was an organizational shift to the MGH Department of Nursing. This provided increased collaboration with oncology nurse colleagues throughout the hospital resulting in improving patient care, practice issues, professional opportunities, participation on committees, and professional development. The patient care activities of the radiation oncology nurses were directed full time to patients receiving radiation treatment, i.e., they did not rotate to other oncology units.

In 1995, Ena Chang transitioned to patient care at the HCL and later at FHBPTC. With the opening of the proton therapy center on campus, Rachel Bolton, a pediatric oncology certified nurse, joined the staff to help care for the growing volume of complex pediatric patients. The Oncology Nursing Society (ONS) established oncology certification in 1985 and Katie Mannix became the first radiation oncology nurse to achieve certification. Currently, 85% of radiation oncology nurses have attained oncology certification. In addition to presentations at ONS and APON, nurses have contributed to professional textbooks and actively participate on committees throughout the MGH such as Cancer Nursing Practice, Patient Education, HOPES Seminars, Radiation Safety, and Quality Assurance. Nurses have achieved recognition through the MGH Clinical Recognition Program; Sheila Brown became the first Radiation Oncology Clinical Scholar. To date there have been three Clinical Scholars and eight Advanced Clinicians. The Nurse Practitioner role was introduced in the department in 2010".

13.3 Social Workers in Radiation Oncology

Eve Malkin prepared this section. Social work began at MGH in 1905 and was the first hospital-based Social Work program in a US hospital. This program was initiated by Dr. Richard Cabot to "make medical care effective" and to "cure consumption." He hired Ida M. Cannon and together they pioneered professional psychosocial care of patients and their families. The service grew and in 1929, at the request of physicians, a social worker was hired to serve patients in the Tumor Clinic. Thus began oncology social work services.

Social workers need skills in problem solving, knowledge of community resources, effective patient advocates, responding effectively to the diverse needs of patients and their families, and implement educational programs. Early social workers in the department were here only part time. These included Debbie Essig, Alice Hatch Jane Calhoun, Ellie Darmon, and Betty Bawdecker worked helped in Cox when needed.

Eve Malkin. Eve (Fig. 13.4) has been the leader in social work in radiation oncology from 1981 to the present. She came into radiation oncology in 1981 on a part-time basis to replace the departing Debbie Essig. Later Eve had a cubbyhole on Cox Ground Level so that patients were easily able to stop in with problems and/or questions.

It became clear that in order to be of the greater assistance to patients, social workers need to follow patients through their course of treatment and often at follow-up visits. At present, Eve spends most of her time at FHBPTC where 10–12 children are under treatment. She has been a valuable leader in this program.

Social workers have traditionally served hospitalized cancer patients. As more cancer treatments shifted to ambulatory settings, social workers were assigned to specialized clinics and to radiation oncology. Currently, there are 15 social workers in Oncology, as well as 3 in the Cancer Resource Room, 1 of whom leads the Network for Patients and Families, plus 1 directing the HOPES program and 2 Resource Specialists for lodging, transportation, and support groups.

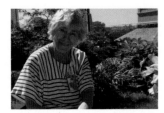

Fig. 13.4 Eve Malkin

13.4 Medical Record Staff

Maintenance of the medical record intact and available for each patient is a critically important clinical function. We have been fortunate in having a quite effective team performing this operation and for Claire Cronin (Fig. 13.5) to serve as the manager of the medical record system. They achieve timely and fuss free provision of medical records to the patient examination rooms. The senior person running the record room is Millie D'hooge. Claire has many other administrative responsibilities with that for medical records being the one with the most direct impact on physician's care of patients.

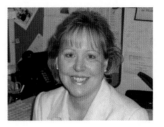

Fig. 13.5 Claire Cronin

Claire and the entire department are impatient for the arrival of the full electronic medical record system, i.e., no looking for a paper chart, viz., similar to the change that has so dramatically changed diagnostic radiology. For this we are dependent on the excellent IT unit of the department and the hospital.

In addition to managing the medical records (file room staff and operation), Claire has responsibility for managing the Patient Service co-coordinators, proton intake manager, and the Cox 3 Office manager. She is justifiably proud of the patient friendly reception team at the Cox Ground and at the FHBPTC.

Claire had worked in pediatric oncology units at the MGH and DFCI. Claire was brought to this department by Connie Stone as a Unit Manager. Connie was an important role model for Claire.

The fact that both of her parents died before the age of 40 were strong factors in her decision to be in the oncology programs of a research hospital.

13.5 Receptionists

The receptionists perform a critically important function in the care of our patients, welcoming them each day and providing extensive support and assistance. We have a wonderful team who greatly ease the patients introduction to the treatment area and their daily visits to the department. These

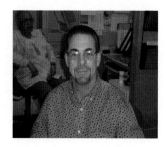

Fig. 13.6 Paul Chase

talented workers are a star in the complex of our patient care groups.

Paul Chase (Fig. 13.6) is the cheerful and positive leader of this group. He has been working at the reception desk for 30 years. He was born in Woburn and graduated from Burlington High school. His connection with the MGH was his mother's treatment here for a malignant tumor of the brain. He worked initially in patient transport and then came into the reception unit. Paul has consistently received the most positive comments of praise by patients.

13.6 Cox Front Door Welcoming Team

A function that is regularly praised by patients and their relatives is the splendid reception at the front door to the Cox building. They cheerfully and easily welcome the patients, assist them into wheel chairs, give directions, make calls for special support, and to park their car. This team is headed by M.C. Callum Moore (Fig. 13.7). He is on the job regularly and manages this delicate operation with grace and ease. We constantly receive highly positive components regarding Moore and his co-workers.

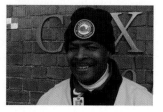

Fig. 13.7 McCallum [Mac] Moore

Chapter 14

Administration

The department in 1970 did not have a designated administrator until 1977. From 1970 to then, administrative functions were performed by Claire Hunt, a billing clerk, and Suit. See Chapter 4 for description of the many functions provided by Claire in the early years.

14.1 Connie Stone 1997–2003, Administrator and Business Manager

Connie was appointed in October 1977 to the newly created position of Business Manager of the department and assist Claire with general administrative functions.

This was one of several such positions established in the hospital at that time to improve financial and general operational relationships between administration and the departments.

Her first assignment was to evaluate the efficiency and accuracy of the difficult billing operations. The entire process was manual, viz., services provided by physicians, physicists, treatment machines, machine shop, and others were recorded on daily logs and these submitted to the department's billing clerk. The charges were transferred onto a billing sheet for each patient and then submitted to the hospital billing services at completion of treatment.

Financial reports and statements were generated on paper and calculated using an adding machine, with a final copy typed by a secretary.

Additionally, she worked with Michael Goitein on the annual proton grant budgets. Due to its growth, he later appointed a proton program business manager. Importantly, Michael brought into the department one of the first computer spreadsheets on the market. Although cumbersome by current standards it was a big improvement in our operation. The arrival of Dr. Rakesh Jain with several of his own grants added to the budgeting process, although he soon hired his own Business Manager.

Concurrently, we engaged Wang Laboratory to develop both a billing and word processing program specific to Radiation Oncology. This was a stand-alone system used for several years before it was finally replaced by the IMPAC systems.

A major change in our financial operation was the joining of MGPO (Massachusetts General Physicians Organization) by our physician group in the 1980s and to commence independent billing by the department. Prior to this, the physicians' charges were bundled into the hospital charges and allocated back to the department to be used for salaries and other direct physician expenses. Working with Ms. Helen Reid from Blue Shield of Massachusetts, we developed pro forma budgets to determine that an independent billing practice would be most beneficial to physician reimbursement. This was definitely the case and provided for a much greater independence in planning our operations from central administration and substantially improved operational efficiency.

Connie also worked with Suit in the planning and budgeting for affiliations with several community hospitals for radiation oncology services. These included Cape Cod Hospital, Waltham Hospital, Mount Auburn Hospital, Emerson Hospital, Jordan Hospital, and South Shore Oncology Center. The arrangement with BMC was in place earlier.

Financial responsibilities included not only the major hospital budgets for the clinical division but those for physics and biology research, viz., research grants.

Connie retired in 2003 and is spending her time quite happily with her granddaughter.

Jennifer [Jackson] Ransom was the departmental administrator for 2 years, 2000–2002.

Nancy Corbett (2002–2007). After a search, Nancy Corbett, the billing coordinator for the department was made Administrative Director. Nancy brought with her a strong business background, billing experience, and an entrepreneurial spirit. Plans for the new Department in B3C were launched during her tenure as well as the MGH facility at Newton Wellesley Hospital. She left the department to assume a senior management position in ProCure.

H.D. Suit, J.S. Loeffler, *Evolution of Radiation Oncology at Massachusetts General Hospital*,
DOI 10.1007/978-1-4419-6744-2_14, © Springer Science+Business Media, LLC 2011

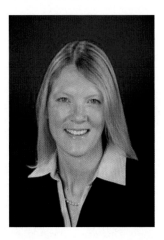

Fig. 14.1 Andrea Beloff Paciello, FACHE, January 1, 2008–present

Andrea (Fig. 14.1) was appointed on January 1, 2008, to provide administrative leadership over the large and growing department. As the complexity of patient care operations, billing, financial management, number of personnel, interactions with industry and other departments of the hospital, operations in affiliated hospitals, and dealing with the diverse regulatory agencies have increased, so has the need for strong administrative leadership of the department.

As Executive Director, Andrea's responsibilities include administration of the $23 M annual operating budget, a $5 M annual capital budget plus additional professional, sundry, and research funds. Her role also includes overseeing roughly 330 FTEs, including the Radiation Therapy team, the Administrative team, the Director of Business Development, and the Finance, Facilities, Grant Managers, as well as administration of the Quality Assurance program.

A key component of the Executive Director position is to work with the management team and staff to ensure smooth patient care operations across all sites. Andrea and the operational management team continually review and problem-solve in response to volume, wait time, and patient satisfaction information, always striving to improve the patient experience. In addition, Andrea works with the team to ensure compliance with and readiness for regulatory and accreditation visits, including those by the Joint Commission, CMS, ACR, DPH, and Radiation Safety.

Andrea also serves an important role in advocating for the department in collaboration with Senior Vice President of Administration, Jean Elrick MD, and in representing the department in negotiations and forums within and outside the MGH, including the Department's relationship with the MGH Cancer Center. Of particular note, the department currently licenses and operates radiation oncology services at Emerson Hospital in Concord, MA, Newton-Wellesley Hospital in Newton, MA, the Mass General/North Shore Center for Outpatient Care in Danvers, MA, and also provides professional services (either physician or physics services or both) at Boston Medical Center, Exeter Hospital, and South Suburban Oncology Center. Seeing the strength of MGH Radiation Oncology, additional institutions frequently express interest in collaborating with the department. Andrea plays a key role in assessing and managing those negotiations.

Andrea is also responsible for managing the space allocated to the department, including leading the planning for additions or renovations of space. Of special importance in the next few years, Andrea is coordinating planning for the relocation of photon patient treatment areas to the MGH's new 10-story patient care tower, which will open during the MGH's bicentennial year in 2011. The patient care space in the Cox Lower Level vacated during the transition will then be converted into a radiation imaging center, and Andrea is coordinating the plans for that project as well.

Finally, a key part of Andrea's role involves identifying areas for improvement – either in the general operations, in structure, in strategy, or in culture – and working with the diverse range of role groups within the department to find and implement short-term and long-term solutions to impact those areas of opportunity.

Andrea is active in the American College of Healthcare Executives, elected last year to serve a 3-year term as the Regent representing ACHE affiliates in Massachusetts. She is a Fellow in the College (FACHE) and Board Certified in Healthcare Management. She serves on the Board of the Healthcare Management Association of Massachusetts, on the Board of the Junior League of Boston, and is a volunteer wish granter with the Make-A-Wish Foundation.

Chapter 15

Affiliated Hospitals

The first affiliations were in the form of a staff participating in Tumor Board meetings and consulting on individual patients. Milford and CC served the Mt. Auburn Hospital and the Waltham Hospital in this capacity for the 1960s. Then we had staff there part time to operate their clinical treatment units. These two were subsequently purchased by Beth Israel-Deaconess hospital system.

Boston University Hospital and Boston City Hospital obtained a Betatron in 1963 under Drs. Aral, Spira, and Shapiro. M. Feldman was the Chief of Radiation Oncology from the early 1970s to 1989. In 1970, there was no machine at MGH with energy above 2 MV, viz., the Van de Graaff. Suit had been using higher energies from a Betatron for 11 years at MDACC and was keen to have access to such a radiation beam for MGH patients. In October 1972, arrangements were completed for our department to utilize the BMC Betatron with their physics and technical staff on a daily basis from 1:30 to 4:30 PM. This continued until our new units were operational in Cox.

Boston Medical Center (BMC) and MGH signed a contract in 1989 for the MGH to be responsible for the radiation oncology staff and that MGH residents would have a formal rotation at BMC. BMC was to continue with the responsibility for physics and technical support.

Thomas Delaney was appointed the Director of the BMC Department of Radiation Oncology in 1992 and continued in that role until 2000 when he moved to MGH. Several medical advances for the BCM program included 1993, IMPAC; 1996 Prostate Seed Implant by A. Zietman; 1996 SRS by A. Taghian and 1998, 3 D Treatment Planning.

In 2000 Lisa Kachnic (a graduate of our residency program) became the new Director of the BMC Department of Radiation Oncology. The program has grown and there are three additional clinicians: Ariel Hirsch, Min Tam Truong, and George Russo, There are positions for two full-time physicists. John Willins is the Head of their physics unit. Technical advances include 2004, IMRT; 2006, Two Varian Image guidance Lin ACCs; Phillips Large Bore Planning CT and Planning PET-CT. A bio sketch of Kachnic is in Chapter 10.

Throughout the period 1989 to present, our residents and now the HROP residents have been consistent in evaluating favorably the rotation at BMC.

We provide physician coverage for South Suburban Oncology Center in an arrangement with Shields Inc. though we do not run the facility. The physicians are employed by us through the MGPO.

MGH worked with the Emerson Hospital in the development of their radiation oncology program, starting with an MGH staff attending their Tumor Board meetings and being available for consultations. The radiation oncology program became a fully licensed facility of the MGH with the formal responsibility for the medical, physics, therapists, nursing secretarial and receptionist staff. The MGH provided the linear accelerator and a series of upgrades, including IMXT. The clinicians are Robin Shoenthaler and John McGrath; the physicists are Tom Harris and Rui Qi.

The path for development of the program at the Newton-Wellesley Hospital in Newton has followed a similar path from consultants frequently available and regular participants in Tumor Board meetings to a fully licensed component of the MGH. The MGH also provided the radiation therapy equipment. The clinicians are Sarah Thurman and Gail Tillman and the physicist is Kjung-Wook Jee. The North Shore Cancer Center is now also a fully licensed part of the MGH department. The clinicians are James McIntyre (a graduate of our residency program) (Head), Margarita Rasca, Derek Chism, Walter Sall, and Daniel Soto. The physicist is Michael Kirk. Quite recently, the MGH has made an agreement with the Exeter Hospital, Exeter, NH, to be responsible for the medical staff. Gary Proulx (a graduate of our residency program) is the radiation oncologist at Exeter; he is an alumnus of our residency program. The arrangements whereby Emerson, Newton Wellesley, and North Shore have become fully licensed components of the MGH department are the result of the active and future oriented leadership of Jay Loeffler.

There are several discussions in progress for additional affiliations. Our history in this regard is that our department has been a significant factor in the development

H.D. Suit, J.S. Loeffler, *Evolution of Radiation Oncology at Massachusetts General Hospital*, DOI 10.1007/978-1-4419-6744-2_15, © Springer Science+Business Media, LLC 2011

of radiation oncology units in several hospitals in this region and they have enjoyed substantial success in providing improved care for cancer patients. As they matured, some have become independent or have been purchased by other medical facilities. These include Waltham Hospital, Mt. Auburn Hospital (Cambridge, MA), and Jordan Hospital. Although they are not currently part of our family, we have contributed to their growth and success.

Chapter 16

Patrons of the Department

16.1 Major Facilities

16.1.1 The Cox Building

Jessie Bancroft Cox, sister of Jane Bancroft Cook, gave money to construct the Cox Building – home of the current Department. The gift was in memory of her late husband, William C. Cox.

16.1.2 Edwin Steele Laboratory

A laboratory for tumor biology research, occupying the entire seventh floor of the Cox building, was established by a gift of Jane Bancroft Cook in honor of her first husband – Andrew Werk Cook.

16.1.3 Francis Burr Proton Therapy Center

Francis Hooks Burr was a prominent Boston attorney who for years worked pro bono to improve health care and higher education in the Commonwealth. Throughout his long career, Mr. Burr helped dozens of civic and corporate organizations, none more so than MGH and Harvard University. Mr. Burr, who never formally retired as an attorney with the Boston firm of Ropes & Gray, where he was a partner, served as a trustee of MGH from 1962 to 1987, with the last 5 years as chairman. He helped raise more than $165 M that helped us build the Ellison and Blake buildings, and he was one of our leaders who met with the leaders of the Brigham, who made the decisions to create Partners HealthCare in 1993. Mr. Burr also served as a fellow of Harvard College from 1954 to 1982 and as senior fellow the last 11 years. He was a major advocate of proton therapy and was an instrumental supporter of H. Suit in his efforts to build a hospital-based facility. Upon his death in November 2004, corporate partners, friends of the family, and his wife made contributions to support the former Northeast Proton Therapy Center. In recognition of his loyalty and generosity to the MGH, the proton therapy center was named in his honor.

16.2 General Support for the Department

16.2.1 Anne G. and Williams C. Bowie

Anne and Williams Bowie for the Anne G. and Williams C. Bowe Endowed Fund gave $4 M in honor of Dr. Chiu Chen Wang for Radiation Oncology at the Massachusetts General Hospital. This 1998 gift was to support the work of the department.

16.2.2 James and Ruth Clark

In 2008, the Clarks gave $15 M to the MGH to support radiation oncology. In recognition of their gift, the Department in Cox LL was named in their honor as well as the new Department to open in 2011 in the Building for the 3rd century. James Clark is the grandson of the founder of the Avon Corporation and has managed several large investment houses in New York and Boston. James and Ruth were both successfully treated by members of the Department.

16.3 Endowed Chairs at Harvard Medical School

In 1986, The Andres Soriano Professorship in Oncology was established. The Chair honors the Filipino industrialist who died at the Massachusetts General Hospital on December 30, 1964, after surgery for cancer. The Chair was endowed

H.D. Suit, J.S. Loeffler, *Evolution of Radiation Oncology at Massachusetts General Hospital*, DOI 10.1007/978-1-4419-6744-2_16, © Springer Science+Business Media, LLC 2011

by the gift of Soriano's sons, Jose and Andreas Soriano II. Herman Day Suit was the Soriano Professor from 1986 to 2000, Dr. Jay Loeffler held the Professorship from 2000 to 2004, and Dr. William U. Shipley is the current incumbent. Dr. Suit is presently the Andres Soriano Distinguished Professor.

The Andrew Werk Cook Professorship was established at the MGH/HMS in 1987 by Jane Bancroft Cook in memory of her late husband. The incumbent is to serve as the Director of the Edwin L. Steele Laboratory of the Department of Radiation Oncology. Mrs. Cook was the youngest child of Hugh Bancroft, former President of the Dow Jones and Company, publishers of The Wall Street Journal and Barron's weekly. Dr. Peter W. Vaupel was the Cook Professor from 1987 to 1989 and Dr. Rakesh Jain is the current incumbent.

On March 2, 2004, the Herman and Joan Suit Professorship was established in honor of the founding Chair of the Department and his wife. The gift was made possible by a substantial gift of the Suit family, their relatives, and loyal graduates of the Department. The Suit Professor will reside with the Chair of the Department. Dr. Jay S. Loeffler is the current incumbent.

The C.C. Wang Professorship in Radiation Oncology was established in 2007 by a major gift of Dr. C.C. Wang, former Professor and Clinical Director of the Department. Additional contributions were made by Dr. Wang's daughter Janice, former graduates of the Department as well as current and former faculty members. Dr. Nancy J. Tarbell, Dean of Clinical and Academic Affairs at HMS, is the first incumbent of the C.C. Wang Professorship.

In October of 2007, Harvard Medical School established the William U. and Jenoit Shipley Professorship in Radiation Oncology to serve full-time at the MGH. The Professorship was established to honor the distinguished career of Dr. Shipley. The financial support of the Chair was made possible by a generous gift of the Shipley and Upjohn families as well as by Dr. and Mrs. Suit, former graduates of the Department and loyal patients of Dr. Shipley. Dr. Anthony Zietman, Director of Education of the Department, is the first incumbent.

16.4 Visiting Committee for the Department

David Crockett was clearly serious that we develop an effective support system among the patrons of the hospital. He established a Visiting committee for our department. He arranged this with the interested support of Ms Jane Claflin. The structure of the committee was that there be serious scientist members who could ask significant questions about our achievements and proposed future studies.

Were the assessment of our work positive by scientists, that would constitute important validity to our work. These would give the financial patrons important basis for evaluating our reports.

Crockett was quite successful in recruiting important patrons and equally valuable were the scientists. The members in attendance at the 1984 meeting are presented here.

16.5 The MGH Radiation Oncology Department Visiting Committee

Members in Attendance for the 1984 Meeting:

Professor Richard Wilson – Physics Department, Harvard University.
Chairman, Radiation Medicine Visiting Committee
Anthony Athanas – Owner of Anthonys Pier 4, Boston, MA.
Mr. Gordon Erickson – Investor in Start up Companies
Mrs. Gordon Erickson.
Mrs. Paul Flinn – Daughter of Mrs. A. Werk Cook.
James W. Fordyce – Vice President, FH Prince & Co., New York.
Roy A. Hammer, Esq. – Hemenway & Barnes.
Salvadore E. Luria – Director, Center for Cancer Research, MIT. Professor Emeritus, MIT. Nobel Prize.
Mrs. Lawrence E. MacElree – Trustee and Daughter of Mrs. Jessie Cox.
Anthony M. Macleaod – Trustee of the Andres Soriano Cancer Research Fund.
Roger Nichols – Director Museum of Science. Professor of International Health
William Preston – Prof. of Physics, Harvard Medical School.
John A. Shane – Chairman and former President of the Boston Biomedical Research Institute.
W. Davies Sohier – Oncologist, Massachusetts General Hospital staff.
Robert A. Weinberg – Professor of Biology, MIT
Ralph B. Williams – Retired Vice President Fiduciary Trust Company, Boston, MA.

Members Not in Attendance:

Howard W. Johnson – Former President, MIT. Honorary Chairman, MIT.
William C. Cox – Executive Director Dow Jones (Europe) and Trustee of the Jessie B. Cox Lead Trust.
Jose M. Soriano – Trustee of the Andreas Soriano Cancer Research Fund

20 Members (7 scientists and physicians):

2 Professors at MIT (Biology Director for Cancer Research)
2 Professors of Physics, Harvard, FAS
1 Director of the Museum of Science
1 Former President of MIT
1 MGH Medical Oncologist.

The Visiting Committee happily continues to meet on a yearly basis. The Department has been quite fortunate in that the members have consistently been highly interested, active, and supportive. Administration continues to be positively involved in the member selection. The new Chair is Steven A. Kosowsky, a highly successful business person. Under his leadership there has been an expanded and effective emphasis on fund raising.

Chapter 17

Special Social Functions

17.1 Summer Picnics

The department organized a long series of lobster picnics-feasts from 1980 to 2001 at the exceptionally generous invitation of Senior Nurse Agnes Fiore. These were held at her Cohasset home. This was a splendid arrangement due to the exceptionally gracious hospitality of Agnes at the site within view of the ocean.

As per phone conversation with A. Fiore, March 20, 2008.

The lobsters were caught early in the morning of the picnic, ~5:00 AM by her favorite lobsterman, Tom Lagrotteria. She relates the history of lobstering in that region as the preserve of descendents of the Portuguese who came to that area during the time of whaling. Her estimate is that there are 25 such families and they continue to dominate this business. For the preparation of the lobsters, her sons served as cooks and general managers. There was, of course, a variety of other foods. There were many who ate more than one lobster. One quite enthusiastic young man ate 5 lobsters plus a few other items. He survived.

For the picnics, there were on average 170 department staff and family. In addition to the food, there were baseball and aquatic sports on adjacent land fronting the beach.

After the retirement of Agnes, the summer picnic parties have been organized at other festive sites, unusually in Boston or close thereto.

17.2 Christmas or New Year Parties

The first Christmas party was in December, 1972. This was held in the laboratory space in Temp II and was quite informal with the various employees bringing in a variety of delicacies. Wine and beer were provided. There was no band or dance music in that minimalist space, but the evening was clearly convivial. Remarks were made by several on several humorous incidents in getting into the new facilities. The subsequent parties have been held in a series of sites to accommodate the larger staff and provide room for music and dancing. These have been in a series of hotels and in several years in restaurants.

In recent years, Anthony Zietman and many of the residents in each class organized the entertainment at the New Year's party. These were diverse and clearly a source of real pleasure and substantial amusement for resident, fellows, and the entire staff. The offerings varied between pantomime, theatrical skits, musicals, and dances. The creativity and originality has been strikingly evident by the absence of repetition, viz., a different entertainment format and content each year.

Figures 17.1 and 17.2 are photos of some of the joy experienced by the department at two recent New Year parties.

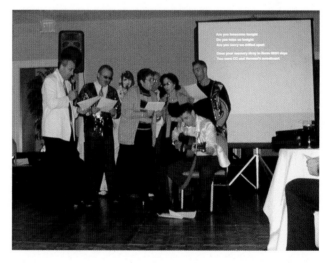

Fig. 17.1 A departmental musical group at a New Year's party. The musicians from left to right are Jay Loeffler, Paul Busse, Diane Lassonde, William Shipley, Alison Brookes, John Coen, and Anthony Zietman

H.D. Suit, J.S. Loeffler, *Evolution of Radiation Oncology at Massachusetts General Hospital*,
DOI 10.1007/978-1-4419-6744-2_17, © Springer Science+Business Media, LLC 2011

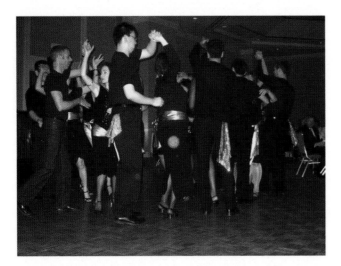

Fig. 17.2 Dancing at the January 2008 department party. Ron Chen, center, and A. Zietman with Alison Brookes. The other dancers are not identified

Chapter 18

Future of the Department of Radiation Oncology at the MGH

18.1 Goal Is to Increase the Complication Free Cure Rate of Cancer Patients

The Department has a 40-year commitment to improving the outcome of cancer patients. As radiation oncologists, we strive to explore physical and biological means to improve local tumor control while minimizing normal tissue complications. The exploration of proton therapy, IORT, IMRT, and brachytherapy are great examples of the physical attempts to improve the therapeutic ratio for our patients. The translational work in the Steele Laboratory is investigating ways to overcome hypoxia and increased interstitial tumor pressure as methods to improve outcome for our patients. We are optimistic that our Department will continue the fundamentally important work moving forward.

18.2 Clinical Care

The disease-specific model established by Herman Suit in the early 1970s has served our patients very well. Having nationally recognized experts in all disease sites has served as a role model for the MGH Cancer Center disease centers. The Department has grown into a large matrix including many MGH radiation oncology community practices. These MGH community services provide outstanding care to our patients from a wide variety of geographic locations throughout a 70-mile radius of the greater Boston area. We continually evaluate further expansion including the potential of facilities outside the northeast and even outside the USA. We are switching our nursing model to that of nurse practitioners (NPs). NPs will allow for more continuity of patient care since our physicians will be seeing patients in the Cox LL, B3C new Department (James and Ruth Clark Department), FBPTC, and the disease-specific clinics in the Yawkey Building. We anticipate that our services will involve more intensive and complicated cases as our community partners take care of more and more "routine cases." Planning and treatment capacity will increase substantially on the main campus with a larger simulation center as well as a 40 ft^2 treatment center with photon/proton delivery systems in B3C. We also anticipate that more and more patients will be treated on clinical trials with the addition of Jose Baselga as the new Chair of Medical Oncology. We expect a 10–15% growth in clinical and physics faculty over the next few years once the new Department is fully operational.

18.3 Teaching and Education

Currently, radiation oncology is the most competitive postgraduate discipline in American medicine. We have enjoyed the position as the top program since the Harvard Radiation Oncology training program was developed nearly 10 years ago. This competitive advantage should provide a steady pipeline of enormously talented young faculty members for years to come. We are also committed to train and educate residents and fellows from a wide variety of global locations. Our experience with our foreign friends has resulted in significant benefits for the Department as well as the institution in general. Under the leadership of Anthony Zietman, we are restructuring our residency program to optimize our residents' exposure to experiences in basic and applied research. The concentration of life science research within the MGH as well as the immediate vicinity of the hospital provide our residents with unparalleled opportunities.

18.4 Research

The research was clearly successful with highly impressive NCI funding for the laboratory research activities in the Steele laboratory, the Charlestown laboratory, and physics and clinical research in the Proton project. The Department

H.D. Suit, J.S. Loeffler, *Evolution of Radiation Oncology at Massachusetts General Hospital*,
DOI 10.1007/978-1-4419-6744-2_18, © Springer Science+Business Media, LLC 2011

secures over $20 M a year in research support. We anticipate expanding our basic efforts in DNA repair. The first new recruit in these efforts is Andy Elia, M.D., Ph.D., a former resident and molecular geneticist who is finishing his second post-doc in the laboratory of Dr. Steve Elledge at HMS. Dr. Elia will commit his full-time efforts to basic research and we will support his efforts to build a substantial research team over the next 5 years. The 15-year commitment of millions of dollars from the federal share pools will facilitate our recruitment capabilities. We are seeking philanthropic support to expand the Steele Lab in the field of translational oncology work. Scientific hypotheses will flow from the lab into the clinic and back to the lab. We have been very successful with these translational projects in the past but we will need to expand rapidly with the new era of biologics, functional imaging, and genomics in oncology. We must be prepared to continue our lead in these efforts moving forward. Under the leadership of Thomas Bortfeld, medical physics research has grown with more independent investigators. The federal share dollars should provide resources for continuous growth and expansions of research themes.

18.5 Financial

The Department has many challenges and opportunities in the years to come. The achievement of innovation and advances in patient care clearly require continued funds adequate for the pursuit of our stated goals. Our definite intent is to have superior care available for some categories of patients every few years. That is, we cannot be satisfied with the level of care today but to make regular and significant gains.

The recently passed US healthcare reform initiative could result in significant financial constraints for insured patients but will provide much needed coverage for the uninsured patients we see and treat. The constant attack by third-party payers and CMS on the technical and professional reimbursement will lead to many changes in our practice by limiting the flexibility of treatment delivery that we enjoy today. We have been very prudent in our use of sundry funds and our MGPO surpluses, thus we will weather the storm as well as any major academic medical center in the USA. Five endowed HMS Chairs will also allow us more security in retention as well as recruiting power moving into the next 10 years.

Appendix

1. The Note of Rev. Bartlett to Several Sympathetic Friends
Provided by Mass Historical Society, May 2010

2. Letter from Rev. Bartlett to his Son 1830

HISTORY OF MASSACHUSETTS GENERAL HOSPITAL

"MARBLEHEAD, *Mass*

Friday Eve, 29, 1830

Taken from Reed W. A memoir of the Reverend John Bartlett. Boston, MA: The Merrymount Press; 1936.

My dear son:

"You ask me to state what I remember of my agency in the commencement of the Massachusetts Hospital and of the McLean Asylum. I believe that I have told that the first measures in the very earliest stage of that concern originated with me. From Nov. 3, 1807 to 1810 I was chaplain at the Almshouse in Boston. Dr. Jno. Gorham was the physician of the staff the first, and part of the second year of my residence, and Dr. Parker (son of the Bishop) the rest of the time. You know that I was ever interested in your profession, and having there a fine opportunity of indulging my taste, I pursued the study of it from the mere love of it. Much of my time was devoted to the sick, but the portion of the diseased which most interested me was the insane. There were generally from 10 to 20 in the house, and although the care was taken of them, which the circumstances of the house would afford, yet there was no proper place for their confinement and rest; a 20-foot building, with several cells opening into a long entry, in each of which cells was a board cabin or berth, with loose straw, a pail for necessary purposes, was their only accommodation. The violent were confined in strait jackets, and the filth and wretchedness of the place were dreadful. At that time there were no places of refuge for the insane in Massachusetts except in a few private houses in the country, owned and managed by Doctors, such as Willard's, of Uxbridge, etc., etc. The mode of managing the insane then was most cruel, and unfavorable to recovery. Whipping, etc., was often resorted to (not at the Almshouse) but in these country places. The physicians at the Almshouse were humane, good men, but the subject of insanity they did not appear to understand; or rather, no facilities were afforded them for the employment of those moral remedies which Pinel and others had so successfully applied in France. This wretchedness of this class of patients and their miserable condition in the Almshouse moved my feelings exceedingly. I gave my mind intensely to the study of the causes and remedies of mania in its various kinds. I went to Philadelphia, N. York, examined the hospitals there, read Pinel and all the accounts I could procure of the Asylums in France, and England. I became deeply convinced of the importance of a similar Asylum in Massachusetts. What

prompted me to action was, several persons of respectability seized suddenly deranged, and brought to the Almshouse, were put in these cells. Among others, a Capt. Jones seized suddenly on Change violently deranged. He was a stranger, commander of a vessel, and instantly put into a strait jacket, and locked up in one of these cells.

"I sat down to my desk and wrote from 15 to 25 billets addressed to some of the wealthiest and most respectable; gentlemen of Boston, requesting them to meet at Conant Hall on the Monday evening following, to take into consideration the importance of adopting some measures for the establishment of a Hospital for the Insane. Among these gentlemen were Sam Smith, Barney Smith, Francis D. Channing, Esq., Thomas Perkins, Col. Joseph May, Drs. J.C. Warren, James Jackson, Jno. Gorham, several others. They met agreeably to notice. Inquired who called them together and why. I gave a representation of the sad condition of the insane, the need of an Asylum, etc. They listened with interest and agreed that something should be done. They adjourned to the next Monday, when they met and formed themselves into a society for the purpose. At these meetings, I was Secretary. ''They adjourned for another week. When they met Doctors Warren, and Jackson, and Gorham suggested the Expediency of uniting with this object, the establishment of a Hospital for the sick. Some fears were expressed that by proposing too much, neither object could be obtained. Consequently, subscriptions were first solicited for the Insane Hospital. Lt. Gov. Phillips subscribed $20,000.

"At this third meeting, I observed to the gentlemen that as I was a young man and little known, it would be better that some other more known should be chosen Secretary. Accordingly they chose Mr. Codman (Richard, I think), son of Stephen Codman, Esq.

Yours in haste,   J. BARTLETT."

3. Circular Written by Drs. Warren and Jackson, August 1810

Warren Circular

Boston, August 20, 1810. Taken from Bodwitch N. History of the Massachusetts General Hospital. 1851. Printed by John Wilson and Son

Sir, - It has appeared very desirable to a number of respectable gentlemen, that a hospital for the reception of lunatics and other sick persons should be established in this town. By the appointment of a number of these gentlemen, we are directed to adopt such methods as shall appear best calculated to promote such an establishment. We therefore beg leave to submit for your consideration proposals for the institution of a hospital, and to state to you some of the reasons in favour of such an establishment.

It is unnecessary to urge the propriety and even obligation of succouring the poor in sickness. The wealthy inhabitants of the town of Boston have always evinced that they consider themselves as 11 treasurers of God's bounty; " and in Christian countries, in countries where Christianity is practised, it must always be considered the first of duties to visit and to heal the sick. When in distress, every man becomes our neighbour, not only if he be of the household of faith, but even though his misfortunes have been induced by transgressing the rules both of reason and religion. It is unnecessary to urge the truth and importance of these sentiments to those who are already in the habit of cherishing them, to those who indulge in the true luxury of wealth, the pleasures of charity. The questions which first suggest themselves on this subject are, whether the relief afforded by hospitals is better than can be given in any other way; and whether there are, in fact, so many poor among us as to require an establishment of this sort.

The relief to be afforded to the poor, in a country so rich as ours, should perhaps be measured only by their necessities. we have, then, to inquire into the situation of the poor in sickness, and to learn what are their wants. In this inquiry, we shall be led to answer both the questions above stated.

There are some who are able to acquire a competence in health, and to provide so far against any ordinary sickness as that they shall not then be deprived of a comfortable habitation, nor of food for themselves and their families; while they are not able to defray the expenses of medicine and medical assistance. Persons of this description never suffer among us. The Dispensary gives relief to hundreds every year; and the individuals who practise medicine gratuitously attend many more of this description. But there are many others among the poor, who have, if we may so express it, the form of the necessaries of life, without the substance. A man may have a lodging; but it is deficient in all those advantages which are requisite to the sick. It is a garret or a cellar, without light and due ventilation, or open to the storms of an inclement winter.

In this miserable habitation, he may obtain liberty to remain during an illness; but, if honest, he is harassed with the idea of his accumulating rent, which must be paid out of his future labours. In this wretched situation, the sick man is destitute of an those common conveniences, without which most of us would consider it impossible to live, even in health. 'Wholesome food and sufficient fuel are wanting; and his own sufferings are aggravated by the cries of hungry children. ?above all, he suffers from the want of that first requisite in sickness, a kind and skilful nurse.

But it may be said, that instances are rare among us, where a man, who labours, with even moderate industry, when in health, endures such privations in sickness as are here described. They are not, however, rare among those who are not industrious; and who, nevertheless, when labouring under sickness, must be considered as having claims to assistance. In cases of long-protracted disease, instances of such a description do occur amongst those of the most industrious class. Such instances are still less rare among those women who are either widowed, or worse than widowed. It happens too frequently that modest and worthy women are united to men who are profligate and intemperate, by whom they are left to endure disease and poverty under the most aggravated forms. Among the children of such families also, instances are not rare of real suffering in sickness. To all such as have been described, a hospital would supply every thing which is needful, if not all they could wish. In a well-regulated hospital, they would find a comfortable lodging in a duly attempered atmosphere; would receive the food best suited to their various conditions; and would be attended by kind and discreet nurses, under the directions of a physician. In such a situation, the poor man's chance for relief would be equal perhaps to that of the most affluent, when affected by the same disease.

There are other persons, also, who are of great importance in society, to whom the relief afforded by a hospital is exceedingly appropriate. Such are generally those of good and industrious habits, who are affected with sickness, just as they are entering into active life, and who have not had time to provide for this calamity. Cases of this sort are frequently occurring. Disease is often produced by the very anxiety and exertions which belong to this period of life; and the best are the most liable to suffer. Of such a description, cases are often seen among journeymen mechanics and among servants.

Journeymen mechanics commonly live in small boarding-houses, where they have accommodations which are sufficient, but nothing more than sufficient, in health. When sick, they are necessarily placed in small, confined apartments, or in rooms crowded with their fellow-workmen. They are sheltered from the weather, and have food of some sort; and these must, in many cases, be the extent of their accommodations. Persons of this description would do well to enter a hospital, even if they had to pay the expense of their own maintenance. In most cases, they would suffer less, and recover sooner, by so doing. When, as sometimes happens, they have knot the means of payment, they become objects of charity; and the welfare to such persons should be considered among the strong motives in favour of "establishing" a hospital. Servants generally undergo great inconveniences, at least when affected with sickness, and oftentimes much more than inconveniences. With so much difficulty is the care of them attended in private families, that many gentlemen would pay the board of their servants at a hospital, in preference to having them sick in their own houses. In some cases, however, neither the master nor servant can afford the expense of proper care in sickness. Not uncommonly, a young girl is taken sick in a large family, where she is the only servant.

She lodges in the most remote corner of the house, in a room without a fireplace. The mistress is sufficiently occupied with the unusual labours which are thrown on her at a time perhaps when she is least fitted to perform them. Under such circumstances, how can the servant receive those attentions which are due to the sick? Of what use is it that the physician leaves a prescription to be put up at the Dispensary? He goes the nest day, and finds that there. has not been time even to procure the remedies which he had ordered; meanwhile, the period in which they would have been useful has passed by, and the incipient disease of yesterday has now become confirmed.

Persons of these descriptions would not be disposed to resort to a hospital on every trivial occasion. But, when afflicted with serious indisposition, they would find in such an institution an alleviation of their sufferings, which it must gladden the heart of the most frigid to contemplate.

There is one class of sufferers who peculiarly claim all that benevolence can bestow, and for whom a hospital is most especially required. The virtuous and industrious are liable to become objects of public charity, in consequence of diseases of the mind. When those who are unfortunate in this respect are left without proper care, a calamity, which might have been transient, is prolonged through life. The number of such persons, who are rendered unable to provide for themselves, is probably greater than the public imagine; and, of these, a large proportion claim the assistance of the affluent. The expense which is attached to the care of the insane in private families is extremely great, and such as to ruin a whole family that is possessed of a competence under ordinary circumstances, when called upon to support one of its members in this situation. Even those who can pay the necessary expenses would perhaps find an institution, such as is proposed, the best situation in which they could place their unfortunate friends. It is worthy of the opulent men of this town, and consistent with their general character, to provide an asylum for the insane from every part of the Commonwealth. But if funds Are raised for the purpose proposed, it is probable that the Legislature will grant some Assistance, with A view to such An extension of its benefits.

Of Another class, whose necessities would be removed by the establishment of a hospital, Are women who Are unable to provide for their own welfare And safety in one of nature's most trying hours. Houses for lying women have been found extremely useful in the large cities of Europe; and, Although abuses may have Arisen in consequence, these Are such as are more easily prevented in a small than in A large town.

There Are many others who would find great relief in A hospital, And many times have life preserved when otherwise it would be lost. Such especially Are the subjects of accidental wounds And fractures Among the poorer classes

of our citizens; And the subjects of extraordinary diseases, in any part of the Commonwealth, who may require the long and careful attention of either the physician or surgeon.

It is possible that we may be asked whether the almshouse does not answer the purposes for which A hospital is proposed. That it does not, is very certain. The town is so much indebted to the liberality of those gentlemen who, without compensation, superintend the care of the poor, that we ought not to make this reply without an explanation. The truth is that the Almshouse could not serve the purpose of A hospital, without such an entire change in the arrangements of it as the overseers do not feel themselves authorized to make, And such as the town could not be easily induced to direct or to support.

The Almshouse receives All those who do not take care of themselves, and who Are destitute of property, whether they be old And infirm, And unable to provide means of assistance; or Are too vicious And debauched to employ themselves in honest labour; or are prevented from so employing themselves by occasional sickness. This institution, then, is made to comprehend what is more properly meant by An Almshouse, A bridewell or house of correction, And a hospital. Now, the economy And mode of government cannot possibly be adapted At once to All these various purposes. It must necessarily happen that in many instances the worst members of the community, the debauched And profligate, obtain Admission into this house. Hence it has become, in some measure, disreputable to live in it; And, not unfrequently, those who Are the most deserving objects of charity cannot be induced to enter it. To some of them, death appears less terrible than a residence in the Almshouse.

It is true that the sick in that house are allowed some greater privileges and advantages than are extended to those in health; yet the general arrangements and regulations are, necessarily, so different from those required in a hospital, that the sick - far from having the advantages afforded by the medical art - have not the fair chance for recovery which nature alone would give them. Most especially they suffer for the want of good nurses. In these officers must be placed trust and confidence of the highest nature. Their duties are laborious and painful. In the almshouse, they are selected from among the more healthy inhabitants; but, unfortunately, those who are best qualified will always prefer more profitable and less laborious occupations elsewhere. It must, then, be obvious that the persons employed as nurses cannot be such as will conscientiously perform the duties of this office.

In addition to what has already been stated, there are a number of collateral advantages that would attend the establishment of a hospital in this place. These are the facilities for acquiring knowledge, which it would give to the students in the medical school established in this town. The means of medical education in New England are at present very limited, and totally inadequate to so important a purpose.

Students of medicine cannot qualify themselves properly for their profession, without incurring heavy expenses, such as very few of them are able to defray. The only medical school of eminence in this country is that at Philadelphia, nearly four hundred miles distant from Boston; and the expense of attending that is so great, that students from this quarter rarely remain at it longer than one year. Even this advantage is enjoyed by very few, compared with the whole number. Those who are educated in 'New England have so few opportunities of attending to the practice of physic, that they find it impossible to learn some of the most important elements of the science of medicine, until after they have undertaken for themselves the care of the health and lives of their fellow-citizens. This care they undertake with very little knowledge, except that acquired from books; - a source whence it is highly useful and indispensable that they should obtain knowledge, but one from which alone they never can obtain all that is necessary to qualify them for their professional duties. With such deficiencies in medical education, it is needless to show to what evils the community is exposed.

To remedy evils so important and so extensive, it is necessary to have a medical school in Now England. All the materials necessary to form this school exist among us. Wealth, abundantly sufficient, can be devoted to the purpose, without any individual's feeling the smallest privation of any, even of the luxuries of life. Every one is liable to suffer from the want of such a school; every one may derive, directly or indirectly, the greatest benefits from its establishment.

A hospital is an institution absolutely essential to a medical school, and one which would afford relief and comfort to thousands of the sick and miserable. On what other objects can the superfluities of the rich be so well bestowed?.

The amount required for the institution proposed may, at first sight, appear large. But it will cease to appear so, when we consider that it is to afford relief, not only to those who may require assistance during the present year or present age, but that it is to erect a most honourable monument of the munificence of the present times, which will ensure to its founders the blessings of thousands in ages to come; and when we add that this amount may be raised at once, if a few opulent men will contribute only their superfluous income for one year. Compared with the benefits which such an establishment would afford, of what value is the pleasure of accumulating riches in those stores which are already groaning under their weight?

Hospitals and infirmaries are found in all the Christian cities of the Old World; and our large cities in the Middle States have institutions of this . sort, which do great honor to the liberality and benevolence of their founders. We flatter ourselves that in this respect, as in all others, Boston may ere long assert her claim to equal praise.

We are, sir, very respectfully, your obedient servants,
James Jackson							John C. Warren

4. Charter Authorizing the Massachusetts General Hospital

In the public Domain

An Act to incorporate certain persons by the name of the Massachusetts General Hospital.

Section 1. Be it enacted by the Senate and House of Representatives in General Court assembled, and by the authority of the same, That James Bowdoin, John Adams, Elbridge Gerry, Theophileus Parsons, William Gray, John Thornton Kirkland, Harrison Gray Otis, Christopher Gore, William Eustis, William, Phillips, John Quincy Adams, Henry Dearborn, Levi Lincoln, Isaac Parker, Joseph B. Varnum, George Cabot, Perez Morton, Thomas Dawes, Thomas Hazard, jun., Thomas Cutts, Israel Thorndike, Mathew Bridge, Samuel Brown, James Perkins, David Tilden, John Lowell, Samuel Dana, Joseph Story, William King, Samuel Fowler, Marshall Spring, Thomas H. Perkins, Thomas C. Amory, Benjamin Bussey, Aaron Hill, William Heath, Thomas Kittredge, James Prince, Benjamin Green, Thomas Melville, Joseph Coolidge, Elias H. Derby, John C. Jones, Jonathan Davis, Jonathan Harris, James Mann, Timothy Childs, Daniel Kilham, Benjamin Crowninshield, Arnold Wells, Jonathan Amory, Robert Hallowell, Andrew Craigie, John Warren, Richard Sullivan, and William Payne, together with such other persons, as may hereafter be admitted members of the Corporation hereinafter created, according to the Bye Laws thereof be, and they hereby are incorporated and made a Body Corporate and Politic, by the name of The Massachusetts General Hospital, and by that name may sue and be sued, and shall have and use a Common Seal, to be by them devised, altered, and renewed at their pleasure.

Section 2 . And be it further enacted, That the said Corporation may take and receive, hold, purchase, and possess, of and from all persons disposed to aid the benevolent purposes of this institution, any grants and devises of lands and tenements, in fee simple, or otherwise, and any donations, and bequests, and subscriptions of money, or other property, to be used and improved for the erection, support, and maintenance of a General Hospital, for sick and insane persons, [which, among its functions may carry on educational Activities and scientific research related to the care of such persons or to the promotion of health and the prevention of disease.] Provided that the income of said Corporation, from its real and personal estate together, do at no time exceed the sum of Thirty thousand Dollars.

Section 3. And be it further enacted, [(T)hat the said Corporation shall be held and obliged to appropriate out of its funds, annually forever, to the support and maintenance of such sick poor, and lunatic persons, as may be received into said Hospital at the request of the legislature, or of any committee or officer appointed as the legislature may here-after provide for the purpose, a sum equal to simple interest on the money, for which the Province-House estate shall be sold; and until the sale thereof, the said Corporation shall be held to keep a correct account of the rents received, to be applied to the maintenance of sick poor, and lunatic persons, who would otherwise be chargeable to the Commonwealth, as soon as the Hospital shall be erected. And in case the said estate shall revert to the Commonwealth, as by the former the amount of said rents shall be paid into the Treasury of the Commonwealth.]

Section 4. And be it further enacted, That in consideration of the obligation aforesaid imposed upon said Corporation in the foregoing section, the estate commonly called the Old Province House, with all the lands under and appurtenant to the same, be, and are hereby given and granted unto said Corporation in fee simple, to be sold at the discretion of said Corporation, and the proceeds thereof to be held and applied as a foundation for a General Hospital.

Section 5 . Be it further enacted, That the said General Hospital, shall be under the direction and management of Twelve Trustees, who shall be chosen annually, and shall remain in office until others are chosen, and qualified in their stead. [eight of which Trustees shall be chosen aforesaid.] [(I)n case of the occurring of any vacancy, by death or res-ignation in the Board of the Trustees of the Massachusetts General Hospital, it shall be lawful, for the remaining Members of the Board, to fill such vacancy; provided, the same shall occur in that part of the Board, chosen by the Corporation. The Governor with the advice and consent of the council, shall annually, as soon as may be after the first Wednesday in February, appoint four trustees of the Massachusetts General Hospital, who shall hold their offices for one year, or until the appointment of their successors; and in case of the occurring of any vacancy by death or resignation among the trustees so appointed, the governor may, with the advise and consent of the council, fill such vacancy].

Section 6. And be it further enacted, That the said Corporation may, at their first, or any subsequent meeting, choose all necessary and convenient officers, who shall have such powers and authorities as the said, Corporation may think proper to prescribe and grant to them, and who shall be elected in such manner, and for such periods of time, as the Bye Laws of said Corporation may provide. And said Corporation may further make and establish such Bye Laws and regulations, for the internal Government and economy of the Hospital, as they may think proper, not repugnant to the Constitution and Laws of this Commonwealth.

Section 7 . And be it further enacted, That the Governor, Lieutenant Governor; the President of the Senate and Speaker of the House of Representatives, with the Chaplains of both Houses for the time being be, and hereby are made and constituted a Board of Visitors of the said Hospital; with authority to visit the same semi-annually, and as much oftener as they may think proper, in order to inspect the estab-lishment, and the Actual condition of the sick, to examine the Bye Laws and regulations,-enacted by said Corporation, and generally, to see that the design of the institution be car-ried into effect, in a careful, tender and effectual manner; and especially to see that the State has its full proportion of patients in the Hospital, as provided in the third section of this Act, and that the said patients are suitably attended to, and comfortably maintained.

Section 8. And be it further enacted, by the authority aforesaid, That in case of the separation of the District of Maine, and the erection of it into a separate State, pursuant to the provisions of the Constitution of the United States, the amount of the sale of the Province House shall be carried into the estimate, with the other public property of the Commonwealth.

Section 9. And be it further enacted, That it shall be law-ful for the said Corporation, at any general meeting of the members thereof, to alter or change the name of said Corporation, either by substituting the name of any distin-guished Benefactor, who may contribute a sum exceeding the amount given by the Commonwealth, or by adding the name of such Benefactor, to the name given to said Corporation by this Act, in case the sum so given by such Benefactor, shall not exceed the sum given by this Commonwealth. And upon such change so as aforesaid made, the said Corporation shall have a right to assume and take such name, and shall have hold and enjoy all the powers and privileges given by this Act, notwithstanding such alteration and change.

Section 10. And be it further enacted,   That   James Bowdoin, Esquire be, and hereby is authorized to call the first meeting of said Corporation, by notification, and therein to appoint the time and place, of said meeting: Provided, that no notification shall be deemed valid unless it be published in all the Newspapers printed in Boston for six weeks in succession.

[(Section 11.) Be it (further) enacted,   That   the Massachusetts General Hospital be, and the said cor-poration hereby is authorized to grant annuities on the life or lives of one or more persons, or for shorter terms of time, on such conditions, and with such security, as the said corporation and the annuitant or annuitants, may agree upon.]

[(Section 12.) Be it further enacted, That if at any time hereafter it shall appear to the Legislature, that the privilege of granting annuities, hereby given to the said corporation, shall be injurious to the public welfare the power of the Legislature to repeal this Act, authorizing such annuities, shall not be denied or impaired; but such repeal shall not effect any engagement to which said corporation may have become a party previous thereto. And it shall be the duty of the Trustees of the said Massachusetts General Hospital to transmit to the Governor and Council of this Commonwealth for the time being, annually, on the first Monday in January of each year, an accurate account of all annuities by them sold or granted, by virtue of this Act, signed by the said trustees or a major part of them, and attested by the Treasurer of the, corporation.]

[(**Section 13.**) The Household Nursing Association, a charitable corporation incorporated under Chapter one hundred and twenty-five of the Revised Laws, is hereby authorized, by acceptance of this Act within one year after its effective date at a meeting of the members duly called for the purpose, to consolidate with The Massachusetts General Hospital, a charitable corporation organized and existing under Chapter ninety-four of the Acts of eighteen hundred and ten, and upon such consolidation The Massachusetts General Hospital shall in all respects be a continuation of, shall have all the powers, privileges and exemptions of, and shall be subject to all duties, liabilities and restrictions provided by law in so far as they relate to both said corporations. Upon such acceptance, and upon acceptance Of this Act within one year after its effective date at a meeting of the members of The Massachusetts General Hospital duly called for, the purpose, copies of the votes of acceptance certified by the clerk or other officer of the respective corporations shall be filed in the Registry of Deeds for Suffolk County and with the state secretary, and the consolidation of The Household Nursing Association with The Massachusetts General Hospital shall thereupon be complete.]

[**Section 14.**) Upon consolidation, all property, real and personal, of The Household Nursing Association and all devises, bequests, conveyances and gifts heretofore and hereafter made to such corporation shall vest in The Massachusetts General Hospital and otherwise shall be held by its subject to the same terms, conditions, limitations and trusts as they are now held by The Household Nursing Association or would have been held but for this Act, and the treasurers of such corporations are hereby respectively authorized to execute, acknowledge and deliver all papers and documents that may be deemed necessary or proper for the purpose of confirming in The Massachusetts General Hospital the record title of the property of The Household Nursing Association.]

[(**Section 15.**) Whatever right or authority is granted or conferred by this Act is hereby declared to be limited to such authority or right as the general court may constitutionally grant or confer, without prejudice to any proceeding that may be instituted in any court of competent jurisdiction to effect the purposes of this Act.

[**Section 16.** And be it further enacted, that the Massachusetts General Hospital may, in the course of its educational Activities, award the degrees of Bachelor of Science in Radiologic Technology, Bachelor of Science in Respiratory Therapy, Master of Science in Dietetics, of Science in Nursing, Master of Science Master in Physical Therapy, and Master of Science in Speech Pathology.]

5. Excerpts of the Translation of W. Roentgen's Paper

On a New Kind of Rays. Nature. 1896;53:274276.

Read before the Würzburg Physical and Medical Society, 1895. (Translated by Arthur Stanton. Nature. 1896;53:274.)

"A discharge from a large induction coil is passed through a Hittorf's vacuum tube, or through a well-exhausted Crookes' or Lenard's tube. The tube is surrounded by a fairly close-fitting shield of black paper; it is then possible to see, in a completely darkened room, that paper covered on one side with barium platinocyanide lights up with brilliant fluorescence when brought into the neighborhood of the tube, whether the painted side or the other be turned towards the tube. The fluorescence is still visible at two metres distance. It is easy to show that the origin of the fluorescence lies within the vacuum tube.

"Lead 1.5 mm thick is practically opaque."

"The preceding experiments lead to the conclusion that the density of the bodies is the property whose variation mainly affects their permeability."

"density alone does not determine the transparency"

	Thickness	Relative thickness	Density
Platinum	0.018 mm	1	21.5
Lead	0.050"	3	11.3
Zinc	0.100"	6	7.1
Aluminium	3.5000	200	2.6

"The fluorescence of barium platinocyanide is not the only noticeable action of the X-rays. It is to be observed that other bodies exhibit fluorescence, e.g. calcium sulphide, uranium glass, Iceland spar, rock-salt, &c."

(2) It is seen, therefore, that some agent is capable of penetrating black cardboard which is quite opaque to ultra-violet light, sunlight, or arc-light. It is therefore of interest to investigate how far other bodies can be penetrated by the same agent. It is readily shown that all bodies possess this same transparency, but in very varying degrees. For example, paper is very transparent; the fluorescent screen will light up when placed behind a book of a thousand pages; printer's ink offers no marked resistance." "If the hand be held before the fluorescent screen, the shadow shows the bones clearly with only faint outlines of the surrounding tissues."

"Pieces of platinum, lead, zinc, and aluminium foil were so arranged as to produce the same weakening of the effect. The annexed table shows the relative thickness and density of the equivalent sheets of metal.

From these values it is clear that in no case can we obtain the transparency of a body from the product of its density and thickness. The transparency increases much more rapidly than the product decreases".

"Of special interest in this connection is the fact that photographic dry plates are sensitive to the X-rays. It is thus possible to exhibit the phenomena so as to exclude the danger of error"

"It is, hence, obvious that lenses cannot be looked upon as capable of concentrating the X-rays; in effect, both an ebonite and a glass lens of large size prove to be without action."

"I have also a shadow of the bones of the hand"

"It is, hence, obvious that lenses cannot be looked upon as capable of concentrating the X-rays; in effect, both an ebonite and a glass lens of large size prove to be without action."

"I have also a shadow of the bones of the hand"

Index

Note: The letters 'f' and 't' following the locators refer to figures and tables respectively.